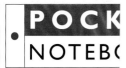

T0202093

Pocket
PSYCHIATRY

Edited by

JUDITH A. PUCKETT, MD
Fellow in Consult Liaison Psychiatry, Massachusetts General Hospital
Clinical Fellow, Harvard Medical School

SCOTT R. BEACH, MD
Program Director, MGH/McLean Adult Psychiatry Residency
Assistant Professor of Psychiatry, Harvard Medical School

JOHN B. TAYLOR, MD, MBA
Assistant Program Director, MGH/McLean Adult Psychiatry Residency
Assistant Professor of Psychiatry, Harvard Medical School

Wolters Kluwer

Philadelphia • Baltimore • New York • London
Buenos Aires • Hong Kong • Sydney • Tokyo

Acquisitions Editor: Chris Teja
Product Development Editor: Ariel S. Winter
Editorial Coordinator: Ashley Pfeiffer
Marketing Manager: Rachel Mante-Leung
Production Project Manager: Bridgett Dougherty
Design Coordinator: Elaine Kasmer
Manufacturing Coordinator: Beth Welsh
Prepress Vendor: TNQ Technologies

Library of Congress Cataloging-in-Publication Data

Names: Puckett, Judith A. (Judith Allison), 1987- editor. | Beach, Scott R., editor. |
    Taylor, John B. (John Bartell), 1983- editor.
Title: Pocket psychiatry / edited by Judith A. Puckett, Scott R. Beach, John B. Taylor.
Description: Philadelphia : Wolters Kluwer, [2020] | Includes index.
Identifiers: LCCN 2019006777 | ISBN 9781975117931
Subjects: | MESH: Mental Disorders | Handbook
Classification: LCC RC454 | NLM WM 34 | DDC 616.89–dc23
LC record available at https://lccn.loc.gov/2019006777

CCS0324

Gowri G. Aragam, MD
Instructor, Department of Psychiatry, Harvard Medical School
Psychiatrst, Psychiatry Academy, Massachusetts General Hospital

Baktash Babadi, MD, PhD
Resident, Massachusetts General Hospital/McLean Hospital Adult
Psychiatry Residency
Clinical Fellow, Harvard Medical School

Jessica E. Becker
Fellow, Massachusetts General Hospital/McLean Hospital Child and
Adolescent Psychiatry
Clinical Fellow, Harvard Medical School

Noor Beckwith, MD
Resident, Massachusetts General Hospital/McLean Hospital Adult
Psychiatry Residency
Clinical Fellow, Harvard Medical School

Ren Belcher, MD
Resident, Massachusetts General Hospital/McLean Hospital Adult
Psychiatry Residency
Clinical Fellow, Harvard Medical School

Nicole M. Benson, MD
Fellow, Massachusetts General Hospital/McLean Hospital Child and
Adolescent Psychiatry
Clinical Fellow, Harvard Medical School

Suzanne Bird, MD
Director, Acute Psychiatric Service, Massachusetts General Hospital
Assistant Professor of Psychiatry, Harvard Medical School

Samuel Boas, MD
Resident, Massachusetts General Hospital/McLean Hospital Adult
Psychiatry Residency
Clinical Fellow, Harvard Medical School

Rahel Bosson, MD
Resident, Massachusetts General Hospital/McLean Hospital Adult
Psychiatry Residency
Clinical Fellow, Harvard Medical School

Allison Brandt, MD, MPhil
Resident, Massachusetts General Hospital/McLean Hospital Adult
Psychiatry Residency
Clinical Fellow, Harvard Medical School

Douglas Brennan, MD
Resident, Massachusetts General Hospital/McLean Hospital Adult
Psychiatry Residency
Clinical Fellow, Harvard Medical School

Joan A. Camprodon, MD, MPH, PhD
Assistant Professor, Department of Psychiatry, Harvard Medical School
Chief, Division of Neuropsychiatry, Department of Psychiatry
Massachusetts General Hospital

Philip Cawkwell, MD
Resident, Massachusetts General Hospital/McLean Hospital Adult
Psychiatry Residency
Clinical Fellow, Harvard Medical School

Kristina Cieslak, MD
Resident, Massachusetts General Hospital/McLean Hospital Adult
Psychiatry Residency
Clinical Fellow, Harvard Medical School

Jacci Clauss, MD, PhD
Resident, Massachusetts General Hospital/McLean Hospital Adult
Psychiatry Residency
Clinical Fellow, Harvard Medical School

Hilary S. Connery, MD, PhD
Assistant Professor, Department of Psychiatry, Harvard Medical School
Clinical Director, Division of Alcohol and Drug Abuse, McLean
Hospital

Julia Cromwell, MD
Resident, Massachusetts General Hospital/McLean Hospital Adult
Psychiatry Residency
Clinical Fellow, Harvard Medical School

Cristina Cusin, MD
Assistant Professor, Department of Psychiatry, Harvard Medical School
Staff Psychiatrist, Department of Psychiatry, Depression Clinical
Research Program, Massachusetts General Hospital

Daniel J. Daunis, Jr., MD
Clinical Fellow, Department of Psychiatry, Harvard Medical School
Fellow, Consultation-Liaison Psychiatry, Department of
Psychiatry, Massachusetts General Hospital

Stephanie Davidson, MD
Fellow, Massachusetts General Hospital/McLean Hospital Child and
Adolescent Psychiatry
Clinical Fellow, Harvard Medical School

Lauren Deaver, MD
Resident, Massachusetts General Hospital/McLean Hospital Adult
Psychiatry Residency
Clinical Fellow, Harvard Medical School

Sam Dotson, MD
Resident, Massachusetts General Hospital/McLean Hospital Adult
Psychiatry Residency
Clinical Fellow, Harvard Medical School

Veronica A. Faller, MD
Resident, Massachusetts General Hospital/McLean Hospital Adult
Psychiatry Residency
Clinical Fellow, Harvard Medical School

Carlos Fernandez-Robles, MD
Assistant Professor, Department of Psychiatry, Harvard Medical School
Assistant Psychiatrist, Department of Psychiatry, Massachusetts General
Hospital

Mark Fusunyan, MD
Resident, Massachusetts General Hospital/McLean Hospital Adult
Psychiatry Residency
Clinical Fellow, Harvard Medical School

Oscar Gerdner, MD
Child and Adolescent Psychiatry Fellow, Child Study Center, Yale
University School of Medicine

Fiona Gispen, MD, MS
Resident, Department of Internal Medicine, Massachusetts General
Hospital
Clinical Fellow, Harvard Medical School

Raphaela Gold, MD
Resident, Massachusetts General Hospital/McLean Hospital Adult
Psychiatry Residency
Clinical Fellow, Harvard Medical School

Zachary Grunau, MD
Resident, Massachusetts General Hospital/McLean Hospital Adult
Psychiatry Residency
Clinical Fellow, Harvard Medical School

Reuben A. Hendler, MD
Resident, Massachusetts General Hospital/McLean Hospital Adult
Psychiatry Residency
Clinical Fellow, Harvard Medical School

Jonathan Henry, MD
Resident, Massachusetts General Hospital/McLean Hospital Adult
Psychiatry Residency
Clinical Fellow, Harvard Medical School

Michael E. Henry, MD
Lecturer, Department of Psychiatry, Harvard Medical School
Director of Somatic Therapy, Department of Psychiatry, Massachusetts
General Hospital

Elisabeth Hill, MD
Resident, Massachusetts General Hospital/McLean Hospital Adult
Psychiatry Residency
Clinical Fellow, Harvard Medical School

Katie Hsih, MD, MPhil
Resident, Massachusetts General Hospital/McLean Hospital Adult
Psychiatry Residency
Clinical Fellow, Harvard Medical School

Alok Kanojia, MD, MPH
Instructor, Department of Psychiatry, Harvard Medical School
Assistant Psychiatrist, Department of Psychiatry/ADATP, McLean
Hospital

Lianna Karp, MD
Resident, Massachusetts General Hospital/McLean Hospital Adult
Psychiatry Residency
Clinical Fellow, Harvard Medical School

Katherine Kilgore, MD
Resident, Massachusetts General Hospital/McLean Hospital Adult
Psychiatry Residency
Clinical Fellow, Harvard Medical School

Katherine A. Koh, MD, MSc
Instructor, Department of Psychiatry, Harvard Medical School
Attending Psychiatrist, Department of Psychiatry, Massachusetts General
Hospital

Ran Li, MD
Resident, Massachusetts General Hospital/McLean Hospital Adult
Psychiatry Residency
Clinical Fellow, Harvard Medical School

Geoffrey Liu, MD
Resident, Massachusetts General Hospital/McLean Hospital Adult
Psychiatry Residency
Clinical Fellow, Harvard Medical School

James Luccarelli, MD, DPhil
Resident, Massachusetts General Hospital/McLean Hospital Adult Psychiatry Residency
Clinical Fellow, Harvard Medical School

Elizabeth N. Madva, MD
Resident, Massachusetts General Hospital/McLean Hospital Adult Psychiatry Residency
Clinical Fellow, Harvard Medical School

David E. Marcovitz, MD
Assistant Professor, Department of Psychiatry and Behavioral Sciences, Vanderbilt University School of Medicine
Medical Director, Addiction Consult Team, Vanderbilt University Medical Center

Michal McDowell, MD, MPH
Resident, Massachusetts General Hospital/McLean Hospital Adult Psychiatry Residency
Clinical Fellow, Harvard Medical School

Andy Melaragno, MD, MS
Resident, Massachusetts General Hospital/McLean Hospital Adult Psychiatry Residency
Clinical Fellow, Harvard Medical School

Flannery Merideth, MD
Resident, Massachusetts General Hospital/McLean Hospital Adult Psychiatry Residency
Clinical Fellow, Harvard Medical School

Meghan Musselman, MD
Resident, Massachusetts General Hospital/McLean Hospital Adult Psychiatry Residency
Clinical Fellow, Harvard Medical School

Maeve O'Neill, MD
Resident, Massachusetts General Hospital/McLean Hospital Adult Psychiatry Residency
Clinical Fellow, Harvard Medical School

Mladen Nisavic, MD
Instructor, Department of Psychiatry, Harvard University
Director for Trainee Education, Addiction Consult Team, Massachusetts General Hospital

Lucy Ogbu-Nwobodo, MD, MS, MAS
Resident, Massachusetts General Hospital/McLean Hospital Adult Psychiatry Residency
Clinical Fellow, Harvard Medical School

Nate Praschan, MD, MPH
Resident, Massachusetts General Hospital/McLean Hospital Adult Psychiatry Residency
Clinical Fellow, Harvard Medical School

Lisa Rosenfeld, MD, MPH
Resident, Massachusetts General Hospital/McLean Hospital Adult Psychiatry Residency
Clinical Fellow, Harvard Medical School

Cordelia Ross, MD
Resident, Massachusetts General Hospital/McLean Hospital Adult Psychiatry Residency
Clinical Fellow, Harvard Medical School

Rachel A. Ross, MD, PhD
Instructor, Department of Psychiatry, Harvard Medical School
Assistant Neuroscientist and Psychiatrist, Department of Psychiatry, Division of Depression and Anxiety Disorders, McLean Hospital

Joshua Salvi, MD, PhD
Resident, Massachusetts General Hospital/McLean Hospital Adult Psychiatry Residency
Clinical Fellow, Harvard Medical School

Tim Shea, MD
Resident, Department of Psychiatry, Massachusetts General Hospital

Leah Shesler, MD
Resident, Massachusetts General Hospital/McLean Hospital Adult Psychiatry Residency
Clinical Fellow, Harvard Medical School

Andrew Skoirchet, MD
Resident, Massachusetts General Hospital/McLean Hospital Adult Psychiatry Residency
Clinical Fellow, Harvard Medical School

Maya Son, MD
Resident, Massachusetts General Hospital/McLean Hospital Adult Psychiatry Residency
Clinical Fellow, Harvard Medical School

Emily Sorg, MD
Resident, Massachusetts General Hospital/McLean Hospital Adult Psychiatry Residency
Clinical Fellow, Harvard Medical School

Renee Sorrentino, MD
Clinical Assistant Professor, Department of Psychaiatry, Massachusetts
General Hospital
Clinical Assistant Professor, Department of Psychaiatry, Harvard Medical
School

Marc Weinberg, MD
Resident, Massachusetts General Hospital/McLean Hospital Adult
Psychiatry Residency
Clinical Fellow, Harvard Medical School

John W. Winkelman, MD, PhD
Professor, Department of Psychiatry, Harvard Medical School,
Chief, Sleep Disorders Clinical Research Program, Department of
Psychiatry and Neurology, Massachusetts General Hospital

Curtis Wittmann, MD
Instructor, Department of Psychiatry, Harvard Medical School
Associate Director, Acute Psychiatry Service, Department of Psychiatry,
Massachusetts General Hospital

Kathryn Zagrabbe, MD
Assistant Professor of Clinical Psychiatry, Department of Psychiatry,
University of Pennsylvania Perelman School of Medicine

Jonathan Zebrowski, MD
Resident, Massachusetts General Hospital/McLean Hospital Adult
Psychiatry Residency
Clinical Fellow, Harvard Medical School

*To my parents, Joanne Hendrick and Frank Puckett,
and my husband, Daniel Restrepo*

Pocket Psychiatry was inspired by the long tradition of the Massachusetts General Hospital medical house officer manual, written annually by residents, for residents. This manual eventually evolved into Pocket Medicine, but the internal version continues to be updated yearly. For me, the tradition and anticipation of writing in the medicine manual highlighted the absence of a concise reference for clinical knowledge and key information for psychiatric trainees. This spurred a similar resident-driven movement to collect, consolidate, and systematically document the approach and management of the most commonly encountered psychiatric conditions.

The first edition of *Pocket Psychiatry* aims to provide a thoughtful starting point and comprehensive reference for clinicians. We have included the latest evidence for pharmacology, psychotherapies, and somatic therapies for the most common conditions general psychiatrists encounter. We encompass aspects of patient care often unique to psychiatry, including places where it overlaps with the legal system, such as involuntary commitment, risk assessment, and capacity assessment. We have also included sections on populations in psychiatry that may require special considerations for treatment because of the population's historic relationship with psychiatry or because the population requires a specialized subset of knowledge. Although our best attempts were made to encompass the most salient aspects of psychiatric care today, we anticipate and welcome suggestions for improvement.

Of course, the evolution and complexity of psychiatric care and research is too vast to summarize in any single textbook. *Pocket Psychiatry* is meant to be a guide for initial evaluation and management that will hopefully inspire and promote further discovery over time. We have made every effort for the recommendations included in this text to be as evidence-based as possible, but recognize that the complexity of the brain and mind highlight the importance of individual clinical judgment.

It has been a privilege to train at Massachusetts General Hospital and McLean Hospital. I am grateful for the tremendous support of fellow house officers, fellows, and attendings who provided advice and support in making this initial resident project a reality. I am grateful to a number of mentors who have not only supported but guided and promoted my clinical and professional growth including Jerry Rosenbaum and Scott Rauch for their leadership and support; Scott Beach and John Taylor, who helped make this reference a reality; Heather Vestal and Joe Stoklosa of the Clinician Educator Program; Kimberly Hartney, without whom I would not be a psychiatrist; Felicia Smith, Nick Kontos, Oliver Freudenreich, and Stuart Beck, who helped guide and focus my interest in education; and Theodore Stern, who supported my growth as a medical writer. I must also give special thanks to my family at work and at home, including: my parents; my husband, Daniel Restrepo, who has been an inspiration through his passion for medical education; and Nicole Benson and Daniel Daunis, for whose friendship and support I cannot express enough gratitude.

I hope *Pocket Psychiatry* will continue to evolve and improve with every edition through the feedback from future and current resident psychiatrists.

JUDITH A. PUCKETT, MD

FOREWORD

When I began 45 years ago as a resident in Psychiatry and found myself in certain social settings, I would dissemble and say I was a neurologist, to avoid making the other persons feel uncomfortable and typically quieting. How the world has changed over the ensuing decades with dramatic reduction of stigma, the appreciation that more than half the population is dealing with psychiatric symptoms and disorders, and that others are in fact intensely interested in our knowledge and expertise as psychiatrists. Truly "no family goes untouched" as we say at Mass General. These days folks draw closer to those who might have knowledge and skill to offer for those who suffer or worry.

A volume like this, that makes all the essential clinical information readily available to students and trainees, puts them at the ready to respond as experts to those who reach out to them. But of course, most importantly, it represents a tool for the bedside and the office, to have right at hand comprehensive and essential information to contribute to excellent care that only accurate and up-to-date information can support and to build a foundation for becoming an excellent physician and expert psychiatrist.

That this volume evolved from the expansion of teaching resources written and organized by one of our residents (JP) for students and trainees is a reason for admiration and pride. The detail and breadth of this volume moreover recommends it even to elders of our profession, indeed all physicians and psychiatrists as well. It is a resource that will truly make for better patient care in any clinical setting.

JERROLD F. ROSENBAUM, MD
CHIEF OF PSYCHIATRY, MASSACHUSETTS GENERAL HOSPITAL
STANLEY COBB PROFESSOR OF PSYCHIATRY
HARVARD MEDICAL SCHOOL

CONTENTS

PSYCHIATRIC ASSESSMENT
Mark Fusunyan, Flannery Merideth, Joshua Salvi, Tim Shea, Marc Weinberg

PSYCHIATRIC DISORDERS
Gowri G. Aragam, Baktash Babadi, Jessica E. Becker, Noor Beckwith, Ren Belcher, Samuel Boas, Allison Brandt, Kristina Cieslak, Julia Cromwell, Daniel J. Daunis Jr., Lauren Deaver, Sam Dotson, Oscar Gerdner, Fiona Gispen, Elisabeth Hill, Katie Hsih, Geoffrey Liu, Elizabeth N. Madva, Andy Melaragno, Flannery Merideth, Meghan Musselman, Lucy Ogbu-Nwobodo, Maeve O'Neill, Nate Praschan, Cordelia Ross, Rachel A. Ross, Leah Shesler, Andrew Skoirchet, Maya Son, Renee Sorrentino, Jonathan Zebrowski

SUBSTANCE USE DISORDERS
Hilary S. Connery, Mark Fusunyan, Zachary Grunau, Jonathan Henry, Katie Hsih, David E. Marcovitz, Maeve O'Neill, Lisa Rosenfeld, Maya Son

SOMATIC THERAPIES
Noor Beckwith, Nicole M. Benson, Joan A. Camprodon, Carlos Fernandez-Robles, Michael E. Henry, Joshua Salvi, Tim Shea

PSYCHOTHERAPIES
Gowri G. Aragam, Stephanie Davidson, Oscar Gerdner, Reuben A. Hendler, Katie Hsih, Lianna Karp, Alok Kanojia, Ran Li, Geoffrey Liu, Jonathan Zebrowski

MEDICATIONS AND SIDE EFFECTS
Gowri G. Aragam, Noor Beckwith, Rahel Bosson, Kristina Cieslak, Cristina Cusin, Sam Dotson, Veronica A. Faller, Katie Hsih, Katherine Kilgore, James Luccarelli, Andy Melaragno, Mladen Nisavic, Nate Praschan, Lisa Rosenfeld, Maya Son, John W. Winkelman

EMERGENCY PSYCHIATRY
Suzanne Bird, Mark Fusunyan, Katie Hsih, Katherine A. Koh, Meghan Musselman, Nate Praschan, Curtis Wittmann

LEGAL ISSUES
Ren Belcher, Douglas Brennan, Raphaela Gold, Meghan Musselman, Marc Weinberg

SPECIAL POPULATIONS
Noor Beckwith, Ren Belcher, Philip Cawkwell, Jacci Clauss, Julia Cromwell, Stephanie Davidson, Sam Dotson, Michal McDowell, Cordelia Ross, Emily Sorg, Kathryn Zagrabbe

ABBREVIATIONS

INDEX

MENTAL STATUS EXAM

The Mental Status Exam (MSE) is regarded as a "moment in time," functioning as a systematic, generally informal depiction of the state of the patient's mental health. It outlines through observation and interview a broad swathe of a person's appearance, behavior, interaction with the environment, and internal mental state. It serves as a portion of the psychiatric interview and, when thoughtfully written, marks a valuable comparison point to previous and subsequent assessments. Aspects of the MSE can have significant legal implications (eg, violent ideations and insight/judgment) and warrant particular consideration. Some of the common components of the MSE and a glossary of terms can be found below.

Components of the Mental Status Exam (Richards M. *The Pocket Guide to the DSM-5 Diagnostic Exam*; 2014; Wenzel A. *The SAGE Encyclopedia of Abnormal and Clinical Psychology*; 2017)	
Appearance	Write with the goal of later being able to reconjure the person's most salient features on physical presentation. Consider gender, apparent age, weight, dysmorphic features, dress, grooming, hygiene, smell, unusual skin markings or accessories, etc.
Behavior	Movement (motor agitation/retardation, fidgeting, tics, tardive dyskinesia, stereotypy), facial expression, eye contact, positioning (sitting, standing)
Attitude/ motivation	Attitude/position toward examiner, does the interviewee seem to express motivation/desire relief from distress or acknowledge distress? Cooperativity vs hostility, suspicion, guardedness, or passivity
Speech/ language	Qualities of speech include rate, tone, volume, rhythm, prosody, articulation, fluency and quantity, unusual use of language (neologisms or words used incorrectly), paucity of speech or poverty of content
Mood	Often includes the interviewee's own words: *"How would you describe your mood today?"* The purpose being to capture an immediate subjective state of the interviewee (Trzepacz and Baker, 1993). Words used may include: euthymic, dysphoric, elevated, elated, irritable, angry.
Affect	Here the examiner evaluates the quality of a patient's emotional state through observation. The clinician also evaluates the interviewee on stability, appropriateness (stated vs apparent emotional state), range, and intensity.
Thought process	Flow and form/coherence of thought (as compared to Thought content, below). A normal thought process is linear, logical, and goal-directed; consider directed vs disorganized; loose association, tangentiality, flight of ideas, magical thinking, inhibition, poverty, circumstantiality, perseverativity, rumination, and preoccupation

(continued)

Components of the Mental Status Exam *(continued)*	
Thought content/ perceptual experiences	SI/HI, *asked explicitly*; violent ideations, paranoia, obsessions, compulsions, delusions (types and definitions listed below), ideas of reference, thought broadcasting/ insertion, and mood congruency/incongruency of psychotic features.
Orientation/ cognition	Awareness of time, place, and identity. General sense of cognitive functioning obtained through conversation; however, additional tests, eg, MMSE/MoCA expand this exam. Educational background
Insight/ judgment	**Insight**: the interviewee's sense of their own disposition/ illness and its effects on their well-being. Does the interviewee attribute their symptoms to a mental disorder or are they unconvinced of a problem? There are a number of validated insight rating scales designed for use in treating psychotic disorders (eg, Beck Cognitive Insight Scale, Markov's Insight Scale) which include examples of insight-based questions. **Judgment**: a person's capacity for reasonable decision-making. In assessment consider proposing a real-life challenge to the interviewee such as a work/home-based scenario and assess planning, self-awareness, safety, and consideration of consequences. Insight and judgment are generally rated as *intact, fair, limited,* or *impaired*. We recommend including additional explanation or examples of limited or impaired insight or judgment, as these labels can impact a patient's capacity to consent for medical care.

Glossary of Terms Related to the Mental Status Exam	
(Limited adaptation from: *Diagnostic and Statistical Manual of Mental Disorders.* 5th ed.)	
Behavior	**Dyskinesia:** distortion of voluntary movements with involuntary muscle activity. **Dystonia:** disordered tonicity of muscles. **Echopraxia:** mimicking the movements of another. **Psychomotor agitation:** excessive motor activity associated with a feeling of inner tension. The activity is usually nonproductive and repetitious and consists of behaviors such as pacing, fidgeting, wringing of the hands, pulling of clothes, and inability to sit still. **Psychomotor retardation:** visible generalized slowing of movements and speech. **Stereotypies, stereotyped behaviors/movements:** repetitive, abnormally frequent, non–goal-directed movements, seemingly driven, and nonfunctional motor behavior (eg, hand shaking or waving, body rocking, head banging, self-biting). **Mannerisms:** repetitive, bizarre, purposeful movements

Glossary of Terms Related to the Mental Status Exam (continued)	
Speech/ language	**Articulation:** movement of facial anatomy (eg, tongue, lips) to make speech sounds. **Fluency:** smooth, lack of hesitancy, effortlessness of speaking. **Incoherence:** speech or thinking that is essentially incomprehensible to others because words or phrases are joined together without a logical and meaningful connection; this disturbance occurs within clauses. In its extreme, called word salad. Lack of education or low intelligence should not be considered incoherence. **Neologism:** creation of new words that are meaningless except to the person coining the term. **Paucity of speech:** alogia, a lack of unprompted content; considered a negative symptom in schizophrenia. **Poverty of content:** speaking without substance; requiring excessive speech to convey a message. **Pressured speech:** speech that is increased in quantity, accelerated, and difficult or impossible to interrupt. Usually it is also loud and emphatic. A person might not require social stimulation or an audience to speak. **Prosody:** the elements of speech connecting words beyond vowel and consonant, eg, intonation, tone, stress, rhythm. **Rate:** subjective estimate of speech units over a given amount of time. **Rhythm:** sense of movement of speech; flow of sound and silence. **Tone:** variation in inflection/pitch while speaking. **Volume:** loudness/softness of speech.
Mood/affect	**Appropriateness:** congruency between normative and actual emotional expression during conversation. **Blunted:** significant reduction in the intensity of emotional expression (greater than constricted). **Constricted/restricted:** mild reduction in range and intensity of emotional expression when talking about emotionally arousing topics. Usually stated as constricted/ restricted to a particular emotion. **Dysphoric:** a condition in which one experiences feelings of discontent, and in some cases indifference to the world around them; less extreme negative mood state than depressed. **Elation:** great happiness. **Elevated:** positive feelings of enthusiasm, well-being, confidence, and/or energy; a component of euphoria. Can be a symptom of mania. **Euphoria:** experience of intense feelings of well-being, elation, happiness, excitement, and joy. **Euthymic:** a normal, tranquil mental or mood state. **Expansive:** an extreme expression of emotion, often accompanied with inflated self-worth, excessive friendliness, grandiosity, or superiority. **Flat:** absence or near absence of any sign of affective expression. **Guarded:** caution in disclosing; filtering one's emotional expression.

(continued)

Glossary of Terms Related to the Mental Status Exam (continued)

	Inappropriate: discordance between affective expression and the content of speech or ideation. **Intensity:** strength of emotional responsiveness, from low to high. **Irritable:** a prolonged state of negative emotion, short temper, crossness, or frustration. Primary mood quality is anger. **Labile:** abnormal variability in affect with repeated, rapid, and abrupt shifts in affective expression (laughing one moment, crying the next). **Range:** totality of emotions apparent during assessment. Terms used to describe range include full, restricted/ constricted, blunted, flat, expansive. **Stability:** consistency of emotional expression within the interview.
Thought process	**Alogia:** see *Paucity of speech*, above. **Circumstantiality:** inability to answer a question or make a point without unnecessary detail. Generally inclusive of excessive information. Usually returns to and completes the original thoughts (contrasting with tangentiality). **Flight of ideas:** a nearly continuous flow of accelerated speech with abrupt changes from topic to topic that are usually based on understandable associations, distracting stimuli, or plays on words. When the condition is severe, speech may be disorganized and incoherent. **Goal directed:** answering questions or speaking with a sense of purpose, without straying off-topic. **Logical:** thought demonstrating rationality in connections between points. **Linear:** sequentiality of thought progression; contrasted with fragmented thinking. **Loosening of associations:** lack of logical relationship between two thoughts expressed in sequence. **Magical thinking:** false belief in causal relationships between actions and events; the erroneous belief that one's thoughts, words, or actions will cause or prevent a specific outcome in some way that defies commonly understood laws of cause and effect. **Perseverativity/rumination:** continuous brooding or worry about past or future negative events. **Poverty of thought:** an overall reduction in the quantity of thought; a negative symptom of schizophrenia, also present in severe depression or dementia. **Preoccupation:** absorption; inability to shift from a particular thought. **Tangentiality:** shifting thoughts and speech away from original topic without return (compare to circumstantiality). **Thought blocking:** sudden cessation in speech without explanation.

Thought content/ perceptual experience	**Compulsion:** repetitive behaviors (eg, hand washing, ordering, checking) or mental acts (eg, praying, counting, repeating words silently) that the individual feels driven to perform in response to an obsession, or according to rules that must be applied rigidly. The behaviors or mental acts are aimed at preventing or reducing anxiety or distress, or preventing some dreaded event or situation; however, these behaviors or mental acts are not connected in a realistic way with what they are designed to neutralize or prevent, or are clearly excessive.
	Delusion: a firmly held false belief based on incorrect inference about external reality despite apparent incontrovertible evidence to the contrary. This belief is not ordinarily accepted by other members of the person's culture (ie, it is not an article of religious faith). Types of delusions:
	of being controlled: a delusion in which feelings, impulses, thoughts, or actions are experienced as being under the control of some external force rather than being under one's own control;
	bizarre: a delusion involving a phenomenon that the person's culture would regard as impossible;
	delusional jealousy: a delusion that one's sexual partner is unfaithful;
	erotomania: a delusion that another person, usually of higher status, is in love with the individual;
	grandiosity: a delusion of inflated worth, power, knowledge, identity, or special relationship to a deity or famous person;
	persecutory: a delusion wherein the individual or someone close to the individual is being attacked, harassed, cheated, persecuted, or conspired against;
	somatic: a delusion of which the main content pertains to the appearance or functioning of one's body;
	thought broadcasting: a delusion that one's thoughts are being broadcast out loud so that they can be perceived by others;
	thought insertion: a delusion that some of one's thoughts are not one's own, but rather are inserted into one's mind;
	thought withdrawal: the delusional belief that thoughts have been "taken out" of a person's mind without permission.
	Homicidal ideations (HI): preoccupation with the killing of another person.
	Ideas of reference: the feeling that causal incidents and external events have a particular meaning that is specific to the person.
	Mood congruency: beliefs in which the content is entirely consistent with affect. Contrasted with mood-incongruent thoughts.

(continued)

	Glossary of Terms Related to the Mental Status Exam (continued)
	Suicidal ideation (SI): preoccupation with killing of oneself, from fleeting thought to detailed planning.
	Obsession: recurrent and persistent thoughts, urges, or images that are experienced, at some time during the disturbance, as intrusive and unwanted and that in most individuals cause marked anxiety or distress. The individual attempts to ignore or suppress such thoughts, urges, or images, or to neutralize them with some other thought or action (ie, by performing a compulsion).
	Paranoid ideation: ideation, of less than delusional proportions, involving suspiciousness or the belief that one is being harassed, persecuted, or unfairly treated.
Orientation/ cognition	**MMSE:** A 30-point questionnaire used to measure cognitive functions such as recall, attention, calculation, orientation, and command-following. Has an 18%, 78% sensitivity for MCI, AD, respectively. 100% specificity for MCI, AD, respectively (M.F. Folstein et al., 1975).
	MoCA: Montreal Cognitive Assessment: a cognitive test of complex visuospatial and executive function, freely available in many languages (www.mocatest.org). Up to 90, 100% sensitivity for MCI, AD, respectively, 87% specificity for MCI, AD, respectively (J Am Geriatr Soc. 53(4):695-699).

NEUROPSYCHIATRIC TESTING

Formal Neuropsychiatric Testing
- Performed by a trained provider to characterize cognitive/emotional functioning, define pt strengths/weaknesses, and clarify diagnosis
- **IQ Testing:** Wechsler Adult Intelligence Scale-IV and Wechsler Abbreviated Scale of Intelligence—Full Scale IQ mean of 100, SD 15
- **Cognitive Tests:** Wisconsin Card Sort Test (WCST; pt sorts deck of cards and is required to shift set during sorting; executive fxn); Conners Continuous Performance Test (CPT; pt clicks mouse or inhibits clicking based on long stream of visual/auditory stimuli; sustained atten); Hopkins Verbal Learning Test (HVLT; pt recalls semantically categorized list of words; memory/learning)
- **Personality Testing:** *Self*-report measures; Minnesota Multiphasic Personality Inventory-2 (MMPI-2, 567 items) and Personality Assessment Inventory (PAI, 344 items); measure personality traits ie, social introversion, neuroticism, suspiciousness; include embedded validity scales to detect overreporting/underreporting of sxs ie, "faking good" and "faking bad" and intentional random answers (J Pers Assess. 1991;57(2):264-277)
- **Psychological Performance Testing:** Formerly "projective" testing; less structured, reveals pt problem-solving style and unique personality characteristics
  - Thematic Apperception Test (pt interprets ambiguous pictures through narrative; may suggest conscious/unconscious motives)
  - Rorschach Inkblot Test; high interrater reliability w/ standardized scoring system (Wiley. The Rorschach: A Comprehensive System. Vol. 1; 1993)

Bedside Neuropsychiatric Testing

- Includes structured and unstructured assessments
- **Mini-Mental State Examination (MMSE):** *Clinician*-rated scale; greater focus on memory and orientation; score <26 indicates MCI; low Sn/high Sp (LR+ >100, LR− 0.8 for MCI) (*J Am Geriatr Soc.* 2005;53(4):695-699)
- **Montreal Cognitive Assessment (MoCA):** *Clinician*-rated scale; score <26 indicates MCI; high Sn/moderate Sp (LR+ 6.9, LR− 0.1 for MCI); greater focus on executive function; higher AUC for individual domains than MMSE; consistently ↓ scores than MMSE (*J Am Geriatr Soc.* 2005;53:695-699; *Movement Disord.* 2010; *J Am Geriatr Soc.* 2017;65:1067-1072)
- **Executive Interview (EXIT-25):** *Clinician*-rated scale; score >15 indicates MCI; correlates w/ level of care (community-dwelling vs nursing home) and behavioral disturbance (*J Am Geriatr Soc.* 1993;40(12):1221-1226)
- **Clock-Draw:** Reliable screen for cog dysfxn; common errors incl perseveration, stimulus-bound, missequencing; errors have anatomical correlates (*J Neuropsychiatry Clin Neurosci.* 2012;24(3):260-265)

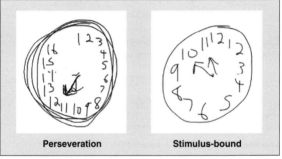

| Perseveration | Stimulus-bound |

Clock-Draw Prompt: "Set the time to ten past eleven."

- **Luria Sequencing:** Exec fxn; can distinguish healthy controls from MCI, MCI from dementia; common errors are missequencing, perseveration, impulsivity (*Int Psychogeriatr.* 2012;23(10):1602-1606)
- **Go/No-Go:** Exec fxn, inhibition; many forms (ie, "When I tap once, you tap once. When I tap twice, you don't tap.")

Cognitive Domains		
Domain	**Description**	**Tests**
Executive function	Decision-making; planning; working memory; inhibition; set shifting	Clock draw; go/no-go; WCST; Luria sequencing
Attention	Sustained attention; selective attention; processing speed	Digit span; days of wk frwd/bkwrd; CPT
Memory and learning	Immediate/recent/long-term memory	HVLT; immediate and delayed recall

(continued)

Cognitive Domains (continued)		
Visuospatial	Visual perception, praxis, spatial awareness, visuoconstruction	Cube copy, line bisection, pantomime, grooved pegboard
Language	Expressive and receptive	Naming; FAS fluency; verbal command
Social cognition	Theory of mind, emotion recognition	TAT; emotion naming

Cognitive Scale Scoring Comparison			
Domain		MMSE	MoCA
Orientation		10 pts (33%) • time/place	6 pts (20%) • time/place
Attention and calculation		5 pts (17%) • "WORLD" backward	6 pts (20%) • Serial 7s • CPT • Digit span
Comprehension/ executive function		4 pts (13%) • 3-step command • Read/obey command	6 pts (20%) • Verbal fluency • Trail-making • Abstraction • Draw clock (numbers, hands)
Naming		2 pts (7%) • Pencil, watch	3 pts (10%) • 3 animals
Learning and memory	Registration	3 pts (10%) • 3 words	0 pts (0%) • 5 words
	Delayed recall	3 pts (10%) • 3 words/>10 s	5 pts (17%) • 5 words/5 min
	Cued recall (opt.)	0 pts (0%)	0 pts (0%)
	Recognition (opt.)	0 pts (0%)	0 pts (0%)
Repetition		1 pt (3%) • 1 short sentence	2 pts (7%) • 2 longer sentences
Visuospatial		1 pt (3%) • Copy int. pentagons	2 pts (7%) • Copy cube • Draw clock (contour)
Writing		1 pt (3%)	n.a.
Total score		30 pts	30 pts

Table above compares points awarded for each cognitive domain in the MMSE and MoCA. Items in **bold** highlight those domains enriched in that test.

Depression

- **Hamilton Rating Scale for Depression (HAM-D):** *Clinician*-rated scale; 17-point version has greater validation; ratings include mild (7–17 pts), moderate (18–24 pts), severe (>24 pts) depression; cutoffs of M ≥ 12 and F ≥ 13 have LR+ of 5.51 and LR− of 0.25 (*Psychosomatics. 2001;42(5):423-428*)
- **Beck Depression Inventory (BDI):** *Self*-reported scale; measure of cross-sectional symptom severity; variable convergent validity; correlation of 0.73 w/ HAM-D (*Clin Psychol Rev. 1988;8:77-100*)
- **Montgomery-Åsberg Depression Rating Scale (MADRS):** *Clinician*-rated scale; designed to be sensitive to effects of antidepressant meds; scores >30–35 indicate severe depression; high correlation w/ HAM-D (r = 0.8–0.9) (*J Affect Dis. 2003;77:255-260*)
- **Quick Inventory of Depressive Symptomatology (QIDS):** Shortened (16-Q) version of IDS; includes both *clinician*-rated (QIDS-C) and *self*-reported (QIDS-SR) scales; QIDS-C has high interrater reliability (κ = 0.96); QIDS-C highly correlated w/ HAM-D (r = 0.92) and less w/ BDI (r = 0.61) (*Biol Psych. 2003;54:573-583*)
- **Patient Health Questionnaire-9 (PHQ-9):** *Self*-reported scale; used as a screening tool to detect depression; scores ≥10 have LR+ 7.33 and LR− for MDD (*J Gen Intern Med. 2001;16(9):606-613*)

Mania (Clinical Trial Design Challenges in Mood Disorders; 2015:105-136)

- **Young Mania Rating Scale (YMRS):** *Clinician*-rated scale; rates severity of each abnormality; can give scores between points on form (esp. when severity of each item does not follow progression given on keys); high interrater reliability for total score (κ = 0.93) and variable for individual items (κ = 0.67–0.95)

Anxiety and OCD

- **Hamilton Anxiety Scale (HAM-A):** *Clinician*-rated scale; rates severity of symptoms; ratings include mild (>17) and moderate-severe (>25–30) anxiety; may be confounded w/ depressive sxs (*J Psychiatric Res. 2017;93:59-63*)
- **Beck Anxiety Inventory (BAI):** *Self*-reported scale; high internal consistency (α = 0.94); not highly confounded w/ depressive sxs (*J Anxiety Disord. 1992;6(1):55-61*)
- **Yale-Brown Obsessive-Compulsive Scale (Y-BOCS):** *Clinician*-rated scale; high internal consistency (α = 0.81); LR+ 2.58 and LR− 0.22 for OCD (*Nord J Psychiatry. 2014;68(8):549-559*)

Psychosis-Related Scales

- **Metabolic Syndrome Screening:** Incorporates objective values to screen for metabolic syndrome; ≥3 of HTN, abd obesity, low HDL, high TG, high FPG indicates metabolic syndrome
- **Abnormal Involuntary Movement Scale (AIMS):** *Clinician*-rated scale; assesses sxs of TD in pts on neuroleptics; includes orofacial movements, extremity/truncal dyskinesia, global severity; follow validated exam procedure

- **Brief Psychiatric Rating Scale (BPRS):** *Clinician*-rated scale; incorporates severity of 24 symptoms; 20% reduction often used a criterion for response to antipsychotics in clinical trials (*Am J Psychiatry.* 2005;162(1):130-136)
- **Positive and Negative Symptoms Scale (PANSS):** *Clinician*-rated scale; assesses positive, negative, and general psychopathology symptoms associated with schizophrenia (*Schizophr Bull.* 1987;13(2):261-276)

Catatonia
- **Bush-Francis Catatonia Rating Scale (BFCRS):** *Clinician*-rated scale; ≥2 positive findings req. for dx of catatonia; ≥3 positive findings w/ LR+ 81 and LR− 0.11 for catatonia (*Psychiatry Res.* 2015;229(3):919-925)

PTSD
- **Trauma Assessment/Checklist:** *Self*-reported scale; inventory of frequency of symptoms of PTSD over the past month

Others
- **Clinical Global Impression (CGI):** *Clinician*-rated scale; measures the global symptom severity in patients with mental disorders; includes an efficacy index for management of psychopharmacology and its side effects

Children
- **Self-Report for Childhood Anxiety and Related Disorders (SCARED):** *Self*-reported scales for both parent and child; scores ≥25 for anxiety d/o; subscales for panic d/o, GAD, separation anxiety, social phobia
- **Revised Children's Anxiety and Depression Scale (RCADS):** *Self*-reported scale for youth; subscales for separation anxiety, social phobia, GAD, panic d/o, OCD, and MDD; T-score conversion based on gender and grade (3–12)
- **Disruptive Behavior Disorders (DBD) Rating Scale:** *Self*-reported scale for parent and teacher; three subscales for ADHD, ODD, and conduct d/o; respondent must choose "pretty much"/ "very much" for significance

NEUROIMAGING

Introduction
- Evidence scant for routine neuroimaging in workup of most psychiatric conditions, as current methods have not consistently delivered data that inform prognosis or alter the course of treatment (*Psychiatry Res Neuroimaging.* 2014; 224(2):104-106).
- In 6200 psychiatric patients with MRI, 1.6% had treatment altering MRI findings; MS and hemorrhage most common (*Harv Rev Psych.* 1995;2(6):297-312).

Suggested Indications for Neuroimaging in Psychiatric Populations (*Am J Psychiatry.* 1984;141(12):1521-1527)
- **Exam:** acutely altered mental status, focal neurologic deficits

- **History**: trauma with loss of consciousness, whole brain radiation, cancer, neurologic comorbidities, late onset of psychiatric symptoms (>50 y), or atypical presentation—may suggest organic cause
- **First episode psychosis:** Controversial, percentage of patients with abnormal/treatment altering imaging findings is low (*Health Technol Assess.* 2008;12(18):iii-iv, ix-163; *Clin Radiol.* 2013; 68(3):245-250). Still, some clinicians advocate for imaging at least once given potential to dramatically influence disease course and prognosis.
- **ECT:** if concern for intracranial pathology

Imaging Modalities		
Modality	**Safety Issues**	**Indications**
Computed tomography (CT)	• Radiation exposure, contrast allergies, renal damage (*N Engl J Med.* 2007;357(22):2277-2284).	Acute cerebrovascular injury, some malignancies, edema, and ventricular or midline structure pathology (ie, herniation, hydrocephalus). **Cheaper and faster than MRI
Magnetic resonance imaging (MRI)	• Contraindicated in those with paramagnetic materials (including pacemakers, metallic joint replacements) in body • Gadolinium may cause nephrogenic systemic fibrosis in patients with renal dysfunction (rare)	Sequences (*Radiographics.* 2006;26(2):513-537): • **T1:** Best for anatomy • **T2:** Best for pathology • **FLAIR:** T2 image with CSF signal subtracted. Very sensitive to pathology, especially periventricular. • **DWI:** Measures water diffusivity—decreased in stroke, abscess, hypercellular tumor, excitotoxicity • **DTI** can provide axonal maps that are used in TBI and presurgical mapping **Outperforms CT as diagnostic tool except for acute hemorrhage and fractures
Functional magnetic resonance imaging (fMRI)	Same as MRI, though no gadolinium	Primarily a research tool. Some clinical use in presurgical mapping. Allows estimate of regional activity based on ratio of deoxy to oxyhemoglobin (*Nature.* 2008;453(7197):869-878)
Positron emission tomography (PET)/single photon emission computer tomography (SPECT)	Radiation dose is similar to CT	Can be used to measure perfusion, metabolic activities (ie, FDG-PET), neurotransmitter systems, or pathologic deposits (ie, amyloid) Clinically useful in dementia and seizures, emerging use in TBI
See also: *Prim Care Companion CNS Disord.* 2013;15(4).		

Clinical Findings in Specific Conditions

- **Alzheimer's disease (FDG-PET):** Temporal and parietal hypometabolism that includes midline structures; spreads to frontal cortex as disease progresses. Spares somatosensory/visual cortices, basal ganglia, and cerebellum (Clin Nucl Med. 2014;39(10):e413-e426).
- **Frontotemporal dementia (FDG-PET):** Hypometabolism in frontal and anterior temporal cortices, cingulate gyri, uncus, insula, basal ganglia, and medial thalamus. Often more pronounced in left hemisphere, which may help distinguish from Alzheimer's (J Nucl Med. 2005;46(2):233-239).
- **Seizures (FDG-PET):** Ictal hypermetabolism and peri/postictal hypometabolism at focus. Useful for surgical planning (Am J Nucl Med Imag. 2015;5(5):416-430).
- **Limbic encephalitis (MRI):** May be normal or show T2-FLAIR hyperintense lesions, especially in the medial temporal lobe. Abnormal imaging more common in HSV encephalitis (95%) vs paraneoplastic (>50% have normal imaging), but MRI alone cannot elucidate etiology (J Clin Neurol. 2016;12(1):1-13; Am J Neurorad. 2017;38(6):1070-1078).

EEG

Background: (Psychophysiology. 2014;51:1062; J Neurol Neurosurg Psychiatry. 2005;76:ii2-ii7; J Clin Neurophysiol. 2016;33:340; Measurement Sci Rev. 2002;2:2; PLoS Biol. 2011;9:3)

Definition: Electroencephalography (EEG) is the recording of electrical activity in the brain.

Clinical EEG Types

- **Routine:** Scalp EEG lasting 20–60 min.
- **Continuous:** Longer-duration EEG monitoring, including sleep-deprived EEG lasting several hours, ambulatory EEG monitoring lasting days to weeks, and inpatient video-EEG monitoring for clinical-electrographic correlation. Sleep deprivation and monitoring across periods of sleep and wakefulness increases diagnostic yield.
- **Polysomnogram (PSG):** Scalp EEG during sleep paired with monitoring of eye movements, muscle activity, and cardiorespiratory parameters; used for evaluation of sleep disorders. Used for diagnosis of sleep apneas, periodic limb movement disorders, narcolepsy, and other sleep disorders.

Normal Rhythms

- **Beta (>12–30 Hz):** Predominant rhythm in normal awake adults with eyes open. Best observed frontally.
- **Alpha (8–12 Hz):** Predominant rhythm in normal adults who are awake with eyes closed. Suppressed in states of anxiety. Best observed over posterior scalp, referred to as posterior dominant alpha (PDA).
- **Theta (4–8 Hz):** Slower activity present in normal awake children and in adults during drowsiness and sleep but is pathological if prevalent in waking states.

- **Delta (<4 Hz):** Observed during "slow-wave sleep" (stages 3 and 4) of non-REM sleep in adults, normal background in infants up to 1 y.

Limitations
- **Spatial:** Scalp EEG may fail to detect abnormal discharges with insufficient synchrony or cortical involvement, as well as those originating from medial and basal cortical areas. Specialized electrode placement ranging in depth from subcutaneous to parenchymal may be performed to improve detection and localization in select cases.

  Temporal: Likelihood of capturing abnormal activity increases with duration of monitoring or repeat studies. For routine EEG, sensitivity for interictal discharges within 24 h of first seizure is roughly 50% and declines afterward.

Application and Interpretation (*J Neurol Neurosurg Psychiatry. 2005;76:ii8-ii12; J Neurol. 2013;260:1092; Semin Neurol. 2003;23:7-46; J Clin Neurophysiol. 2004;21:307-318; J Clin Neurophysiol. 2006;23:340; J Neurol Neurosurg Psychiatry. 2005;76:ii2-ii3; Neuropsychobiology. 1992;26:126*)

DDx of Altered Mental Status: Particular findings or lack thereof may help prioritize certain diagnostic categories and can be suggestive of specific etiology in some contexts. Routine EEG is sufficient for most situations and in terms of diagnostic logistics is often available before brain MRI.
- **Normal:** EEG is typically normal in psychiatric disorders, as well as in certain states of apparent nonresponsiveness such as locked-in syndrome. In catatonia, grossly abnormal EEG may increase suspicion for neuromedical etiology.
- **Diffuse/generalized slowing:** Background slowing into theta or delta range is a nonspecific abnormality, often seen in delirium. Frontal intermittent rhythmic delta activity (FIRDA) is similarly nonspecific if symmetric. Anti-NMDAR encephalitis is associated with rhythmic delta activity known as "extreme delta brush," though diffuse slowing remains the most common presentation.
- **Focal slowing:** Focal theta or delta range slowing is suggestive of abnormal cortical activity due to structural lesion (CVA, prior surgery, tumor, TBI, infection, congenital malformation etc) or functional abnormality (ie, partial seizure with postictal slowing).
- **Epileptiform discharges:** EDs typically have sharper morphology than normal background and include spikes and sharp waves which can occur in various permutations with slow waves. In the evaluation of altered mental status, isolated EDs may suggest propensity for or recent occurrence of seizure events. Electroclinical criteria exist for diagnosis of nonconvulsive status epilepticus, an important mechanism for altered mental status. Please see the Seizure chapter for more information.
- **Triphasic waves (TWs):** Consists of a positive polarity sharp wave bounded by two negative sharp waves. Classically associated with uremic and hepatic encephalopathy in adults, but more generally suggestive of severe toxic-metabolic delirium.
- **Periodic epileptiform discharges:** EDs recurring at regular interval, which are further classified as lateralized/focal or bilateral. Controversy exists whether periodic EDs are actually seizures. Lateralized or focal discharges are suggestive of subacute to acute

hemispheric lesion, including CVA, tumor, and infection with temporal localization suggestive of HSV encephalitis. Bilateral discharges can occur with catastrophic global cerebral injury, most often hypoxic encephalopathy.

- **Periodic sharp-wave complexes:** Occur in most patients with CJD often with clinical emergence of myoclonus, and becomes generalized with disease progression. Can also be seen in delirium due to lithium or baclofen intoxication, as well as subacute sclerosis panencephalitis (SSPE).

Other Common Applications
- Video-EEG monitoring is used in specialized epilepsy units to guide medication changes and localize epileptic foci for surgical intervention.
- EEG can be used to assess depth of procedural anesthesia or sedation during mechanical ventilation.
- EEG can also yield prognostic information in coma and persistent vegetative state, as well as contribute to criteria for brain death.
- EEG is the subject of ongoing research regarding potential biomarkers for psychiatric diagnosis and prediction of treatment response.

EEG and Psychiatric Therapeutics (Am J Psychiatry. 2002;159:111; Human Psychopharmacol. 2003;18:643; Epilepsia. 2006;47:2072; J Clin Psychopharmacol. 2010;30:312; J Clin Psychopharmacol. 1984;4:263; Depression Anxiety. 2000;12:160-161)
- **Antipsychotics:** Clozapine is associated with dose-dependent background slowing and incidence of epileptiform discharges even within therapeutic dose range. Of other commonly used agents, olanzapine is most comparable in terms of EEG profile.
- **Sedative-hypnotics:** Diffuse theta or delta range slowing heavily intermixed with beta activity in the setting of decreased level of consciousness is suggestive of sedative-hypnotic intoxication.
- **Mood stabilizers:** Marked EEG changes can occur with lithium at toxic and normal therapeutic levels, including triphasic waves, generalized slowing, and epileptiform activity suggestive of NCSE. EEG changes are typically subtle with AEDs at therapeutic levels, but background slowing can be observed with toxicity.
- **Antidepressants:** EEG changes are typically subtle but dose-dependent background slowing and paroxysmal epileptiform discharges are seen with TCAs and bupropion.
- **ECT:** Interictal EEG may exhibit background slowing for several weeks after treatment. Prefrontal slowing is associated with antidepressant effect, while left frontotemporal slowing is associated with cognitive deficits.

ATTENTION-DEFICIT/ HYPERACTIVITY DISORDER

Definition and Clinical Features

- Significant impairment from symptoms of *inattention*, *hyperactivity/ impulsivity*, or *both*

Inattentive Symptoms
Lacks attention to detail/careless errors
Problems sustaining attention in tasks or play
Seems not to listen when spoken to
Starts but fails to follow through on tasks
Difficulty organizing tasks/materials and managing time
Lengthy mental tasks avoided
Loses important materials and belongings
Easily distracted by unrelated stimuli (external/internal)
Forgetful regarding activities
Hyperactive/Impulsive Symptoms
Fidgets/taps/squirms in seat
Trouble staying in seat in environments where this is the norm
Runs/climbs inappropriately (in adolescents/adults, manifests as inner restlessness)
Finds it hard to play or relax quietly
Appears to others as if "driven by a motor"
Talks too much
Verbal tendency for blurting things out
Trouble waiting one's turn
Interruptive and intrusive
Duration/Symptom Threshold
Symptoms must be present prior to 12 y/o, in ≥2 settings (school, work, home, socially, etc), with clear functional impairment. Symptoms cannot be due to another psych condition
For ≥6 mo, ≥6 inattentive symptoms OR ≥6 hyperactive/impulsive sx OR ≥6 of each type (combined). N.B. only need ≥5 of each if ≥17 y/o

Am Psychiatry Assoc. 2013.

Epidemiology and Pathogenesis

- In childhood, most commonly diagnosed neurobehavioral disorder
- Prevalence: estimated 7.2% in ≤18 y, up to 4.4% in adults (*Pediatrics.* 2015;135(4):e994; *Am J Psychiatry.* 2006;163(4):716)

- M>F, at least 2:1. Differences in prevalence by gender may be explained by higher levels of hyperactive/impulsive symptoms in boys prompting sooner referral to care (NCHS Data Brief. 2015;201; J Am Acad Child Adolesc Psychiatry. 2010;49(3):217)
- Genetic transmission: Highly heritable, 1st-degree relatives of patients with ADHD have 5- to 10-fold greater risk than gen. pop of developing ADHD
- No clear causative factors; association reported with prenatal insults/exposures (eg, maternal smoking/alcohol use), premature birth, low birth weight, and exposure to environmental toxins (Nat Rev Dis Primers. 2015;1:15020)
- **Pathophysiology**
  - Multiple brain regions and pathways implicated
  - Compared to unaffected controls, ADHD associated with delayed maturation of cerebral cortex and overall reduction in cortical volume by 3–5%
  - In experimental conditions, reward-processing altered, default-mode network connectivity disrupted (Nat Rev Dis Primers. 2015;1:15020)

Evaluation

- Clinical diagnosis based on patient and caregiver report (if applicable). Validated rating scales (eg, Vanderbilt and Connors) administered to parents, teachers, and other caregivers very helpful. In adults, often helps to use a standard self-report scale based on DSM criteria
- Differential diagnosis: ODD, learning disorders, ASD, intellectual disability, reactive attachment disorders, anxiety, and mood disorders (includes MDD, BPAD, IED, DMDD), substance use disorders
- Comorbid disorders: ODD (up to 65%), conduct disorder (~15%), bipolar disorder (up to 21% in some ADHD cohorts), substance use disorders; other less common comorbidities include ASD, tic disorders/Tourette syndrome, OCD (Br J Psychiatry. 2011;198(3):195; J Am Acad Child Adolesc Psychiatry. 1996;35(9):1193; Clin Psychol Rev. 2011;31(3):328)

Nonpharmacologic Treatment

- Should be first-line treatment in preschool-aged children (age < 6). Various behavioral approaches have been studied, including psychoeducation, organizational skills training, CBT, parent training, school-based interventions. Most successful when combined with pharmacologic treatment (Nat Rev Dis Primers. 2015;1:15020; https://www.nature.com/articles/nrdp201520)

Pharmacologic Treatment

- **Preschool-aged children:** treat with nonpharmacologic treatments first, medications when symptoms severe
- **Children/adults:** stimulant medications first-line treatment
- **Stimulants:** amphetamine or methylphenidate, prescribed in short-, intermediate-, and long-acting forms, is first-line treatment
  - Screen for preexisting cardiac conditions, family history of sudden cardiac death—refer to cardiology prior to initiation of treatment
  - During treatment, monitor blood pressure/heart rate. Monitor for disrupted sleep, decreased appetite, mood changes (irritability, mania), psychosis, tics

- Long-term stimulant treatment may attenuate neural deficits in ADHD (*J Clin Psychiatry.* 2013;74(9):902)
- **Nonstimulant FDA-approved medications:** (*Am Psychiatry Assoc.* 2016; *Textbook of Child and Adolescent Psychiatry, Ch. 35*)
  - *Atomoxetine*: can be helpful for stimulant nonresponders, comorbid anxiety disorders, tic disorders; **NOTE:** black box warning for increased SI in children/adolescents
  - *Alpha-2 agonists*: long-acting *clonidine* and *guanfacine*, primarily for hyperactive/impulsive symptoms, useful with comorbid tic disorders. Short-acting versions also commonly used, not FDA approved
- **Off-label medications:** *Bupropion (NDRI)* and *modafinil (wake-promoting agent)* improve symptoms of ADHD. *Tricyclic antidepressants* have demonstrated effectiveness in studies over placebo; however, less commonly used due to prominent adverse effect profile

ADJUSTMENT DISORDERS

Definition and Clinical Features (*Clin Pract Epidemiol Ment Health.* 2009;5:15; *Neuropsychiatr Dis Treat.* 2018;14:375-381)
- The emergence of psychiatric or behavioral symptoms within 3–6 mo of a discernible stressor, leading to maladaptive behaviors or decrease in functioning without reaching the level of another diagnosis
- Types (with…):
  - Depressed mood
  - Anxiety
  - Mixed anxiety and depressed mood
  - Disturbance of conduct
  - Mixed disturbance of emotions (depression, anxiety symptoms) and conduct
  - Unspecified
- Diagnostic features:
  - Common stressors: romantic relationship ending, loss of a job, financial difficulties
  - Can be recurrent or continuous stressors: chronic illness, unsafe home environment
  - Can be diagnosed following the death of a loved one when not normal grief reaction and not persistent complex bereavement disorder

Epidemiology and Pathogenesis (*World Psychiatry.* 2011;10(1):11-18; *Eur Psychiatry.* 2000;15(3):190-195; *Indian J Psychol Med.* 2013;35(1):4-9)
- Three times as common as MDD in medically ill inpatients (13.7 vs 5.1%)
- Most common diagnosis in hospital psychiatric consultation settings
- Prevalence in primary care settings is 11–18%, psychiatric ED 17.1% and inpatient psychiatry 9%

- Shorter interval between appearance of symptoms and suicide attempt than in other disorders (<1 mo)
- Pathophysiology not known, though likely neurochemical changes in response to stress

Evaluation (Clin Practice Epidemiol Meant Health. 2009;5:15)
Differential Diagnosis
- Presence of a primary mood or anxiety disorder takes precedence
- Consider MDD, PTSD, acute stress disorder, personality disorders (however, adjustment disorder can be diagnosed acutely in patients with comorbid personality disorder), psychological factors affecting a medical illness, normative stress reactions, normal bereavement, persistent complex bereavement disorder

Risk Factors (Neuropsychiatr Dis Treat. 2018;1:375-381)
- Acute traumatic event, previous trauma, some evidence for female gender increasing risk

Nonpharmacological Treatment (Neuropsychiatr Dis Treat. 2018;1:375-381)
- Psychotherapy is the treatment of choice, though no clear evidence for specific therapy, given limited trials, variability in stressors; supportive therapy most commonly used
- Therapy aims should include:
  - Reducing maladaptive responses and promoting coping utilizing individual strengths
  - Exploring stressor and ways to reduce stressor
  - Supporting use of family and community resources

Pharmacological Treatment (Neuropsychiatr Dis Treat. 2018;1:375-381; World Psychiatry. 2011;10(1):11-18)
- Consider treatment with antidepressants if symptoms are severe, but limit duration and always include psychotherapy; no studies to support antidepressant treatment

Special Populations (Indian J Psychol Med. 2013;35(1):4-9)
- Adolescents with adjustment disorder may be at increased risk of developing major psychiatric illness (only 44% well at 5 y follow-up vs 71% of adults)

GRIEF AND BEREAVEMENT
Definition and Clinical Features
- Acute or normal grief is a normal reaction to loss of a loved one
- Acute grief becomes **complicated grief** when grief responses occur more days than normal and persist for >12 mo in adults (>6 mo in children)

Types of Grief Reactions
- Anticipatory grief: occurs in anticipation of an impending loss
- Four stages of normal grief (National Cancer Institute. 2014)
  1. Numbness-disbelief
  2. Separation distress
  3. Depression-mourning
  4. Recovery

Symptoms of Acute vs Complicated Grief	
Acute Grief	**Complicated Grief**

• Yearning for and seeking proximity to the deceased
• Loneliness
• Crying, sadness, anger, guilt, anxiety upon confrontation of reminders of the loss
• Somatic symptoms (physical sensations, disrupted sleep or appetite)
• Persistent thoughts and memories of the deceased
  • Can include hallucinations but illusions more common
• Feeling drawn to things associated with the deceased (*Acta Psychiatr Scand.* 1993;87:72-80)
• Social withdrawal
• Confusion about one's identity, feeling lost without the deceased
• Disbelief and shock
• Numbness
• Impaired attention, concentration, memory
Nb: consider relevant cultural setting, religious group, or developmental stage when assessing expected norms for grief
	Any symptoms of acute grief that are intense, prolonged, and disabling, plus:
	• Difficulty accepting the deceased has died
	• Disbelief that the person is dead
	• Distressing memories of the deceased
	  • Hallucinations more common
	• Anger, bitterness about the loss
	• Maladaptive appraisals about oneself in relation to the deceased
	• Excessive avoidance of reminders of the loss
	• Desire to die to join the deceased
	• Distrust of others
	• Feeling isolated
	• Belief that life is empty or has no meaning
	• Difficulty engaging in activities, pursuing relationships, planning for future

DSM-5

Epidemiology and Pathogenesis
- **Acute grief:** lifetime prevalence of 57%, associated with increased risk of mortality (*Am J Epidemiol.* 2012;176(4))
- **Complicated grief:** lifetime prevalence of 2.4–4.8% and 7% among the bereaved (*JAMA.* 2013;310(4):416-423), F>M, most often diagnosed in psychiatric settings

Evaluation
- **Risk factors for complicated grief** (*Death Stud.* 2010;34(8):673-698)
  - Older age (>61 y)
  - Female gender
  - Low SES
  - Non-Caucasian race
  - History of anxiety or depression
  - Loss of a spouse or child
  - Difficult circumstances (unexpected, violent) of death of a loved one
- **Type of loss matters**
  - Type of relationship lost (eg, loss of a child can lead to more intense and lasting grief) (*Aust N Z J Psychiatry.* 1998;32:235)
  - Timing of loss
  - Loss from a chronic or terminal illness

- **Psychiatric comorbidities:** MDD, PTSD, anxiety disorders (particularly GAD and panic disorder) (*J Clin Psychiatry.* 2001;62(11):884)
- **Differential diagnosis:** normal grief, PTSD, MDD, demoralization
- **Suicidality**
  - Suicidal ideation and behavior occurs in 40–60% of those with complicated grief after controlling for comorbidities (*J Clin Psychiatry.* 2006;67(2):233)
  - Risk factors for suicidality: prior psychiatric history, active comorbid psychiatric illness, less social support, female gender, non-Caucasian race, death of a loved one by suicide

Nonpharmacologic Treatment

- **Acute grief**
  - Typically does not require clinical intervention
  - Screening and treatment of comorbidities, as grief can precipitate or worsen psychiatric illness
- **Complicated grief**
  - Education
  - Close outpatient monitoring (q1–4wk)
  - Psychotherapy (CBT, behavioral activation, complicated grief therapy)

Pharmacologic Treatment

- **Acute grief**
  - Psychotropics are not recommended
- **Complicated grief**
  - Addition of citalopram to therapy found to be no more effective than placebo with therapy (*JAMA Psychiatry.* 2016;73:685)

ANXIETY DISORDERS

Definition and Clinical Features

- Anxiety is a feeling of worry, nervousness, or unease, often about something in the future with an uncertain outcome. Anxiety is a common experience for all, but can be classified as a disorder when it becomes persistent, impairing, and excessive

Quick Diagnostic Algorithm of Anxiety

- Associated with medical illness? **Anxiety due to general medical condition**
- Temporally related to substances? **Substance-induced anxiety disorder**
- Excessive daily worry about various issues? **Generalized anxiety disorder**
- Prominent fear of embarrassment or scrutiny? **Social anxiety disorder**
- Anxiety bound to specific triggers? **Specific phobia**
- Recurrent, unexpected panic attacks? **Panic disorder**
- Anxiety about having a panic attack or losing control in a place where escape is not possible? **Agoraphobia**

- Related to trauma?
  - With reexperiencing of event? **Acute/PTSD**
  - Related to major psychosocial stressor but not meeting threshold for another anxiety disorder? **Adjustment disorder**
- Also evaluate for obsessive–compulsive, mood, and psychotic disorders, which can all have prominent symptoms of anxiety

Epidemiology and Pathogenesis
- 12-month prevalence—22.2%; lifetime prevalence—33.7%
- Age: can present at any age, and varies significantly by diagnosis, but median age of onset is 11 y old, and 95% onset by age 51 (*Arch Gen Psychiatry.* 2005;62(6):617; *Int J Methods Psychiatry Res.* 2012;21(2):169-184)
- Sex: 3:2 female to male ratio (*Arch Gen Psychiatry.* 1994;51(1):8)
- See disorder-specific chapters for details of pathogenesis. Generally, anxiety is thought to be related to a hypersensitivity and overgeneralization of fear

Evaluation
- Comprehensive history, especially highlighting:
  - Timing and onset of anxiety symptoms
  - Assessment of comorbid mood symptoms and substance use
  - History of trauma or recent major psychosocial stressor
- Anxiety disorders have similar medical differential diagnosis (see table Organic Differential Diagnosis for Panic Disorder below). Especially consider organic etiology when:
  - Onset is after age 35
  - There is no family history of anxiety
  - No recent psychosocial stressor, but new onset symptoms
  - Lack of avoidance behavior
  - Poor effect of anxiolytic medication

Treatment
- Generally, therapy and pharmacotherapy are both effective separately and together in anxiety disorders
- SSRIs or SNRIs are typically first-line for treatment of primary anxiety disorders
- Symptomatic management of severe anxiety with benzodiazepines or other short-term anxiolytics (gabapentin, hydroxyzine, atypical antipsychotics) can be used as needed, typically short term
- If due to medical condition or substance use, address underlying cause in conjunction with symptomatic treatment
- See specific chapters for more detailed summary of treatment options

PANIC DISORDER AND AGORAPHOBIA

Definition and Clinical Features
Panic: Abrupt surge (within minutes) of intense anxiety, with multiple physical (eg, sweating, palpitations) and cognitive (eg, impending doom, fear of dying) symptoms
- Rapidly increasing symptoms, peaking in minutes, lasting 5–10 min, often without trigger
- Can present with depersonalization, difficulty speaking, concentrating
- Presyncopal symptoms are common, syncope is possible though rare

- Patients often flee the situation, sometimes present to the ED
- Anticipatory anxiety and avoidance of situations that might cause panic, or where panic would be problematic
- Frequency varies, between and within individual (eg, weeks or months with daily or weekly attacks, separated by months without attacks)

Diagnostic criteria:
- Multiple, recurrent and unexpected panic attacks
- Presence of at least 4 symptoms
  - Somatic: tremor, GI upset, presyncope, palpitations, tachycardia, tremors, diaphoresis, and extremity tingling
  - Cognitive: intense fear of losing control or death
- Anticipatory anxiety (excessive worry about future panic attacks)
  OR avoidance of situations that might precipitate panic
    Panic attack specifier: Panic attacks alone are not diagnostic of panic disorder and can present in many medical and psychiatric conditions. A panic attack "specifier" is added to a diagnosis to indicate panic (eg, depression with panic attacks)
    Agoraphobia: anxiety about and avoidance of situations that would be difficult to leave. Previously a specifier of panic disorder, now a separate DSM diagnosis
    Diagnostic criteria:
- Significant fear in situations where escape would be difficult, such as:
  - Public transit (cars, buses, trains, etc)
  - Open spaces (parking lots, bridges)
  - Enclosed places (stores, theaters)
  - Crowds or standing in lines
  - Leaving home alone
- These situations are actively avoided or tolerated with distress
- Symptoms present for at least 6 mo
- Not attributable to another anxiety disorder

Epidemiology and Pathogenesis
- 12-month prevalence—2.7%; lifetime prevalence—4.7%
- Age: can present at any age, but median age of onset is 24 y old, and 95% onset by age 56 (*Arch Gen Psychiatry.* 2005;62(6):617; *Int J Methods Psychiatry Res.* 2012;21(2):169-184)
- Sex: F:M 2:1 (*Arch Gen Psychiatry.* 1994;51(1):8)
- In the primary care setting, might be as high as 6.8% (*Ann Intern Med.* 2007;146(5):317)

Etiology and Risk Factors
Genetic
- 1st-degree relatives of individuals with panic disorder have significantly higher rates of panic disorder themselves (*Arch Gen Psychiatry.* 1994;51(5):383-394)
- Twin studies estimate a heritability of 40% (*Am J Psychiatry.* 2001;158(10):1568)

Neurobiology
- Proposed theory that hyperactive circuits between amygdala and hypothalamus are the root of panic that propagates widely (*Am J Psychiatry.* 2000;157(4):493-505)

- Substances can induce panic: GABA blocking (flumazenil, caffeine); dopamine release (cocaine, amphetamines); α_2-adrenergic antagonist (yohimbine); or rapid shift of serum pH (tachypnea, bicarbonate)

Evaluation
- Screening questions:
  - Ever experienced an abrupt surge of intense fear?
  - Felt severe anxiety with racing heart, sweating, difficulty breathing, dizziness, or other physical symptoms?
- Due to another medical condition (see table below)
- Due to substances or another medication (stimulants, caffeine, steroids, phenytoin, see table below)
- Panic due to another mental disorder (eg, panic attacks in social settings due to social anxiety disorder, in the context of flashback due to PTSD, or due to paranoia in psychosis)

Risk Factors
- Childhood adversity including trauma or abuse
- Major stressor in the past 12 mo, especially loss, threat, medical illness (*Depress Anxiety*. 2010;27(8):716-730)
- Panic attacks are strongly comorbid with anxiety, depressive, impulse-control, and substance use disorders

Organic Differential Diagnosis for Panic Disorder	
Cardiovascular Diseases	
• Anemia • Angina • Arrhythmias	• Hypertension • Mitral valve prolapse
Pulmonary Diseases	
• Asthma • Pulmonary embolus	• Hyperventilation
Neurological Diseases	
• Cerebrovascular disease • Epilepsy (specifically temporal lobe epilepsy)	• Transient ischemic attack • Stroke • Migraine
Endocrine Diseases	
• Addison disease • Carcinoid syndrome • Cushing syndrome	• Hyperthyroidism • Pheochromocytoma • Premenstrual syndrome
Drug Intoxication	
• Amphetamines • Amyl nitrite • Anticholinergics • Cocaine	• Hallucinogens • Marijuana • Nicotine • Theophylline

(continued)

Organic Differential Diagnosis for Panic Disorder (continued)	
Drug Withdrawal	
• Alcohol • Antihypertensives (eg, clonidine, B-blockers)	• Opioids • Sedative hypnotics

Adapted from Sadock, et al. Synopsis of Psychiatry: Behavioral Sciences/Clinical Psychiatry. 2015.

Treatment
- Discuss patient's preference for psychotherapy and/or pharmacotherapy
  - Both are reasonable first-line treatment independently or together

Psychotherapy
- Cognitive behavioral therapy for panic is effective and may have more lasting benefit than pharmacotherapy (*JAMA.* 2000;283(19):2529)
- Self-directed CBT guides and mobile apps exist, and while evidence supporting them is limited, they can be used as adjunct treatment
- If poor response after course of CBT, recommend pharmacotherapy

Pharmacotherapy
- SSRIs are first-line
  - Patients with panic are often sensitive to activating effects
- Avoid SSRIs that are particularly activating (eg, fluoxetine)
- Start low (eg, half the normal starting dose), and titrate up slowly
- If good response, continue at least 8 mo before discontinuing
- If poor response after 6 wk at therapeutic dose, switch to SSRI
- If partial response, augment with low-dose benzodiazepine
  Benzodiazepines can be used during initiation of SSRI or as backup to abort panic
- In patients with comorbid substance use when benzodiazepines should be avoided, consider gabapentin, pregabalin, or mirtazapine
- In severe cases, benzodiazepines can be used as SSRI becomes therapeutic
- Discontinue benzodiazepine as soon as possible

GENERALIZED ANXIETY DISORDER
Definition and Clinical Features
- Chronic, excessive worry, that is hard to control and causes distress or impairment
- GAD is highly comorbid with other psychiatric diagnoses
  - Often precedes and predicts future MDD
  - Comorbidity rates: social AD 23%, specific phobia 21%, MDD 42% (*Am J Psychiatry.* 1993;150(8):1216)
  - Lifetime prevalence of substance use disorders (often alcohol and benzodiazepines) in patients with GAD is ~50% (*J Clin Psychiatry.* 2010;71(9):1187-1195)
- Typically, gradual onset, with subsyndromal symptoms initially
- May present primarily or exclusively with somatic symptoms (poor sleep, fatigue, headache) with unexplained, chronic physical concerns

- Thought to be a chronic illness, with some periods of improvement and relapse
- Earlier onset → worse prognosis
- Diagnostic criteria:
  - Excessive, persistent anxiety more than half the days of the past 6 mo
  - Worry about a variety of content and situations
  - With at least 3 physical symptoms (fatigue, restlessness, poor concentration, irritability, tense muscles, poor sleep)
  - Symptoms present for at least 6 mo (though often a lifelong condition)

Epidemiology and Pathogenesis
- 12-month prevalence—2.7%; lifetime prevalence—4.7%
- Age: median age of onset is 31 y old, and 95% onset by age 66, but can present at any age; latest average age of onset of all anxiety disorders (Arch Gen Psychiatry. 2005;62(6):617; Int J Methods Psychiatry Res. 2012;21(2):169-184)
- Sex: 2:1 F:M (Arch Gen Psychiatry. 1994;51(1):8)

Genetics
- Common heritability with major depressive disorder (Br J Psychiatry Suppl. 1996), and the personality trait "neuroticism" (Am J Psychiatry. 2004;161(9):1581-1587)
- "Short-short" (S-S) allele of the serotonin transporter polymorphic region is significantly more common in patients with GAD than in controls (Psychiatr Genet. 2005;15(1):7-11)

Neurobiology
- Effectiveness of both GABA and serotonergic medications for GAD suggests abnormalities in these neurotransmitters, but studies have been inconsistent
- Other studies implicate α_2, norepinephrine, CCK
- GAD may also be understood as an overgeneralization of classically conditioned fear (Bio Psychol. 2014;75(11):909-915)

Evaluation
- Screening questions:
  - GAD-2 screen: in the past 2 wk how often have you
    - Felt nervous, anxious, or on edge?
    - Been unable to stop or control worry?
  - Are you a worrier?
  - Do you worry that you worry too much?
  - Do you play the "what if" game?
- Screen other anxiety disorders, especially panic and social anxiety disorder
- Assess substance history (including nicotine and caffeine), family history of anxiety, and screen for any recent stressful events or trauma
- Anxiety/panic due to another medical condition (see table Organic Differential Diagnosis for Panic Disorder below)
  - Especially with atypical, late-onset, or new physical sx
  - TSH, CBC, BMP, tox screen
  - >40 with cardiac symptoms → EKG

Risk Factors
- Childhood adversity including trauma or abuse
- Parental overprotection, childhood history of separation anxiety disorder
- Female sex, poverty, recent adverse events, chronic medical illness
- Major stressor in the past 12 mo, especially loss, threat, medical illness *(Depress Anxiety. 2010;27(8):716-730)*

Nonpharmacologic Treatment
- Discuss patient's preference for psychotherapy and/or pharmacotherapy
- No significant difference in efficacy of psychotherapy vs meds in GAD *(Psychol Bull. 2005;131(5):785)*
- CBT-based psychotherapy is effective short-term treatment of GAD *(Cochrane Database Syst Rev. 2007)*
- Self-directed CBT guides and mobile apps exist, and while evidence supporting them is limited, they can be used as adjunct treatment
- General approach is exposure, not reassurance, and cognitive restructuring
- If poor response after course of CBT, add pharmacotherapy

Pharmacologic Treatment
- Stronger preference for pharmacotherapy when depression is comorbid

SRIs (SSRIs and SNRIs) Are First-Line
- No SRI has been shown to have higher efficacy than any other
- Choose based on any drug interactions, adverse effect profile
- If good response, continue at least 12 mo before discontinuing
- If poor response after 6 wk at therapeutic dose, switch to SSRI
- If partial response, augment with low-dose benzodiazepine

Benzodiazepines
- Efficacious but risk of tolerance/dependence, and rebound anxiety. Should be cautious/avoided in patients with substance use disorders
- In cases of significant impairment at presentation, benzodiazepines can be used while SSRI becomes therapeutic

Buspirone
- Partial 5-HT agonist is sometimes effective. Similar to SSRIs takes weeks for full effectiveness, but few side effects. Often used for SSRI augmentation

Pregabalin/Gabapentin
- Consider in patients with comorbid substance use when benzodiazepines should be avoided
- Pregabalin is approved for GAD in the EU but not in the US, is often well-tolerated, and has low abuse potential. Gabapentin is a cheaper, more accessible alternative for many but has some abuse potential

Treatment-Refractory
- In treatment-refractory cases, other medications can be tried (tricyclics, atypical antipsychotics, hydroxyzine, anticonvulsants), but are

not first line due to adverse effects and no evidence of greater efficacy. Used for target symptoms (eg, hydroxyzine for PRN in pt with SUD, SGA for insomnia)

SOCIAL ANXIETY DISORDER

Definition and Clinical Features

Excessive fear of embarrassment, scrutiny, or humiliation; that they will be negatively evaluated by others

- Physical symptoms in social or performance settings
- Often with good insight, knowing they are irrationally anxious, which can lead to anticipatory anxiety of social situations
- Strongly comorbid with other anxiety, substance, and mood disorders, especially atypical depression
- High risk of subsequent development of a substance use disorder, especially alcohol (Arch Gen Psych. 2004;61(8):807-816)
- Highly comorbid with avoidant personality disorder (J Affective Disord. 2013;145(2):143-155)

Diagnostic Criteria

- Significant anxiety in at least one social situation (eg, performing, meeting people, public speaking, dating, using public restrooms, eating in front of people, starting conversations)
- Fear of humiliation or embarrassment, either offending others or leading to rejection
- Provoking situations are avoided or intensely uncomfortable
- The fear is excessive, given the actual risk of the situation

Epidemiology and Pathogenesis

- 12-month prevalence—6.8%; lifetime prevalence—13.0%
- Age: onset as early as age 5, but median age of onset is 13 y old, and 95% onset by age 34 (Arch Gen Psychiatry. 2005;62(6):617; Int J Methods Psychiatry Res. 2012;21(2):169-184; N Engl J Med. 2006;355(10):1029)
- Sex: Somewhat more common in women than in men, but less so than all other anxiety disorders (J Psychiatr Res. 2011;45(8):1027-1035)
- May be related to autonomic arousal (tachycardia, tremor, GI upset), that is overresponsive in public situations and leads to positive feedback (J Abnorm Psychol. 1995;104(1):224)

Evaluation

- Screening questions:
  - Feared that people will notice you blush or appear anxious?
  - Felt sweaty, faint, or racing heart in social situations?
  - Had thoughts of being humiliated, embarrassed, or rejected?
  - Avoided or left social situations early?
  - Had stage fright?
  - Had difficulty or avoided using public restrooms?
- History focused on settings that trigger symptoms, and situations that are comfortable (eg, close friends or family)
- Fear of embarrassment in assessment itself often leads to minimizing symptoms or reluctance to disclose symptoms
- Early childhood abuse is a risk factor for SAD, thought to be via modulation of HPA-axis (Biol Psychol. 2010;83(1):1)

Treatment (N Engl J Med. 2006;355(10):1029)
- CBT and pharmacotherapy are evidence-based treatments
- Both are effective and choice should be made based on patient preference
- 67% respond to treatment

Nonpharmacologic Treatment
- CBT targeted at anticipatory negative thoughts and behaviors by cognitive restructuring and therapeutic exposure
- Often done in courses of 12–16 wk of weekly psychotherapy

Pharmacologic Treatment
SSRI and SNRIs Are First-Line
- Response rate is 50–80% after 8–12 wk
- No evidence of SSRI better than SNRI in head-to-head trials
- Initiate at half the usual effective dose and increase after 1 wk
- After 4 wk, increase again, and initial trials should be at least 12 wk

Benzodiazepines
- Limited evidence, but can be used in those who cannot tolerate SRIs, have residual symptoms, or when urgent symptom reduction is necessary
- Preference for longer-acting (eg, clonazepam) at scheduled, divided doses
- Not recommended as monotherapy and should be avoided in patients with comorbid substance use diagnoses

Other Medications
- Gabapentin and pregabalin are superior to placebo; less effective than SRIs
- The MAOI phenelzine has been shown to be effective but is used only for treatment refractory disease, given interactions and adverse effects

AUTISM SPECTRUM DISORDER

Clinical Features (Pediatr Rev. 2014;35(2):62; APA, Diagnostic & Statistical Manual of Mental Disorders. 5th ed.; 2013)
- **Definition:** ASD refers to a continuum of neurodevelopmental d/o's marked by early-onset deficits in social communication and interaction combined w/ restricted, repetitive patterns of behaviors, interests, and activities that manifest first few years of life
- **Core deficits:**
   Social communication and interaction: Common presenting complaint is language deficit (delay, regression) at 18–24 mo. of age. Other language problems may include difficulty initiating/sustaining dialogue, flattened prosody, echolalia. Difficulties understanding and using language nuance (eg, sarcasm) and nonverbal communication (eg, body language, posture, gesture) are common. Difficulty w/ social reciprocity, incl. perspective-taking, sharing, empathizing,

maintaining joint attention. May avoid eye contact. Absence of protoimperative pointing (to get a desired object) by 18 mo. is a red flag, though more sensitive is the absence of protodeclarative pointing (to draw another's attention to an object)

Restricted, repetitive behaviors: Strong desires for rigid routine (w/ distress upon deviation) are common. Related difficulties are seen w/ sleep onset and maintenance, restricted food preferences, sensory hyper- and hyposensitivities. These sx are often isolating for pt and a source of stress for caregivers. Repetitive motor movements (eg, hand flapping, intense preoccupation w/ parts of an object) are also frequently seen

- **Asperger disorder:** Controversial term still used in ICD-10 to refer to a syndrome similar to that described herein for ASD but w/ absence of significant language or cognitive delay; per DSM-5, now encompassed under dx of ASD along w/ other historical neurodevelopmental d/o's (eg, pervasive developmental disorder, not otherwise specified) lacking sufficient evidence for diagnostic distinctiveness
- **Severity and intellectual disability:** Level 1 severity (requiring support) to Level 3 severity (requiring very substantial support). Of kids w/ ASD, ~50% have severe ID, 35% have mild–moderate ID, and remaining 20% have IQ WNL
- **Comorbidity:** Of kids w/ ASD, 2 of 3 may meet criteria for ADHD; 20–25% have a seizure disorder; affective, attentional, anxiety, and obsessive–compulsive sx and tics may be seen

Epidemiology and Pathogenesis (Nat Rev Genet. 2017;18(6):362; Exp Neurobiol. 2016;25(1):1)

- Prevalence estimated around 1–2% w/ 2–3 × more M than F; increasing prevalence in the last 20 y at least partially resulting from increased recognition, earlier diagnosis, and expanded diagnostic criteria
- ASD is a multifactorial disorder resulting from genetic and nongenetic factors

    Genetic risk factors: Etiological heterogeneity, variable penetrance, and genetic pleiotropy characterize the genetics of ASD, for which 100's of gene variants have been identified w/ highly variable risk effects and associations w/ other disorders, though common neurobiological pathways are being identified (incl. gene mutations involved in synaptogenesis and axon motility)

    Nongenetic risk factors: Advanced parental age (incl. paternal age) is associated w/ higher risk for ASD. Birth complications associated w/ trauma and ischemia have been linked to dev't of ASD. Maternal obesity, diabetes, and C-section are weakly associated w/ risk for ASD. Associations reported w/ maternal C-section and maternal SSRI use are likely confounded by indication. Current evidence suggests maternal smoking and ART are unrelated to risk of ASD. Despite historical public concern, there is no evidence for vaccines or thimerosal as contributing factors (Mol Autism. 2017;8:13).

Evaluation (*JAACAP*. 2014;53(2):237; *Pediatr Rev*. 2014;35(2):62)

- **Screening:** All children 18–24 mo should be screened for ASD per Am Acad Pediatr (2007), and age-based screening instruments (ITC, M-CHAT, CAST) are typically used in pediatric primary care settings; psychiatric evaluation of all kids should probe for ASD sx
- **Comprehensive diagnostic workup:** Indicated following a positive screen to make a definitive diagnosis; r/o sensory/perceptual impairments, alternative diagnoses on the ddx that may account for presenting sx; and identify any comorbid d/o's that may affect tx or genetic counseling

  Diagnosis of ASD is clinical and based on standard psychiatric assessment and DSM-5 criteria using hx and MSE supplemented by evidence-based diagnostic tools w/ caregiver report and direct observation measures (eg, ADOS-2)

  Medical workup includes hearing screen, PE (neuro exam, growth parameters, r/o dysmorphia and neurocutaneous lesions w/ Wood lamp), genetic testing (karyotype, fragile X testing, chromosomal microarray), and further evaluation (eg, EEG, metabolic labs) based on particular history or exam findings

  Psychological assessment guides tx planning and includes measures of cognitive and intellectual capacity, adaptive skills, identification of strengths and weaknesses

  Communication assessment, OT and PT evaluations are also useful for Dx and tx planning

Nonpharmacologic Treatment (*JAACAP*. 2014;53(2):237; *Pediatr Rev*. 2014;35(2):62)

- Structured behavioral and educational interventions are associated w/ better outcomes in ASD
- **Behavioral:** Applied Behavioral Analysis (ABA) programs use behavioral techniques to reinforce adaptive behavior and are effective for academic, coping, communication, social and vocational skills; CBT for anxiety and anger in pts w/ high-functioning ASD can be useful
- **Communication:** Coordination w/ SLP; programs to enhance social reciprocity and pragmatic language skills for pts w/ fluent speech; sign language, picture exchange, voice output aids, etc, for those w/ nonfluent or absent speech
- **Educational:** Special education or regular classroom w/ IEP or 504 plan to secure access to supports, services in school; effectiveness shown for 2 structured educational models (incl. Early Start Denver Model)
- **Complementary and Alternative Medicine (CAM):** Despite very limited empirical support for its use, CAM for ASD is highly prevalent among pts and families; therefore, clinicians must specifically inquire about CAM to provide education, r/o drug interactions and adverse effects

Pharmacologic Treatment (*JAACAP*. 2014;53(2):237; *Pediatr Rev*. 2014;35(2):62; *Autism Spectrum Disorder in Children & Adolescents: Pharmacologic Interventions*. UpToDate)

- Growing evidence for utility of specialist pharmacotherapy for clearly defined target sx or comorbid d/o's, though must r/o occult medical

causes (eg, constipation, pain) and optimize nonpharmacologic interventions
- Combining pharmacotherapy w/ parent training is moderately more efficacious than meds alone for reducing serious behavioral disturbance
- While the goal is to help pt adjust and engage w/ educational interventions, given the language deficits in ASD, clinician observation, caregiver report, and rating scales may be useful in guiding assessment of response to pharmacotherapy
- **FDA indications for ASD-associated irritability (aggression, SIB, etc):**
  Risperidone (ages 5–16): For pts weighing 15–20 kg, initial dose 0.25 mg/d PO × ≥4 d → may increase dose to 0.5 mg/d, which should be maintained × ≥14 d (doses ranging from 0.5 to 3 mg/d have been studied; in trials, therapeutic effect plateaued at 1 mg/d). For pts ≥20 kg, initial dose 0.5 mg/d PO × ≥4 d → may increase dose to 1 mg/d, which should be maintained × ≥14 d → if insufficient response, may increase by 0.5 mg/d at ≥2 wk intervals (doses ranging from 0.5 to 3 mg/d have been studied; in trials, therapeutic effect plateaued at 2.5 mg/d [3 mg/d in pts >45 kg]). May do QD or BID dosing. Following clinical response, consider gradually decreasing to lowest effective dose (Lexicomp, Risperidone: Drug information)
  Aripiprazole (ages 6–17): Initial dose 2 mg PO QD × 7 d → 5 mg PO QD; subsequent dose increases may be made in 5 mg increments every ≥7 d (up to max. 15 mg/d) (Lexicomp, Aripiprazole: Drug information)
  For repetitive behaviors, consider fluoxetine (or other SSRI) despite lack of high-quality evidence
  For sleep disturbance, melatonin may be beneficial
- **Comorbid d/o's:** Generally, consider similar factors as when treating pts without ASD, but "start low and go slow" since pts w/ ASD may respond to very low doses or may require standard pediatric doses
  ADHD: May consider stimulants (most—though still limited and mixed—data for methylphenidate), alpha-agonists or atomoxetine; kids w/ ASD may have smaller effect sizes and more adverse effects at lower doses than kids without ASD
  Anxiety: May consider SSRI despite mixed evidence for SSRI in kids w/ ASD and either anxiety or OCD (incl. recent systematic review showing no effectiveness) (Cochrane Database Syst Rev. 2010;8(8):CD004677)
  Depression: Consider SSRI or SNRI for clear sx of depression despite limited data
  Catatonia: May occur in 1 of 7 adolescents and young adults w/ ASD and should be ruled out in any marked reduction of movement, vocalization; limited data available support tx w/ BZDs and/ or ECT (Eur Child Adolesc Psychiatry. 2008;17:327)
- **Adults w/ ASD:** For repetitive behaviors, SSRI are more efficacious in adults and older adolescents than in younger children, who may exhibit more behavioral activation w/ SSRI (Dialogues Clin Neurosci. 2012;14(3):263)

AUTOIMMUNE SYNDROMES

Basic Concepts

Blood-Brain Barrier (BBB) (Neuroimmunomodulation. 2012;19:121-130)

> *Function*: Protect CNS from bugs, toxins, etc. Directly make immuno-modulatory proteins
>
> *Structure:* Choroid plexus ependymal cells and brain vascular endo-thelial cells. Constitutive and inducible expression of tight junc-tions modulates permeability
>
> *Permeability:* Includes (1) passive diffusion of lipid-soluble molecules; (2) constitutive and inducible cytokine transporters (altered in dz); (3) regulated leukocyte diapedesis (transmigration) into CNS (altered in dz); and (4) gross violation in trauma and surgery

Special Features of CNS Immunology (Neurotherapeutics. 2016;13:685-701; Annu Rev Pathol. 2018;13:379-394)

> *Glial cells (neuroglia):* Includes *microglia* (CNS-resident tissue macro-phages w/ roles in recovery from injury) and *astrocytes* (support cells w/ innate excitability/neurotransmission capabilities, synaptic maintenance roles, neurocrine fx, and antigen-presenting fx)
>
> *Glymphatic system:* A glia-dependent network analogous to the lymphatic system in the periphery. Processes and drains CNS interstitial fluid

Key Cytokines and Pathways (Janeway's Immunobiol. 9th ed.; 2016; Acta Neuropathol. 2015;129:625-637; Pharmacol Res. 2009;60:85-92; Neuropeptides. 1985;5:371-374; Immunobiology. 2011;216:579-590)

> *TNF-α:* Many roles incl acute phase rxn, pyrogen, lymphocyte regula-tion. Made mainly by macrophages; neurons and glia can also make it. Involved in nl synaptic plasticity, memory and healing. Dysregltn thought to cause excitotoxicity; implicated in neurovascular dysfx and demyelination. Dysregltn observed in Alzheimer's, TBI, MDD, SCZ, Parkinson's. +Dysregltn in IBD; notably, *bupropion* is potent antiTNF and is a/w improvement in IBD sx. (Int Immunopharmacol. 2006;6:903-907)
>
> *IL-1:* Pyrogen, leukocyte activation/recruitmt, acute and chronic inflamm. Produced mainly by macrophages and dendritic cells; also by microglia and astrocytes. Receptors on leukocytes as well as neurons and astrocytes. Involved in regulation of HPA axis, neuro-transmission, synaptic plasticity. Dysregltn has been found in CVA, TBI, mood and psychotic d/o's
>
> *IL-6:* Function incl pyrogens, acute phase, lymphocyte differentiation. Leukocytes produce it, as well as neurons and glia. Can modulate CNS ion channels, glial differentiation/fx, and BBB permeability. ↑↑↑ in: MS, dementia, TBI, MDD and SCZ
>
> *IL-17:* Function incl neutrophil recruitmt and defense from fungi/extracell bacteria. Produced mainly by T-cells; receptors on leuko-cytes, as well as neurons and most neuroglia, which may make it as well. Dysregltn found in RA, SLE, IBD, psoriasis, MS, as well as SCZ
>
> *Kynurenine pathway:* Carried out in CNS and periphery. Metabolizes tryptophan variably (in response to signaling milieu) thru several

possible pathways that generate neurotransmitters w/ effects ranging from neuroprotective to neurodegenerative. Dysregltn seen in MDD, BPAD, SCZ, OCD, CVA, CNS infections, and many other neuropsy dz

Endocannabinoids (EC): Initially discovered roles in memory/amnesia and pain; EC receptor activity likely the 1° mechanism of acetaminophen. (*J Neurosci.* 2018;38:322-334) Receptors on leukocytes → regulate cytokines, neuroprotection, innate+adaptive imm

Endorphins and enkephalins: Endogenous opioids. Pain regultn. Receptors also found on lymphocytes, w/ various fx incl: promote NK cell activity and suppress T cell proliferation

Hypothalamic–pituitary axes: End-organs incl adrenals, thyroid and gonads. Key roles in stress-response, energy metab, growth and developmt, libido/reprod, global homeostasis

Clinical Relevance

Roles of Immunity in Classical Psychopathology (*J Neuroinflammation.* 2013;10:43; *Psychosom Med.* 2016;78:389-400; *Nat Rev Immunol.* 2017;16:22-34)

Immunological abnormalities have been found in mental illness *for over 100 y* (*Zeitschrift für die gesamte Neurologie und Psychiatrie.* 1914;25:341-377)—yet they remain cryptic

*Example—**MDD:*** Speculation about inflammatory component. (*Aust N Z J Psychiatry.* 2017;51:23-31) Much study examines CRP as possible marker, but studies have varied widely in results. (*Brain Behav Immun.* 2018;pii:S0889-1591(18)30232-0) Some monoclonal antibodies for rheum dz have antidepressant effect *independent of* rheum dz sx change. (*Mol Psychiatry.* 2018;23:335-343) Some antidepressants affect cytokines and signaling pathways; unclear if this is mechanism of action

Roles of Psychopathology in Autoimmune Disease (*Clin Pract Epidemiol Ment Health.* 2006;2:24)

Overlap syndromes: Several conditions w/ unclear 1° cause, but a/w immune abnls, are frequently comorbid both w/ each other and w/ psych dz. For example, SEID, fibromyalgia, IBS (see dedicated chapters)

Causation vs common cause/vulnerability: Retro cohort study (>100 k people) showed having a trauma/stress-related d/o to be significantly a/w ↑ risk of later autoimmune dz compared w/ matched indiv w/o trauma/stress-related d/o, and w/ full siblings. (*JAMA.* 2018;319:2388-2400) Prospective cohort study (>50 k ppl) showed that PTSD sx → ↑ risk of later rheumatoid arthritis dx, independent of smoking. (*Arthritis Care Res.* 2016;68:292-298)

Modulating severity: Lower mental health measures a/w ↑ pain+disability, ↓ treatment response in rheumatoid arthritis. (*Psychosom Med.* 2017;79:638-645)

Neuropsychiatric (NP) Presentations With Identified Immunologic Etiologies

Three areas are discussed in depth in the sections that follow, around which clinical experience and evidence are most robust: autoimmune encephalitis, NP manifestations of systemic autoimmune diseases, and NP effects of immunotherapies

Neuropsychiatry of Systemic Autoimmune Conditions				
Condition	**Notable Specific Signs/Sx**	**Diagnosis**	**Freq.**	**Refs.**
SLE	Many including, more rarely: **Psychosis, catatonia,** mvmt d/o, CVA, sz, FND	Serum: ANA (screen w/ sens/spec ~90/90%); anticardiolipin; lupus anticoag; anti-β2-glycoprotein; antiribosomal P (possibly a/w psychosis); ↓C3 and C4 (flare) Rad: MRI brain/spine	50%	1–3
Rheumatoid arthritis	Rare: **Meningitis, cerv spine dz,** visual dysfx, ataxia, cranial neuropathy	Serum: RF, CRP, anti-cyclic citrullinated peptide CSF: RF (specific) Rad: MRI w/ meningeal focus	Rare	2
Sjögren syndrome	Common: **Fatigue** (non-speci but ++sensi), **dorsal root (sens) ganglion-pathy**	Serum: anti-Ro/SSA, anti-La/SSB Path: salivary gland biopsy (Rad: MR abnl even w/ no sx)	60%	1,2
Celiac disease	Rare: Memory loss, psychosis, ataxia, sz, neuropathy	Clin: gluten restrict (also the treatment) +/– rechallenge Serum: anti-TTG, antigliadin, antiendomysial Path: duodenal biopsy	50%	6,7
Pernicious anemia	Common: **Neuropathy, paresthesia** Uncommon/rare: **Memory loss,** myelopathy	Serum: levels of B_{12} **and** methylmalonic acid **and** homocysteine (↑ sens); anti-intrinsic factor; ↑ gastrin Rad: MRI brain/spine	Most	8

Neuropsychiatry of Systemic Autoimmune Conditions *(continued)*				
Condition	**Notable Specific Signs/Sx**	**Diagnosis**	**Freq.**	**Refs.**
Sarcoidosis	Rare: **Meningoencephalitis**, psychosis, cranl neuropthy	*Path:* periph +/− CNS biopsy *CSF:* ↓ gluc; ↑ ACE, protein *Rad:* MRI w/ cranial nv root, meninges, pituitary, and/or hypothalamus focus	10%	9
Psoriasis	**Nonspecific but common:** Anx, mood d/o, insomnia	Clinical +/− biopsy	30%	10
IBD	Uncommon: CVA, neuropathy	*Path:* intestinal biopsy	30%	11
Multiple sclerosis	Rare: **Pseudobulbar** affect, **"euphoria sclerotica"** (unusual/ overoptimism)	*CSF:* oligoclonal bands, anti-aquaporin-4, anti-MBP *Rad:* MRIs (over time)	All	12
Vasculitis (eg, ANCA, Behçet's, 1° CNS)	Variable: **Sudden vision loss**, FND, CVA	*Serum:* ANCA, RF, ESR, CRP, cryoglobulins *Path:* vascular or brain biopsy *Rad:* MR/CT/XR angio	30%	1,13,14
PANDAS	All: **rapid-onset OCD and/or tic d/o** (Sydenham chorea = related mvmt d/o)	*Serum and CSF:* antibasal ganglia, antithalamic	All	15

Note: Most of the above disorders are *also* associated with several more nonspecific neuropsychiatric symptoms such as headache, fatigue, depressed mood, anxiety, sleep disturbance, and cognitive dysfunction. The "Freq'" column includes these nonspecific symptoms when providing an approximate percentage of patients with a given condition that may be expected to have neuropsychiatric symptoms. The "Notable Specific Signs/Sx" given above may occur much more rarely. Among these, **bold** indicates relatively **specific** associations.

References: (1) *J Neuropsych Clin Neurosci.* 2011;23:90-97; (2) *Semin Neurol.* 2014;34:425-436; (3) *Drugs.* 2016;76:459-483; (4) *JAMA.* 2014;311:1547-1555; (5) *Br J Pharmacol.* 2017;174:345-369; (6) *NEJM.* 2016;374:1875-1883; (7) *Gastroenterology.* 2005;128:S92-S97; (8) *Handbk of Clin Neurol.* 2014;120:915-926; (9) *Innov Clin Neurosci.* 2012;9:10-16; (10) *Medicine.* 2016;95:e3816; (11) *South Med J.* 1997;90:606-610; (12) *Int Rev Psychiatry.* 2010;22:14-21; (13) *Ann Neurol.* 1993;33:4-9; (14) *J Neurol.* 2007;254:1187-1189; (15) *J Neuroinflamm.* 2013;10:43

Neuropsychiatric Manifestations of Systemic Autoimmune Diseases

General Diagnostic Considerations

Highly prevalent, yet also dx of exclusion (eg, r/o infection). Screen if +PMHx/FHx autoimm dz. Often 1st sx of dz. **Red flags**: other dz activity, FNDs, atypical sx/course

Investigations: Labs may be nonspecific. EEG often nonspecific, but slowing suggestive of encephalopathy raises index of suspicion for organic cause, as do high inflammatory markers (eg, ESR, CRP, ANA, RF). Imaging abnormalities, if present, warrant scrutiny (?cause, ?neurotopographic relation to sx). When considering LP, consider pre- and posttest probabilities, as well as local resources and time-to-results

General Management Considerations

Overall, treat the underlying disorder if possible, while managing sx

Disease modification: Treat underlying d/o w/ rheumatologist and/or neurologist (eg, corticosteroids, IVIg, plasmapheresis, immunomodulators, cytotoxics, biologics)

Corticosteroids (CS): The age-old conundrum is *"Too much or too little?"*—ie, are CS causing/contributing to neuropsych sx, and/or are more CS required acutely for dz tx? The answer is rarely clear; review of sx time course and MAR are mandatory

Psych Tx: Can treat neuropsychiatric symptoms as for primary illness

Neuropsychiatric Effects of Immunotherapies (for Cancer and Autoimmune Dz) (Am J Psychiatry. 2014;171:1045-1051; Neurology. 2013;80:1430-1438; Pediatr Blood Cancer. 2009;52:293-295; Brain Res Bull. 2017;131:93-99; Semin Neurol. 2014;34:467-478; Microbiol Spectr. 2017;5(2); Malar J. 2016;15:332; Semin Arthritis Rheum. 2011;41:524-533; Curr Opin Pharmacol. 2016;29:97-103; J Clin Psychiatry. 2016;77:275-276; Mol Psychiatry. 2018;23:335-343; Curr Opin Neurol. 2017;30:659-668; Palliat Support Care. 2017;15:499-503; Biomark Res. 2018;6:4)

- Coadministration of most of the below therapies (which is common) → ↑↑ in the risks listed
- **Corticosteroids**

    Examples: prednisone (Deltasone), methylprednisolone (Solu-Medrol), dexamethasone (Decadron), hydrocortisone (Solu-Cortef), budesonide (Entocort EC, Uceris)

    Adverse effects (AE): many incl mania (M > F), depression (F > M), SI/SA (↑ w/ older age), psychosis, anx/panic (↑ w/ younger age), agitation, delirium (M > F), hyporexia, insomnia

    Risk: *Most* pts have mild/moderate AE; severe AE occur ~16/100 person-yrs. Dose-dependent; ↑↑ risk if taking ≥**40 mg** of prednisone-equivalent/day. ↑ w/ psych hx. ↑ w/ prior CS-AE. Time of onset highly variable (hyperacute, to months into tx). PPx psychosis/delirium w/ antipsychotics if CS necessary and pt has hx/high risk

    Beneficial effects: ↑↑ mood, energy and appetite (may be good for anorexic/cachectic pts)

- **Conventional immunomodulators and disease-modifying drugs**
  - **Examples:** Antimetabolite (methotrexate/MTX, azathioprine [Imuran], leflunomide [Arava], teriflunomide [Aubagio], mercaptopurine [Purinethol], mycophenolate mofetil [CellCept, Myfortic]), *cytokine modulator* (hydroxychloroquine [Plaquenil], sulfasalazine, tofacitinib [Xeljanz]), *antineoplastic* (cyclophosphamide [Cytoxan], mitoxantrone [Novantrone]), *T-cell modulator* (fingolimod [Gilenya], glatiramer [Copaxone, Glatopa])
  - **Adverse effects:**
    - *Class:* malaise, opportunistic infections including progressive multifocal leukoencephalopathy (JC virus), posterior reversible encephalopathy syndrome, immune reconstitution inflammatory syndrome, malignancy
    - *Intrathecal MTX:* leukoencephalopathy
    - *Hydroxychloroquine:* vivid dreams/nightmares, psychosis, dissociation, SI/SA

- **Biologic Immunomodulators**
  - **Examples:** Anti-TNF (infliximab [Remicade], adalimumab [Humira], golimumab [Simponi], etanercept [Enbrel], certolizumab [Cimzia]), *other anticytokines* (anakinra [Kineret], canakinumab [Ilaris], rilonacept [Arcalyst], tocilizumab [Actemra], ustekinumab [Stelara], secukinumab [Cosentyx]), *T/B-cell modulators* (rituximab [Rituxan], ocrelizumab [Ocrevus], belimumab [Benlysta], abatacept [Orencia], alemtuzumab [Lemtrada], natalizumab [Tysabri]), *interferons* (α [Multiferon], β-1a [Avonex, Rebig, Plegridy], β-1b [Betaseron, Actoferon], γ [Actimmune])
  - **Adverse effects:**
    - *Class:* Acute infusion rxn (HA, fever, malaise); + similar risks as conventionals above
    - *Anti-TNFs* → panic/anxiety/SI acutely after infusion; central and/or periph demyelination (well-known assoc; may be explained by baseline ↑demyelin risk a/w autoimm dz itself)
    - *Interferons* → neuroveg depression (ppx/tx: SSRI)
  - **Beneficial effects:**
    - *Class:* ↑ energy, ↑ sleep quality
    - *Anti-TNF and anti-IL-6:* antidepressant effects independent of autoimmune dz sx improvemt. (*Mol Psychiatry.* 2018;23:335-343) (There is also interest in tocilizumab [anti-IL-6] for SCZ, though a recent RCT was negative. (*Neuropsychopharmacology.* 2018;43:1317-1323))

- **Immune checkpoint inhibition (ICI) and chimeric antigen receptor T-cells (CART)**
  - **Examples:** ipilimumab (Yervoy), nivolumab (Opdivo), pembrolizumuab (Keytruda), atezolizumab (Tecentriq), avelumab (Bavencio), durvalumab (Imfinzi)
  - **Adverse effects:**
    - *ICI* → fatigue (25%); anorexia (9%); 0.1–0.2% meningo/encephalitis, neuropathy
    - *CART* → ~35% have AEs incl anx, HA, tremor (common); sz, resprtry deprsn (rare)

AUTOIMMUNE ENCEPHALITIS

(Ann Neurol. 2018;83:1661-1677; NEJM. 2018;378:840-851; Semin Neurol. 2018;38:330-343; Lancet Neurol. 2016;15:391-404; Curr Psychiatry Rev. 2011;7:189-193; Psychosomatics. 2017;58:228-244; Autoimmunity Rev. 2016;15:1129-1133; Neurology. 2003;60:712-714; Ann Long-Term Care: Clin Care Aging. 2015;23:25-27; J Clin Endocrinol Metab. 2002;87:489-499)

Clinical Features

Autoimmune encephalitis (AE) sx progress over days-wks; can be longer depending on antibody (Ab). Prodrome in ~60% (fever, malaise, HA, N/V, URI). Sx can be psych only

Limbic encephalitis (general): Focal encephalitis of medial temporal lobes (usually bilateral). P/w psychiatric sx/behavior change (range from personality changes to delirium), cognitive dysfxn, seizures (often complex partial), anterograde amnesia; +/− hyperthermia, endocrine disturbance, hypersomnia

Specific Ab Presentations:

Anti-NMDA receptor (NMDAR) encephalitis: More often diffuse encephalitis, but can p/w limbic encephalitis only. P/w initial panic/anxiety, followed by behavior change (irritability, agitation, aggression), insomnia, psychosis (hallucinations, delusions); later progresses to speech dysfunction, dyskinesia, memory deficits, catatonia, autonomic instability, sz, ↓ consciousness. *80% present to psychiatric provider first, 40% psychiatrically hospitalized at initial presentation*

Anti–voltage-gated potassium channel (VGKC) encephalitis: Various Ab targets possible (LGI1, Caspr2, etc)

LGI-1: presents as limbic encephalitis with seizures (generalized tonic-clonic possible); *faciobrachial dystonic seizures* (brief, synchronous arm and ipsilateral facial twitch) are pathognomonic

Caspr2: presents with *muscle hyperexcitability, fasciculations* ("bag of worms" under skin); can also p/w insomnia, dysautonomia, delirium

Anti-dipeptidyl-peptidase–like protein-6 (DPPX) encephalitis: Presents with amnesia, delirium, psychosis, and/or depression, as well as dysautonomia presenting as *sev diarrhea, gastroparesis, bladder dysfxn, or temperature dysrgltn*

Anti-GABA encephalitis: Rapidly progressing severe delirium, *treatment-refractory seizures*, often requiring medically induced coma. Can also p/w limbic encephalitis

Antiglycine encephalitis: Progressive encephalomyelitis with *rigidity and myoclonus*. Can p/w limbic encephalitis

Steroid-responsive encephalopathy assoc w/ autoimmune thyroiditis (SREAT): (Formerly Hashimoto encephalopathy) Convulsions (47%), confusion (46%), memory impairment (43%), speech disorder (37%), gait disturbance (27%), persecutory delusions (25%), myoclonus (22%), coma (15%), depression (12%)

Epidemiology and Pathogenesis

General: Prevalence equivalent to infectious encephalitides, ~11.6/100,000. Incidence ~0.8/100,000; tripled btwn 1995–2005 and 2006–2015. Higher rates in African-Americans than Caucasians. ? HLA Class II genes. FHx of autoimmune disease may be present

Limbic encephalitis: Age >45 y; sex predominance varies by antibody

NMDAR AE: Age <45 y; 4:1 F:M; a/w ovarian teratoma and testicular carcinoma

SREAT: Prev <2/100 k. Median 52 y/o. 3:1 F:M. a/w autoimmune/ Hashimoto thyroiditis, but only 20% of SREAT cases have overt thyroid disease

Pathogenesis: Triggers often not found but can include tumors (*paraneoplastic*; presumed common antigen in CNS) and viral encephalitis (eg, HSV; presumed BBB injury). Common associated tumors: small cell lung, breast, neuroblastoma, prostate, bladder, teratoma, thymoma, lymphoma, gynecologic

AE Autoantibody Types (Semin Neurol. 2018;38:330-343; NEJM. 2018;378:840-851; Psychosomatics. 2017;58:228-244)	
Intracellular	**Cell Surface**
Antibody itself likely not pathogenic	Antibody is likely pathogenic
Marker of T-cell–mediated neuronal damage	Targets involved in neuronal signaling and synaptic plasticity (glutamate, GABA, glycine, VGKC)
Poorly responsive to immunotherapy	Responsive to immunotherapy
Limited recovery	Brain atrophy, irreversible damage possible
Examples: AGNA, amphiphysin, ANNA-1 (Anti-Hu), GFAP, GAD-65, Anti-Ma2 (Ta)	*Examples:* NMDAR (GluN1), AMPAR, CASPR2, DPPX, GABAaR, GABAbR, LGI-1, mGluR5, VGCC

Evaluation

Differential Diagnosis: Infectious encephalitis, primary psychotic disorder, primary mood disorder (mania or depression), anxiety disorder, Creutzfeldt–Jacob disease, stroke, dementia

Workup:

Imaging: MRI FLAIR abnormalities (cortical, subcortical, or cerebellar for anti-NMDA; usu. bilateral medial temporal lobes for limbic encephalitis). PET appears more sensitive than MRI, most often see hypometabolism. May be negative earlier in course. Can also consider imaging for tumors (eg, mediastinum, lungs, gonads)

Serum+CSF: Lymphocytic pleocytosis common in CSF, +/− oligoclonal bands or elevated IgG index. Neuronal autoAb usu. found in CSF, even if CSF studies otherwise nl. Serum and CSF Ab findings may differ depending on causal Ab, so CSF testing is preferred; eg, ~14% of antiNMDAR cases have Ab present only in CSF. AE panel Ab (rather than individual Ab) testing available. Seronegative AE is possible (ie, Ab yet to be discovered). No clear guidelines on when to order panel, so utilize clinical judgment. Not currently recommended as standard first-episode psychosis workup unless other clues

SREAT: Serum>CSF in sensitivity; 10% population has Abs; TSH unhelpful

EEG: Focal *abnormalities* possible (eg, sz, epileptiform discharges). Anti-NMDAR a/w *extreme delta brush pattern.* SREAT: 82% are abnormal—diffuse slowing (70%) and/or epileptiform activity (14%)

Treatment

1. **Immunotherapy:** 1st line is steroid pulse (eg, methylprednisolone 1 g/d IV ×5 d), IVIG, or plasmapheresis (the latter 2 particularly for cell surface Ab, since Ab are pathogenic). 2nd line is rituximab or cyclophosphamide. Acute and maintenance treatment necessary (at least 6 mo); no clear guidelines for treatment type/duration, based on clinical judgment/expert opinion

2. **Remove immunologic trigger, if known:** Demographic-specific cancer screening

3. **Psych sx mgmt:** No consensus. Sedating agents may be helpful (BZDs, valproic acid). Pts have *increased risk for catatonia and NMS, so use antipsychotics sparingly.* ECT can be helpful for psychiatric symptoms (eg, psychosis, catatonia); *not* curative

Prognosis: Recovery varies by AE type, ~70–80% with no/mild residual sx @ 24 mo if treated. Lower tx response rate for intracellular Ab type. Spontaneous improvement is rare; can be fatal or disabling if no tx. Recurrence is not uncommon, even if a presumptive causal tumor is removed. SREAT: death 5%, complete recovery 25%, and partial neurologic recovery ~70%; relapses in 15%

BIPOLAR DISORDER

Clinical Features

- Characterized by episodes of mania or hypomania +/− one or more episodes of depression
- Mood episode at onset is usually major depression
- Psychotic symptoms may be present
- Patients typically have more and longer depressive episodes than episodes of mania/hypomania

Subtypes	
Bipolar I	One lifetime manic episode +/− major depressive episodes
Bipolar II	One lifetime hypomanic episode + one lifetime major depressive episode
Cyclothymia	Several episodes with hypomanic and depressive symptoms that do not meet full criteria for MDD and that alternate for ≥ 2 y
Rapid cycling	One lifetime manic or hypomanic episode + 4 episodes of depression, mania, or hypomania in 1 y

Epidemiology and Pathogenesis

- Bipolar spectrum disorders affect 2.4% of world pop (*Arch Gen Psychiatry.* 2011;68(3):241-251)
- Average age of onset is 21 y (*Psychol Med.* 1997;27:1079-1089)
- Prevalence is similar across racial groups
- Among the 20 leading causes of disability worldwide (*Lancet.* 2012;380:2163-2196)
- Associated with mortality rate 2-3x higher than gen. pop (*Lancet.* 2002;359:241-247)

Evaluation (*Diagnostic and Statistical Manual of Mental Disorders.* 5th ed.; 2013)

- Screen for current or past episode of mania/hypomania by asking if euphoric or irritable mood + DIGFAST symptoms (**D**istractibility, **I**ndiscretions, **G**randiosity, **F**light of ideas, **A**ctivities, **S**leeplessness, **T**alkativeness)
- Sample questions
  Were your thoughts moving so fast that you couldn't keep up with them? (F)
  Did you sleep very little or not at all and still feel full of energy? (S)
  Did anyone tell you that you spoke so fast that they couldn't get a word in? (T)
  Did you start several projects but not complete any of them? (D, A)
- Mania/hypomania often egosyntonic and often not readily disclosed → screen specifically

Criteria for Mood Episodes	
Mania	If irritable mood, 4 DIGFAST sx If euphoric mood, 3 DIGFAST sx Sx last ≥1 wk or hospitalized Psychotic sx may be present
Hypomania	Same as above, but ≥4 d, <1 wk No psychotic symptoms
Mixed	Full criteria for mania or depression met + features of opposite episode type

- **Psychiatric differential diagnosis:**
  - Borderline personality disorder (BPD): often confused w/ Bipolar II d/t overlap of sx: impulsivity, affective instability, aggression, depression, SI. Mood disturbance in BPD is typically in response to interpersonal stressors and less episodic. Mood episodes last hours to days in BPD as opposed to days to months in BPAD. Mood stabilizers and SGAs helpful in both Bipolar II and BPD (*Curr Opin Psychiatry.* 2014;27(1):14-20; *Handbook of Good Psychiatric Management for BPD.* 2014)
  - Schizoaffective disorder: mood episodes + persistence of psychotic symptoms for ≥2 wk in the absence of manic, mixed, or depressive episode
  - Common comorbidities: anxiety, substance use, ADHD, cluster B personality disorders
  - Eval for secondary causes of mania: Substances (corticosteroids, stimulants [cocaine, amphetamines], fluoroquinolones, dopamine

agonists), MS, R-sided subcortical or cortical lesion w/ links to limbic system, seizures, hyperthyroidism, Cushing syndrome (Arch Gen Psychiatry. 1978;35(11):1333-1339)

- Use of antidepressants may induce mania in those w/ or w/out diagnosis of bipolar disorder (6–8% of pts dx with MDD will switch to hypomania/mania); risk is higher with TCAs and younger pts (J Affect Disord. 2013;148(1):129-135; Acta Psychiatr Scand. 2010;121(6):404-414)
- Screen specifically for EtOH and other substance use, as this may cloud accurate dx and there is high comorbidity (J Affect Disord. 2016;206:331-349)
- Safety eval: ↑ risk for suicide (33–50% attempt; 10–19% complete), esp. during depressive and mixed episodes + anxiety (Clin Trials. 2014;11:114-127; J Affect Disord. 2012;143:16-26)

Nonpharmacologic Treatments (Lancet. 2013;381(9878):1672-1682)
- Goals
  1. Treat acute phase + prevent relapse (catch new episodes early)
  2. Enhance tx adherence (address insight/reluctance to lose mania sx, med SE)
  3. Promote regular sleep pattern, general health (social rhythm/sleep disruption → mania)
  4. Target functional impairment (↑ alliance + adherence)
  5. Involve family (notice sx earlier, limit access to cars/finances/other triggers for reckless behavior)
- Education: about course of illness, episode triggers, stressors (ongoing b/c insight variable)
- Optimum management → integration of pharmacotherapy with targeted psychotherapy (Bipolar Disord. 2013;15:1-44)
- Strong evidence for: CBT, family-focused therapy, interpersonal and social rhythm therapy

Pharmacologic Treatments (Lancet. 2013;381(9878):1672-1682)

Medication Treatment		
Phase	**First Line**	**Second Line**
Acute mania	• Lithium OR valproate (VPA) +/− antipsychotic[a] +/− BZD[b] • Antipsychotic alone[a] • Taper and discontinue antidepressants, steroids, stimulants	• Carbamazepine • Oxcarbazepine • Lurasidone • Asenapine
Breakthrough mania	• Check med serum levels (Li, VPA)[c] • +/− antipsychotic/BZD to Li or VPA • ECT	
Mixed episode	• Atypical antipsychotic (olanzapine, quetiapine) • VPA monotherapy	• Lithium • ECT

Medication Treatment (continued)		
Phase	**First Line**	**Second Line**
Acute depression	• Lithium (+/– lamotrigine), VPA • Quetiapine • Olanzapine + fluoxetine • Taper and discontinue steroids, β-blockers, varenicline, statins, OCPs, hormone replacement	• Lurasidone • ECT • Use of SSRIs, SNRIs, TCAs, MAOIs controversial
Breakthrough depression	• Ensure levels of meds are therapeutic • Add antipsychotic • ECT	• Use of SSRIs, SNRIs, TCAs, MAOIs controversial
Maintenance	• Lithium[d] • VPA, lamotrigine, olanzapine, aripiprazole, quetiapine	

[a]First-line antipsychotics: olanzapine, risperidone, haloperidol, aripiprazole, quetiapine, ziprasidone.
[b]Taper BZDs as stabilized, taper antipsychotics (if being used adjunctively) after 3–6 mo. stable/no psychotic sx.
[c]↑ Li secretion during mania, therapeutic level when euthymic may need to be ↑ for breakthrough.
[d]Shown to ↓ risk of suicide by >50%.

Use of Select Mood Stabilizers					
Agent	**Dosing**	**Labs**	**Level**	**Main SE**	**Others**
Lithium	*Initial:* 300–600mg *Target:* 900–1800 mg	Baseline BUN/Cr, TSH, EKG, hCG, Li level (w/ dose ↑) Li, BUN/Cr q3–6mo TSH q1yr	0.6–1.2 mEq/L (trough) >1.5 toxic >2 life threat[a]	Tremor GI upset Polydipsia Polyuria Wt gain Sedation	Long-term use (>10 y), 10–20% will have renal insufficiency May cause hypothyroidism Avoid thiazide diuretics, ACE/ARB, NSAIDs
VPA	*Initial:* 250–500mg *Target:* 1000–2000 mg	Baseline LFTs, CBC, hCG LFTs/CBC q3–6mo VPA level w/ Δ clin state	50–120 mcg/mL	GI upset ↑ LFTs Pancreatitis Tremor Dizziness Sedation Wt gain Alopecia Pltlet dysfx	↑ lamotrigine levels, so ↓dose of both meds if combine Also ↑aspirin, warfarin, diazepam, clonazepam, carbamazepine Caution or avoid in women of child-bearing age d/t neural tube defects

(continued)

Use of Select Mood Stabilizers (continued)					
Agent	Dosing	Labs	Level	Main SE	Others
Lamo-trigine	*Initial:* 25 mg *Target:* 100–400mg	None	Not com-monly used	Headache Nausea SJS/TEN[b] Other rash	If pt is on lamo-trigine + VPA, must ½ the dose of both

[a]May require hemodialysis.
[b]Slow titration decreases risk; can occur at any time during tx.
Adapted from *Med Clin North Am.* 2010;94:1141-1160.

Special Populations: Pregnancy and Children

- VPA and carbamazepine cause neural tube defects and irreversible cog. impairment; lithium associated with cardiac defect (Ebstein anomaly), though risk is low and is likely overstated (*Ment Health Clin.* 2017;7(6):255-261)
- Antipsychotics likely safe: 1st gen. may be preferable due to more data on safety than 2nd gen (*Ment Health Clin.* 2017;7(6):255-261)
- ECT useful and safe for severe depression or mania in pregnancy (*Obstet Gynecol.* 2009;114(3):703)
- In children, limited data, but some evidence supports lithium, VPA, carbamazepine +/– augmentation with antipsychotic or BZD. Psychotherapy and psychoeducation play important role in tx (*J Am Acad Child Adolesc Psychiatry.* 1997;36:10)

BIPOLAR DEPRESSION

Clinical Features

- Bipolar depression is distinct from unipolar depression and responds differently to medications. The FDA separately approves medications for unipolar and bipolar depression
- No traditional antidepressants (eg, TCAs, SSRIs, SNRIs) have shown convincing efficacy or received approval for bipolar depression. Used to be prescribed in combination with a mood stabilizer, but this approach has fallen out of favor. All currently approved bipolar anti-depressants are second-generation antipsychotics
- Causes the majority of morbidity in bipolar affective disorder, yet evidence base is much more limited than other psychiatric disorders leading to greater controversy in its treatment

Off-label Mood Stabilizers

- Likely efficacious, but their evidence base is considerably smaller than that of the approved antipsychotics. Confirming that mood stabilizers are at adequate doses is a reasonable first-line treatment for bipolar depression
- **Lithium:** Associated with robust decreases in completed suicides (OR 0.13, 0.03–0.66) and all-cause mortality (OR 0.38, 0.15–0.95) in a meta-analysis of 48 RCTs (n = 6674) targeting a variety of long-term mood disorders including bipolar affective disorder. Evidence for bipolar depression specifically is largely from old, very small trials (*BMJ.* 2013;346:f3646)

- **Lamotrigine:** An individual patient-level meta-analysis of 5 RCTs (n = 1072) showed a NNT of 11 for lamotrigine (100–400 mg QD) over placebo (*Br J Psychiatry.* 2009;194:4)
- **Valproate acid (Depakote):** One small meta-analysis of 4 RCTs (n = 142) demonstrated a small effect size (SMD −0.35, −0.69 to −0.02) (*J Affect Disord.* 2010;122:1)

FDA-Approved Medications

- **Olanzapine/fluoxetine combination (OFC):** Most effective agent in a network meta-analysis of 29 RCTs (n = 8331). Olanzapine monotherapy is likely also effective based on multiple RCTs. In one RCT with 833 patients with bipolar 1, remission occurred in 49% on OFC vs 33% on olanzapine monotherapy vs 25% on placebo at 8 wk. Cheaper and more flexible dosing when prescribed separately (*Acta Psychiatr Scand.* 2014;130:452; *Arch Gen Psychiatry.* 2003;60:1079)
- **Quetiapine:** Robust evidence base and probably the best evidence for depression in bipolar 2. Shown to be more effective than placebo, lithium, and paroxetine in the EMBOLDEN I/II trials (n = 1542), which enrolled patients with bipolar 1 and 2 (NNT = 7–8 for response and remission, 300 and 600 mg arms equivalent). These trials were industry funded and limited by low doses of active comparators (*J Clin Psychiatry.* 2010;71:150; *J Clin Psychiatry.* 2010;71:163)
- **Lurasidone:** Smaller evidence base but also effective. Main RCT randomized patients with bipolar 1 depression to 20–60 mg (n = 166), 80–120 mg (n = 169), and placebo (n = 170) and showed a NNT of 5–7 for response and remission at 6 wk with no dose response observed between the active arms (*Am J Psychiatry.* 2014;171:160)
- Four negative RCTs are available demonstrating no efficacy for aripiprazole (*J Clin Psychopharmacol.* 2008;28:13) or ziprasidone (*J Clin Psychopharmacol.* 2012;32:470)

Unipolar Antidepressants

- **Treatment emergent affective switching:** Unipolar antidepressants may lead to mania in patients with underlying bipolar disorder, although this risk when used atop a mood stabilizer is controversial. All patients with a major depressive episode should be screened for prior manic and hypomanic episodes (*Acta Psychiatr Scand.* 2008;118:337; *Am J Psychiatry.* 2014;171:1067)
- **Bupropion and paroxetine:** These agents may have a lower risk of inducing mania than other unipolar antidepressants. They were therefore used in the NIMH funded landmark STEP-BD trial where they showed no efficacy over placebo but also no risk of mania when prescribed atop an approved mood stabilizer (*NEJM.* 2007;356:1711)
- **TCAs and venlafaxine:** These agents likely have the highest risk of inducing mania and should generally be avoided in patients with bipolar disorder (*Am J Psychiatry.* 2004;161:1537; *Am J Psychiatry.* 2006;163:232)

Alternative Therapies

- **Electroconvulsive therapy (ECT):** In CORE-II, 220 patients with depression were randomized to 3 electrode configurations and had equal remission/response rates irrelevant of unipolar (170) or bipolar (50) diagnosis. ECT produced an 80% response rate with an average of 6 sessions *(Acta Psychiatr Scand. 2010;121:431)*

- **Psychotherapy:** In STEP-BD, 293 patients were randomized to intensive psychotherapy (n = 163, either CBT, family-focused therapy, or interpersonal and social rhythm therapy) or a brief psychoeducational control condition (130) with better year-end recovery in the active conditions (64.4 vs 51.5%). There were no differences between the 3 active therapy types *(Arch Gen Psychiatry. 2007;64:419)*

FDA Approved Medications for Bipolar Depression			
Generic	Start (mg/d)	Goal (mg/d)	Nota Bene (NB)
Quetiapine	50	300–600	300 and 600 mg arms equivalent in the EMBOLDEN I/II trials Rapid outpatient titration scheme well-tolerated in trials: 100 mg/night to reach 300 mg by 4 d or 600 mg by 8 d
Olanzapine/ fluoxetine	6/25	6–12/25–50	Olanzapine monotherapy also effective but less than combination Also known as OFC (olanzapine/fluoxetine combination therapy)
Lurasidone	20	20–120	Must be taken with food (at least 350 cal) Only one of these three not also approved for unipolar depression

CATATONIA AND RELATED SYNDROMES

Definition and Clinical Features *(World J Psychol. 2016;6(4):392; Arch Gen Psychiatry. 2009;66(11))*

- Catatonia is a syndrome; all catatonia spectrum disorders characterized by deficits in motor and behavior
- Originally described in 1874 by Kahlbaum; considered subtype of dementia praecox by Kraepelin; inappropriately associated with schizophrenia alone (as opposed to mood disorders + medical conditions) until the 1990s
- Subtypes
  - **Stuporous/retarded:** immobility, mutism, staring, rigidity
  - **Excited:** prolonged psychomotor agitation
  - **Malignant:** acute onset catatonia with fever, abnormal blood pressure, tachycardia, tachypnea, severe rigidity; can be fatal
- **Delirious mania** *(J Psychiatr Pract. 2013;19(1):15-28)*
  - Abrupt onset of mania (more acute than typically seen in mania) and delirium

- ◦ Both manic and delirious symptoms wax and wane over the course of hours to days
- Most commonly described in young females
- Features of excited AND malignant catatonia typically present
- Large lapses of episodic memory
- Associated features include denudativeness, inappropriate toileting, and water obsession (*J Affect Disord.* 2008;109(3):312-316)

Epidemiology and Pathogenesis (*World J Psych.* 2016;6(4))

- Mechanism not clear
- Possible mechanisms include disruption in basal ganglia-thalamocortical tracts due to decreased dopamine and/or GABA interneuron regulation of dopamine activity
  - ↓ dopamine activity in motor circuit (rigidity), anterior cingulate-medial orbitofrontal circuit (akinetic mutism), lateral hypothalamus (hyperthermia, dysautonomia), and lateral orbitofrontal circuit (imitative, repetitive behaviors)
- Evolutionary models suggest catatonia may reflect ultimate fear response in humans (*Psychological Rev.* 2004;111(4))

Evaluation (*Acta Psychiatr Scand.* 1996;93(2):129-136)

- ≥ 2 of first 14 signs of BFCRS, remainder conveys severity
- DSM requires 3 of 10 symptoms
- **Catalepsy:** spontaneous maintenance of posture; **echophenomena:** repetition of examiner's words or movements; **stereotypies:** repetitive purposeless movements; **mannerisms:** bizarre purposeful movements; **negativism:** contrary behavior; **waxy flexibility:** ability to mold patient's limbs, with initial resistance; **automatic obedience:** exaggerated cooperation; **mitgehen = anglepoise lamp:** arm raising with light touch despite contrary instruction; **gegenhalten:** resistance proportional to strength of stimulus; **ambitendency:** motorically stuck in indecisive movement

> **Bush-Francis Catatonia Rating Scale (BFCRS)**
> (*Acta Psychiatr Scand.* 1996;93(2):129-136)
>
> 1. Excitement
> 2. Immobility/stupor
> 3. Mutism
> 4. Staring
> 5. Posturing/catalepsy
> 6. Grimacing
> 7. Echopraxia/echolalia
> 8. Stereotypy
> 9. Mannerisms
> 10. Verbigeration
> 11. Rigidity
> 12. Negativism
> 13. Waxy flexibility
> 14. Withdrawal
> 15. Impulsivity
> 16. Automatic obedience
> 17. Mitgehen
> 18. Gegenhalten
> 19. Ambitendency
> 20. Grasp reflex
> 21. Perseveration
> 22. Combativeness
> 23. Autonomic abnormality

- Consider underlying etiology:
  - Primary catatonia = psychiatric etiology (mood disorders ~20% of patients experience catatonic sx, psychotic disorders ~10%, autism spectrum ~17%, neurodevelopmental)
    - ◦ Reports in PTSD, personality disorders, conversion disorder

- Secondary catatonia = medical etiology ~50% of all cases of catatonia in acute medical and surgical settings (seizures, PRES, CNS infection, Wernicke encephalopathy, SLE) (Psychosomatics. 2018;59:337)
- Workup with aim to clarify underlying etiology, severity of catatonia (Psychosomatics. 2011;52:561):
  - Labs: CBC+diff, BMP, LFTs, Ca, Mg, Ph, CPK (when ↑, incr risk of malignant), UA, serum and urine tox, iron studies (↓ serum iron = risk factor for catatonia, conversion to malignant), HIV, RPR
  - Consider EEG, imaging in most cases
  - Consider paraneoplastic panel, ANA, LP in certain cases
  - Lorazepam challenge—2 mg IV, with BFCRS scores pre and 30m-1h post can be diagnostic; if response to challenge equivocal, use likelihood of catatonia as guidance (Gen Hosp Psychiatry. 2017;48:1-19)

Bedside Exam for Catatonia (Modified From MGH Handbook General Hospital Psychiatry. 2018:256)

1. Observe from outside room for 30–60 s
2. Begin a conversation with the patient
3. While conversing, scratch head/gesture exaggerated manner to provoke echopraxia
4. Examine for cogwheeling/alternate force
5. Attempt repose
6. Ask patient to extend arms. Place one finger beneath hands and attempt to raise hands, instructing patient to not raise arms to test for Mitgehen
7. Extend your hand, telling the patient not to shake your hand to test for ambitendency
8. Reach into pocket, instructing the patient to stick out his/her tongue because you want to stick a pin in it to test for automatic obedience

---

Nonpharmacologic Treatment (Prim Care Companion CNS Disord. 2018 4;20(1))

- Supportive care: hydration, nutrition, anticoagulation (risk of DVT/PE), aspiration precautions

Pharmacologic Treatment

- Discontinue contributing medications (dopamine blockade, ie, antipsychotics, antinausea/promotility agents), restart needed medications (ie, benzodiazepine if patient withdrawing, pro-dopaminergic Parkinson's agent, clozapine if precipitated by clozapine withdrawal) (J Psychiatry Neurosci. 2016;41(6):E81; Gen Hosp Psychiatry. 2017;48:17)
- Once patient responds to lorazepam challenge (see above), place on standing (typically 2 mg q6–8h) lorazepam; do not hold for sedation (Gen Hosp Psychiatry. 2017;48:1-19)
- IV lorazepam preferred due to ease of admission, quick onset of action, longer effective length of action (Prim Care Companion CNS Disord. 2018 4;20(1))
- Definitive treatment is ECT
  - Delirious mania, malignant catatonia indications to move quickly to ECT from pharm treatment
  - Bilateral placement with brief pulse is recommended
  - Most patients improve in 1–4 treatments

- Delirious mania: high-dose benzodiazepines are first line; start with 2–4 mg lorazepam. If responds to lorazepam, 6–20 mg daily in divided doses. Low threshold to move quickly to ECT if not responding (*J Psychiatr Pract. 2013;19(1):23*)
- Among antipsychotics, clozapine appears most likely to be beneficial and least likely to do harm (*J Psychiatry Neurosci. 2016;41(6):E81*)

Treatment Algorithm for Catatonia (*Gen Hosp Psychiatry. 2017;48:16*)

Step 1: Trial lorazepam for 2–3 d, at doses of minimum 6–8 mg daily
Step 2: Trial of ECT for > 6 sessions (at minimum 3× per week)
Step 3: Add amantadine 100 mg or memantine 10 mg daily, titrate over 3–4 d to max dose of amantadine 600 mg daily or memantine 20 mg daily
Step 4: Add carbamazepine 300–600 mg daily or valproate 500–1500 mg daily
Step 5: Add aripiprazole 10–30 mg, olanzapine 2.5–10 mg, or clozapine 200–300 mg daily, each dose given in combination with lorazepam (no antipsychotics if signs of malignant catatonia)

SEROTONIN SYNDROME

Definition and Clinical Features (*Cleve Clin J Med. 2016;83(11)*)
- Toxic syndrome due to serotonin excess
- Risk increased with using >1 serotonergic agents (drugs that ↓ serotonin breakdown, ↓ serotonin reuptake, ↑serotonin precursors or agonists, ↑serotonin release, inhibit CYP2D6 and CYP3A4). Common offenders include SSRIs, SNRIs, TCAs, St John's wort, linezolid, opioids, antiepileptics, antiemetics, stimulants
  - Classically involved combination of MAOI and another serotonergic agent but rarely seen today
  - Risk also increased with overdose on serotonergic agents
- Syndrome consists of **autonomic dysfunction** (diaphoresis, ↑HR, ↑temp, mydriasis, ↑bowel sounds, diarrhea, flushing), **neuromuscular excitation** (myoclonus, clonus, hyperreflexia, hypertonicity, rigidity), **altered mental status** (delirium, agitation, anxiety, lethargy, coma)
  - Quick onset (<24 h) and quick resolution (<24 h after removing offending agent)
  - Symptoms of catatonia (stuporous or excited) often present
  - Severe illness can lead to DIC, rhabdomyolysis
- Differentiate from NMS by offending agent, acute onset, hyperreflexia, clonus, though there may be significant overlap

Epidemiology and Pathogenesis
- Based on data from 2010 to 2013, incidence 1.38–10.5 per 1000 patient-years. Highest incidence in those prescribed >5 serotonergic agents or a combination of MAOI and serotonergic agent (*Prim Care Companion CNS Disord. 2017;19(6)*)
- Pathophysiology unclear; based on rat models, thought to reflect 5-HT1A overstimulation (hyperactivity, hyperreflexia, anxiety) and 5-HT2A overstimulation (hyperthermia, poor coordination, and neuromuscular excitability) (*Neuro Endocrinol Lett. 2014;35(4):267*)

Evaluation

- Hunter criteria used for diagnosis
  - May miss mild to moderate cases
    (*BMC Neurology. 2016;16(97):4*)
- Workup: CBC, blood cultures, BMP, LFTs, Ca, CK (uncommonly elevated), urine myoglobin, ABG, coags, serum and urine tox. Imaging not recommended

> **Hunter Criteria**
> (*QJM. 2003;96(9)*)
>
> Patient must have taken a serotonergic agent and have 1 of following:
> - Spontaneous clonus
> - (Inducible clonus or ocular clonus) + (agitation or diaphoresis) OR (hypertonia + fever)
> - Tremor + hyperreflexia

Nonpharmacologic Treatment (*Cleve Clin J Med. 2016;83(11):815*)

- Remove offending agent; syndrome self-limited, with resolution of symptoms often in <24 h
- Supportive measures: antipyretics/cooling blankets, respiratory/CV support, IV fluids

Pharmacologic Treatment

- Anticonvulsants if seizures, antihypertensives PRN
- Benzodiazepines for management of agitation, muscle rigidity (*Cleve Clin J Med. 2016;83(11):816*)
- Cyproheptadine theoretically binds serotonin receptor to block additional serotonergic toxicity; not recommended, as no clear efficacy established, not FDA approved (*Curr Treat Options Neurol. 2016;18:39*)

NEUROLEPTIC MALIGNANT SYNDROME

Definition and Clinical Features (*Am J Psychiatry. 2007;164(6); Neuropsychiatr Dis Treat. 2017;13*)

- Fever, severe muscle rigidity, autonomic dysfunction (↑HR, ↑BP, ↑temp, diaphoresis, nausea, vomiting, cardiac arrhythmia), mental status change (mutism, stupor)
- Idiosyncratic and temporally related to use of dopamine blocking agent or removal of dopaminergic agent
- Many consider NMS to be a subtype of malignant catatonia
- 16% of cases develop within 24 h after antipsychotic tx, 66% within 1st week
- Rhabdomyolysis most common complication (30.1%) (*Neurocrit Care. 2016;24:102*)
- **Atypical NMS:** Can refer either to NMS with atypical features or NMS caused by atypical antipsychotics (which may also be more likely to have atypical features)
  - Though previously thought to be lower risk, atypical antipsychotics can induce NMS (*BJPsych Bull. 2017;41(4)*)
  - NMS with certain atypical antipsychotics may present less frequently with rigidity, tremor, and fever, more frequently with diaphoresis
  - Seen with clozapine (less rigidity), olanzapine (EPS and fever can be absent), aripiprazole (less hyperthermia and delirium)
  - Many cases of so-called atypical NMS may represent nonmalignant catatonia induced by antipsychotics

Epidemiology and Pathogenesis

- Incidence 0.2–3.23%, decreased from in recent years due to awareness and shift to atypical antipsychotics (Neuropsychiatr Dis Treat. 2017;13:162)
- 3:2 M:F. May be related to increased muscle mass in men, increased antipsychotic exposure in men (Acta Psychiatr Scand. 2017;135:405)
- Decreasing mortality over time; 7.6% with use of typical neuroleptics, 3.3% with use of atypical neuroleptics (Neurocrit Care. 2016;24:100)
- Pathogenesis unclear; related to sudden decrease in dopamine. Proposed theory in schizophrenia: proinflammatory cytokines activate a cascade → neurotoxin production → dopamine degraded, decreased dopamine biosynthesis, increased free radicals → impaired mitochondrial electron transport chain → muscle cell damage, hyperreflexia, and electrolytes (K, Phos) and proteins (myoglobin, creatine, CK) leak into blood stream (Neuropsychiatr Dis Treat. 2017;13:162)

Evaluation (Neuropsychiatr Dis Treat. 2017;13:161-175)

- Risk factors: parenteral administration of dopamine blocking meds, higher titration rates, higher total dose, history of catatonia or NMS, withdrawal from GABAergic medication/substance, agitation, dehydration, exhaustion, basal ganglia disorders (Lewy body dementia, Parkinson's, Wilson's, Huntington's, tardive dystonia)
- Ddx: neuro infection (meningitis, encephalitis, tetanus), autoimmune encephalitis, seizure, CNS vasculitis, systemic infection, thyrotoxicosis, drug/toxin intoxication or withdrawal, acute dystonia, porphyria
- Workup: CBC (usually leukocytosis, thrombocytosis), blood cultures, BMP, LFTs (↑ due to muscle damage), Ca, CK (usually > 1000 IU/L), serum iron (often low), urine myoglobin, ABG, coags, serum and urine tox. Imaging not recommended

Nonpharmacologic Treatment

- Discontinue offending drug, provide supportive measures in addition to pharmacotherapy as below. After discontinuation, syndrome is self-limited (7–10 d) but can be lethal if not treated

Pharmacologic Treatment

- **Benzodiazepines** should be used aggressively. Offer IV lorazepam 1–2 mg q4–6h. Doses of up to 24 mg daily of lorazepam may be needed
- **ECT** if not responding to benzodiazepines. Consider swift move to ECT if no improvement after 24–48 h (Curr Treat Options Neurol. 2016;18:39)
- Dopaminergic agents (**bromocriptine, amantadine**) may reduce time to recovery and decrease mortality, but carry significant risk of psychosis and should be used as second-line after benzos
- **Dantrolene** useful in cases with extreme hyperthermia (temp ≥ 40°C), rigidity, tachycardia (HR ≥ 120). Rigidity and hyperthermia rapidly reversed but can recur after dantrolene discontinued (Am J Psychiatry. 2007;164(6):874). Primarily acts as a muscle relaxant, which is also accomplished by benzos. Dantrolene can impair respiratory, cardiovascular, and hepatic function
- Rechallenge with antipsychotic should not occur for at least 2 wk. Risk of recurrent NMS at least 30%. Consider transition to lower potency or 2nd-generation antipsychotic (Ann Pharmacother. 2016;50(11):979)
- Beware of depot antipsychotics, which may prolong syndrome

CHRONIC PAIN

Definition and Clincal Features

- Defined as persistent pain, either continuous or recurrent, that affects a patient's well-being, level of function, and quality of life; >3 mo in duration. Note that only noncancer pain will be discussed in this chapter
- Clinical features vary by condition. Headaches and musculoskeletal pain (back/neck) are most common. Other common pain includes arthritis, neuropathic pain, chronic abdominal pain, chronic pelvic pain (women>men), fibromyalgia (Prog Neuropsychopharmcol Biol Psych. 2018;87:159-167). Features of common conditions include the following:

  Chronic migraines: Episodic uni- or bilateral headaches, typically characterized by severe throbbing, likely the result of neurovascular abnormalities resulting in multimodal sensory pathology. Associated with photo/phonophobia and often nausea (Pract Neuro. 2015;15:411-423).

  Chronic back pain: Multiple etiologies possible, including muscular strain, herniated disc, spondylolysis, spondylolisthesis, connective tissue disease. Roughly 70% of back pain is self-limited, and suspected etiology can guide management (AAFP. 2009;79:1067-1074).

  Postherpetic neuralgia: Reactivation of varicella zoster virus in adulthood along one to several dermatomes results in shingles; 10% of patients continue to experience pain for >3 mo and burning and allodynia in the same distribution despite resolution of the rash (usually 2–4 wk) (Drugs Aging. 2012;29:863-869).

  Diabetic neuropathy: Symmetric, distal, progressive polyneuropathy related to chronic hyperglycemia and subsequent cellular changes in peripheral nerves; the most common polyneuropathy worldwide (30–50% of pts with diabetes) (Front Neuro. 2017;8:825).

  Trigeminal neuralgia: Characterized by lightning-like shocks (usually episodic, occasionally with background pain) in a unilateral distribution of the trigeminal nerve. May be idiopathic or caused by a structural lesion (Therap Adv Neuro Disorders. 2010;3:107-115).

Epidemiology and Pathogenesis

- Estimates of prevalence vary widely, with most studies citing prevalence between 20–40% (Curr Med Res Opin. 2012;28:1221-1229). In the United States, CDC estimates that 20% of adults live with chronic pain, with as many as 8% experiencing "high-impact" chronic pain with major reductions in QoL (MMWR. 2018;67:1001-1006)
- **Modifiable risk factors:** anxiety, depression, chronic disease (CAD, COPD), smoking, obesity, disrupted sleep, unemployment (Br J Pain. 2013;7:209-217)
- **Nonmodifiable risk factors:** female sex, increasing age, low socioeconomic status, history of abuse/violence, family history (Br J Pain. 2013;7:209-217)
- **Pain physiology** (Med Clin North Am. 2016;100:31-42): Peripheral nociceptors depolarize to painful stimuli, travel through first-order sensory neurons in the dorsal root ganglia to ascending second-order neurons of the dorsal horn, which then provide input to the spinal

cord and thalamus via the spinothalamic tract. The thalamus relays information to the cortex (resulting in awareness of pain) and the limbic system (resulting in emotional response to pain) via third-order neurons. Both descending inputs from the cortex and spinal interneurons provide regulation and reduce depolarization of the ascending pathway

- **Pathophysiology** (Med Clin North Am. 2016;100:31-42): Neuropathic pain involves peripheral nerve damage resulting in inflammatory cytokine release. This leads to ectopic signal generation, enhanced nociceptor depolarization, and impaired inhibitory signals within the brainstem. At the level of the brain, damaged neurons become sensitized to inputs rather than desensitized. This reason for this is unclear, but it is likely that this sensitization process is shared by both chronic neuropathic and nonneuropathic pain

Evaluation
Interview

- Pain description: provocative/palliative factors, quality, region/radiation, severity, timing (PQRST). Can use **pain rating scales** including numeral rating scale (0–10), visual analog scale (VAS), verbal rating scale, pain maps (pencil in location of pain), Brief Pain Inventory (BPI) (includes impact of pain on quality of life), McGill Pain Questionnaire (SF-MPQ-2) (includes prior treatment trials), many others
- Associated symptoms: swelling, ROM, strength, sensation, color/temperature changes, sweating, skin/nail/hair growth, spasm, nausea

Characteristics of Pain		
Type	**Quality + Associated Sx**	**Examples**
Neuropathic	Burning, shooting/stabbing, numb, allodynia, hyperalgesia, coolness	Sciatica, diabetic peripheral neuropathy, postherpetic neuralgia, MS, poststroke, trigeminal neuralgia, fibromyalgia
Muscular	Diffuse aching	Back pain, skeletal muscle pain, myofascial pain
Inflammatory	Heat, redness, swelling, history of injury	Inflammatory arthropathies, infection, tissue injury, post-op
Mechanical/Compressive	Aggravated during activity, relief during rest	Muscle/ligament strain/sprain, disk or facet degeneration, compression fracture, renal calculi, visceral pain from tumor/cyst compressing tissue
Headache	Variable	Migraine, tension-type, hemicranias continua, medication overuse, daily persistent, chronic cluster, etc

*Note that pain may fit more than one category Am Fam Physician. 2010;82 (4):434-439.

- Impact on function: social functioning, mood, relationships, occupation, sleep, exercise, ADLs
- Consider tracking the so-called 6 "**dreaded D's**": disability, depression, deconditioning, dependence on opioids, dysfunctional relationships, drinking (and other substance use)
- If >3, usually refer to physical medicine and rehabilitation for ongoing management *(Phys Med Rehabil Clin North Am.* 2015;26(2):185-199)
- Past treatment: Providers, diagnostic studies, pharmacologic and nonpharmacologic management (including complementary medicine, procedures)
- Social and psychological factors: Personal and family history, support system, comorbid psychiatric illness (see *Relationship to Psychiatry* section below), substance use disorder
- Expectations: Patient goals, understanding, willingness to be active participant in care

Physical Exam
- Complete physical exam, including detailed neurological and musculoskeletal exams
- Note splinting, compensatory movements, gait, consistency throughout visit

Diagnostic Testing
- Consider lab tests, plain films and MRI, electromyography, and nerve conduction studies

Relationship to Psychiatry
- Individuals with chronic pain 4× as likely to have anxiety or depression than those without (OR 4.1) *(JAMA.* 1998;290:147-151), with severity of psychiatric disorder positively associated with pain severity *(Gen Hosp Psych.* 2012;34:534-540). Substance use disorders also positively associated with chronic pain, particularly headache, back/neck pain, fibromyalgia *(Prog Neuropsychopharm Biol Psych.* 2018;87:159-167)
- About 1 of 3 patients receiving opiates report depression and/or anxiety *(J Subst Abuse Treat.* 2007;33:303-311)
- Prevalence of suicidal ideation among those with chronic pain estimated between 5 and 50%, with prevalence of suicide attempts estimated between 5 and 14%. Risk factors for death by suicide among those with chronic pain include severe pain, longer duration, sleep-onset insomnia, helplessness/hopelessness about pain, desire to escape pain, catastrophizing and avoidance, problem-solving deficits *(Psychol Med.* 2006;36:575-586)
- Prevalence and intensity of chronic pain **less** among those with schizophrenia (higher pain threshold in schizophrenia poorly understood; pain insensitivity may serve as prodromal predictor for susceptibility for schizophrenia) *(Prog Neuropsychopharm Biol Psych.* 2018;87:159-167)
- Individuals with dementia less likely to report pain, though may be underrecognized/undertreated due to difficulties with assessment *(Age Ageing.* 2004;33:496-499)

Chronic Pain Management

- Currently available treatments provide *on average* a 30% reduction in pain with minimal improvements in physical and emotional functioning (but highly variable by condition/individual patient) *(Lancet. 2011;377(9784):2226-2235)*. Optimal outcomes result from multidisciplinary approach including education, nonpharmacologic, and pharmacologic strategies

Nonpharmacologic

- Can be separated into physical, psychoeducational, and procedural interventions
- **Physical** interventions include aerobic exercise, PT/OT, yoga, tai chi, qigong, massage, acupuncture, chiropractics/osteopathic manipulation, heat/cold, ultrasound, transcutaneous electrical nerve stimulation (TENS)

  Of physical interventions, most consistent evidence for exercise and PT, acupuncture, mind-body practices *(Agency for Healthcare Research and Quality (US); 2018. Report No: 18-EHC013-EF. PMID: 30179389)*
- **Psychoeducational** interventions include CBT, ACT, mindfulness-based stress reduction, biofeedback, relaxation therapy, individual or group psychotherapy

  Of psychoeducational interventions, most consistent evidence for CBT and mind-body practices *(Agency for Healthcare Research and Quality (US); 2018. Report No: 18-EHC013-EF. PMID: 30179389)*
- **Procedural** interventions include spinal cord stimulation, deep brain stimulation, nerve blocks/ablation, botulinum toxin (botox) injections, trigger point injections, facet injections, epidural steroid injections, intrathecal pumps, surgery is also being investigated as treatment for MDD

  Note that botox *(Iran J Public Health. 2017;46(7):982-984)* and DBS *(J Clin Invest. 2013;123(11):4546-4556)* are also being investigated as treatments for MDD

Pharmacologic

- Evidence varies with etiology and condition. If associated with specific condition (eg, autoimmune, infectious, visceral), best is management of underlying condition
- Should be used as *adjunct* to nonpharmacologic therapy
- Best practices of pharmacologic therapy *(AFP. 2010;82:434-439)*
  1. Shared decision-making between prescriber and patient
  2. Goal to improve function and quality of life (not just pain)
  3. Consideration of age, comorbid conditions (psychiatric, neurological)
  4. Use synergistic agents rather than multiple agents in the same class
- **Classes of agent**

  Antiepileptic drugs (AEDs): Effective for neuropathic pain. Most commonly used are **gabapentin** (good choice if co-occurring AUD) and **pregabalin** (more predictable absorption, faster onset of analgesia, and faster titration of dosing *(J Pain. 2008;9:1006)*). Pregabalin commonly first-line for fibromyalgia; **topiramate** commonly used in migraines; **carbamazepine/oxcarbazepine** first-line in trigeminal neuralgia

Antidepressants: TCAs and SNRIs effective in neuropathic pain (*J Neuro Neurosurg Psych.* 2010;81:1372) and fibromyalgia (*Neuropsych Dis Treat.* 2006;2:537-548), particularly in patients with co-occurring depression (*J Affect Disord.* 2015;184:72-80). Most commonly prescribed are **amitriptyline** and **duloxetine**. **Doxepin** has a topical formulation that avoids systemic side effects

Nonnarcotic analgesics: **Tylenol** is the preferred agent, often used in conjunction with opioids to reduce total daily opiate dose. Doses should not exceed 4 g (less in the elderly, <2 g in patients with cirrhosis as Tylenol overdose is associated with acute liver failure). **NSAIDs** also commonly used in the treatment of chronic musculoskeletal pain; providers must be aware of adverse effects (particularly in elderly) including increased bleeding risk, renal failure, gastric ulcer. Topical formulations avoid adverse GI effects (*Cochrane.* 2012;12:CD007400)

Antispasmodics: Used in conditions associated with muscle spasm (eg, multiple sclerosis, low back pain). Commonly prescribed agents include **baclofen**, **tizanidine**, and **carisoprodol** but use is limited by risk of CNS depression and abuse. Patients with severe muscular spasticity (MS, cerebral palsy, spinal cord injury) may benefit from implantation of an intrathecal baclofen pump (*Ont Health Technol Assess Ser.* 2005;5:1-93)

Topical agents: **Topical lidocaine** and **topical capsaicin** recommended for well-localized pain, such as diabetic neuropathy, postherpetic neuralgia, and HIV neuropathy

Marijuana and CBD oil: Low-level evidence in support of marijuana and THC/CBD agonists in neuropathic pain, insufficient evidence for use in other types of pain (*Ann Intern Med.* 2017;167:319)

Narcotic analgesics: A 2015 systematic review was unable to establish efficacy in the use of opioids for chronic pain but found increased incidence of adverse events, including overdose, abuse, and sequelae of falls (*Ann Intern Med.* 2015;162:276)

DELIRIUM

Definition and Clinical Features

- Acute disturbance in attention, awareness, and cognition +/− motor/behavioral/emotional Δ that is a physiological consequence of another medical condition
- Develops over hours to days and can persist for days to months
- Most common cognitive disturbances incl inattention, disorientation, executive dysfxn, ↓ short-term memory
- Perceptual disturbances: VH > AH; tactile hallucinations suggestive of delirium 2/2 substance use
- Delusions: more vague than in primary psychosis; often persecutory (ie, medical team purposefully causing harm)

- **Major subtypes** (Psychiatry Clin Neurosci. 2014;68(4):283-291):
  - Hyperactive: Presents w/ mood lability, delusions, hallucinations, and agitation in addition to fluctuating cognitive sx
  - Hypoactive: Presents as withdrawn, blunted affect, thought process abnormalities (eg, slowed processing speed), and language disturbance; most common subtype among hospitalized elders (Am J Geriatr Psychiatry. 2017;25(10):1064-1071)
  - Mixed: Fluctuating sx of both hyper- and hypoactive subtypes

Epidemiology and Pathogenesis

- Affects ~50% hospitalized pts >65 y/o: ↑ mortality, institutionalization, predicts future ↓ cognition (Lancet. 2014;383(9920):911-922)
- Affects 1 in every 5 pts in the general hospital (BMJ Open. 2013;3(1):1-9)
- Up to 87% of critically ill develop delirium in the ICU (Crit Care Med. 2001;29(7):1370-1379)
- Multiple underlying mechanisms/theories of pathogenesis: neuroinflammation, neuronal aging, oxidative stress, neurotransmitter perturbation, neuroendocrine/glucocorticoid response, diurnal dysregulation, network disconnectivity (Am J Geriatr Psychiatry. 2013;21(12):1190-1222)

Evaluation

- **Determining the underlying cause of delirium is key**
- Always consider life-threatening causes, ie, WWHHHHHIMPS (Handbook of General Hospital Psychiatry. 7th ed.; 2017:84)

Life-Threatening Causes of Delirium—WWHHHHHIMPS
Withdrawal (from GABA-agonists, etc)
Wernicke encephalopathy
Hypoxia
Hypotension
Hypertensive emergency
Hypoglycemia
Hypo- or hyperthermia
Intracerebral hemorrhage
Meningitis/encephalitis
Poisoning
Status epilepticus

- Medications can cause/worsen delirium: BZDs; anticholinergics; narcotics; steroids; sympathomimetics; TCAs; immunosuppressives; antibiotics; antiarrhythmics
- Many underlying conditions are associated with delirium; consider a systematic approach to differential

- **Risk factors:** older age (*Lancet.* 2014;383(9920):911-922); dementia w/ 40% of demented in hospital developing delirium (*Crit Care Clin.* 2008;24(4):657-722); medical illness (ICU > wards > home; ↑ # active medical problems→ ↑ delirium risk); systemic inflammation (burns, long bone fxr, major surgery)

Common Causes of Delirium	
Vascular	CVA, intracranial bleed, PRES
Infectious	PNA, UTI, sepsis, HIV, Lyme, encephalitis/meningitis
Endocrine	Hypo-/hyperthyroidism, Cushing's/Addison's, Parathyroid
Metabolic	Hepatic/renal failure; electrolyte imbalance; acid/base disturbance
Autoimmune	SLE, Hashimoto encephalopathy, MS
Cardiopulm disease	PE, heart failure, cardiopulmonary arrest
Trauma	Heat stroke, burns, postoperative change
Intoxication	Sedatives, opioids, ketamine, tranquilizers
Vitamin deficiency	Thiamin, niacin, B_{12}
GABA-ergic withdrawal	EtOH, sedative/hypnotics
Neurological	Complex-partial Sz, brain tumor, postictal state

- Physical exam and history (incl prior records) guide evaluation—aim for targeted testing
- **Neuro exam:** focus on DTRs and primitive reflexes; pupils and EOM; muscle tone (gegenhalten, cogwheeling, clonus); strength; assess for multifocal myoclonus (sometimes described as the most common neuro finding in delirium), asterixis; also look for frontal release signs
- **Cognitive exam:** consciousness (GCS); tests of attention (days of week or months of year frwd/bkwrd), short-term memory, *executive function*
  - Clock draw: Instruct pt to draw the face of a clock on a blank sheet of paper, write in all the numbers, and set the time to 10 past 11; note any perseveration (ie, drawing numbers beyond 12, multiple clock face circles, etc), mis-sequencing, stimulus-bound responses (ie, setting time to 11:50)
  - Luria sequencing: Instruct pt to mimic your hands in fist, edge, palm pattern; then have pt do on her own
- **Common lab tests:** CBC; BMP; LFTs; TSH; drug levels (ie, lithium, AEDs); serum and urine tox screen; UA and UCx; blood gas

- EKG; CXR; consider LP in rare cases
- **Head imaging:** MRI more sens than CT for stroke, WM damage, tumors
- **EEG:** generalized slow-waves (↓ alpha, ↑ theta and delta waves) diagnostic but also seen in moderate to severe dementia; can r/o underlying sz disorder
- **Confusion Assessment Method and CAM-ICU:** symptom scale for RN/nonpsych clinicians; 94–100% sens, 90–95% spec (*Ann Int Med.* 1990;113(12):941-948)
- **Delirium Rating Scale and DRS-Revised-98:** Dx confirmation and severity rating; DRS-R-98 can be administered serially (*J Neuropsychiatry Clin Neurosci.* 2001;13(2):229-242)

Nonpharmacologic Treatment (*Lancet.* 2014;383(9920):911-922)
- Most effective approach for preventing and ↓ delirium
- Preserve sleep/wake cycle; lights on in the day/off at night; minimize nighttime disruptions
- Improve sensory input; glasses; hearing aids
- Frequent reorientation; clocks; calendars
- Mobilize pt (PT, OT)
- Promote adequate nutrition/fluid intake

Pharmacologic Treatment
- The treatment for delirium is reversal of the underlying cause; antipsychotics may help control delirium sxs of agitation and psychosis and are most effective in hyperactive delirium or hypoactive delirium w/ perceptual disturbance
- **Neuroleptics:** Gold standard = haloperidol IV (↓ EPS than PO/IM but can ↑ QT; overall risk of Torsades is low (*Ann Intern Med.* 1993;119(5):391-394)); chlorpromazine IV (↑ α-blockade → ↓ CO); risperidone PO/IM; olanzapine PO/IM; quetiapine safest in PD, LBD (*Lancet.* 2015;386(10004):1683-1697); minimal evidence for prophylactic antipsychotics in non–critical care settings (*J Am Geriatr Soc.* 2005;53(10):1658-1666); prophylactic antipsychotics in ICU do not reduce mortality (*JAMA.* 2018;319(7):680-690)
- **BZDs:** For tx of GABA-ergic withdrawal delirium only; o/w can worsen delirium
- **Mood stabilizers:** limited evidence; valproic acid shown to ↓ lability, agitation, and hyperactivity (*J Crit Care.* 2017;(37):119-125); caution in liver dz
- **Melatonin receptor agonists:** may promote sleep/wake regulation; no evidence of prophylactic benefit (*Ann Pharmacother.* 2017;51(1):72-78; *Cochrane Database Syst Rev.* 2016;11(3):CD005563)
- **Stimulants:** low-dose methylphenidate → ↑ cognition and activity in cancer pts w/ hypoactive delirium (*J Psychiatry Neurosci.* 2005;30(2):100-107)

Clinical Features (Nat Rev Dis Prim. 2016;2:16065)

- **Major depressive episode:** (1) 5/9 sx of SIGECAPS (at least 1 either depressed mood or loss of interest/pleasure); (2) occurs most of the day, nearly every day, for at least 2 wk; (3) must reflect change in functioning
  - Mean episode duration 13–30 wk; 70–90% recover within 1 y
  - Atypical depression: has different symptoms (2 of 4)—hypersomnia, hyperphagia, leaden paralysis, rejection sensitivity
- **Major depressive disorder (MDD):** disorder marked by recurrent major depressive episodes
- **Persistent depressive disorder (dysthymia):** (1) depressed mood for most of the day, more days than not, for >2 y (2) 2/6 sx of change in appetite, change in sleep, low energy, low self-esteem, poor concentration, feelings of hopelessness (3) during 2-y period, never been without sx for > 2 mo at a time

SIGECAPS
S—sleep (↑/↓)
I—interest (↓)
G—guilt
E—energy (↓)
C—concentration (↓)
A—appetite (↑/↓)
P—psychomotor sx
S—suicidality

- **Other depressive disorders:**
  - Disruptive mood dysregulation disorder
  - Premenstrual dysphoric disorder
  - Substance/medication induced depressive disorder
  - Depressive disorder due to another medical condition
- **Common to all depressive disorders:** sad, empty, or irritable mood + somatic and cognitive changes that limit function

Epidemiology and Pathogenesis (Nat Rev Dis Prim. 2016;2:16065; Lancet. 2012;379(9820):1045-1055)

- **MDD:** 12-month prevalence (2012–2013) = 10.4%, lifetime prevalence = 20.6% (JAMA Psychiatry. 2018;75(4):339); 2:1 women:men; may occur at any age
  - Recurrent major depressive episodes occur in 85% of those with single major depressive episode
  - Highly correlated with diabetes, cardiac disease, obesity
  - Mortality risk in persons with MDD is 2× the general population; standardized mortality ratio for suicide is 21:1 for males, 27:1 for females (compared w/ nondepressed general population)
- **Dysthymia:** lifetime prevalence = 3–6%; early onset, chronic course
- Genetics: no identification of single candidate gene → likely polygenic with interaction between genetics and environment; MDD has been associated with genes for glucocorticoid receptor, monoamine oxidase, and genes responsible for regulation of metabolism
- Molecular studies: genetic variants in growth factors, proinflammatory cytokines, and regulation of HPA axis have been implicated
- Neural systems: functional abnormalities evident in subcortical systems (emotion and reward processing), medial prefrontal and anterior cingulate cortical regions (emotion processing and regulation), and lateral prefrontal cortical systems (cognitive control of emotions)

Evaluation (Nat Rev Dis Prim. 2016;2:16065)

- Useful screening questions: (1) Do you feel depressed? (2) Has there been any change in your self-esteem?
- Ddx: (1) psychiatric: bipolar depression, adjustment d/o w/ depressed mood, seasonal affective d/o, early neurocognitive d/o, personality d/o, psychotic d/o prodrome; (2) medical: meds (steroids, BZD), thyroid dysfunction, OSA, delirium, Huntington dx, neurologic d/o (MS, epilepsy), infection (mono/flu/HIV/syphilis/Lyme), cancer, postsurgical, stroke
- Severity of sx guides treatment of MDD: **mild:** minimum sx required, sx distressing but manageable, minor impairment in functioning; **moderate:** number, intensity, functional impairment between mild and severe; **severe:** number of sx in substantial excess of minimum required, sx distressing and unmanageable, marked interference with functioning
- **Psychotic depression:** mood component more severe + delusions, hallucinations in 10–20%. Delusions can be *mood congruent* (themes of guilt, death, personal inadequacy) or *mood incongruent* (content of delusions independent of depressive theme)
  - 14% of those with MDD have history of episode with psychotic features; 25% of those hospitalized with depression have psychotic features (Cochrane Database Syst Rev. 2015;7:CD004044)
- Severity of sx guides treatment: **mild:** active monitoring, individual guided self-help, exercise, healthy diet, sleep hygiene, therapy; **moderate:** therapy alone/meds alone/both; **severe w/o psychosis:** antidepressant +/− therapy +/− ECT; **severe w/ psychosis:** antidepressant + antipsychotic +/− ECT
  - Mild-moderate depression can be treated in **collaborative care** settings (PCP + case management + consulting mental health specialist) with improved outcomes as compared with usual care (Cochrane Database Syst Rev. 2012;10:CD006525)
  - Psychotherapy + pharmacotherapy more effective than either alone (J Affect Disord. 2016;194:144-152)
- **Maintenance treatment:** aim to prevent relapse/recurrence, regular monitoring, consider ongoing antidepressant tx, psychotherapy

Nonpharmacologic Treatment
- **Psychotherapy:** CBT as effective as antidepressant med for mild-moderate severity, possibly severe depression (JAMA Psychiatry. 2015;72(11):1102-1109); multiple meta-analyses show psychological therapies (CBT, IPT, supportive therapy, psychodynamic therapy) equally efficacious in acute tx of depression (Nord J Psychiatry. 2011;65(6):354-364)
- **Light therapy:** morning light tx, efficacious in seasonal affective dx, may be beneficial in MDD; side effects (uncommon) incl headache, eye strain, blurred vision, insomnia, mania (rare) (J Affect Disord. 2015;182:1-7)
- **ECT:** most effective and rapid tx in severe depression; indicated for severe depression, inability to eat/drink, high suicide risk, high distress, psychotic depression, depression with catatonia, previous response, patient choice, treatment refractory depression; 6–12 tx, generally 3×/wk, followed by 2×/wk or weekly; adverse

effects include headache, delirium, cognitive effects (generally resolve a few weeks after tx course concludes) (Am J Psychiatry. 2012;169:1238-1244)

Pharmacologic Treatment

- Minimal evidence to suggest any antidepressant more efficacious than any others. Choose based on side effect profile, drug interactions—generally SSRIs (escitalopram, sertraline) best tolerated antidepressant (Lancet. 2009;373:746-758)
  - Atypical depression may preferentially benefit from MAOI
- Start antidepressant, titrate to therapeutic dose
  - If poorly tolerated OR not effective (after 4-wk trial), switch to alternate antidepressant based on tolerability and drug interactions (Psychiatr Serv. 2009;60(11):1439-1445)
  - When effective, continue for 6–9 mo, or longer for recurrent depression (National Institute for Health and Care Excellence, 2016)
- Strategies for **treatment refractory major depression** (Nat Rev Dis Prim. 2016;2:16065)
  - Reevaluate diagnosis, consider bipolar depression
  - High-dose drug therapy or combination therapy
  - ECT
  - Add lithium
  - Add levothyroxine
  - Add second-generation antipsychotic (aripiprazole, olanzapine, quetiapine, and risperidone common)
  - Add bupropion, venlafaxine, or mirtazapine to SSRI
- **Dysthymia**
  - Pharmacotherapy is 1st-line tx, no evidence for psychotherapy as monotherapy for dysthymia; antidepressants w/ higher margin of efficacy in dysthymia than MDD (J Clin Psychiatry. 2011;72:512)
  - Most antidepressant classes effective, with full range recommended dose as MDD
  - Antidepressant tx should continue for >2 y (National Institute for Health and Care Excellence, 2016)

DISSOCIATIVE DISORDERS

Clinical Features

- Dissociative disorders are characterized by disrupted integration of consciousness, memory, identity, perception, body representation/control, appearance, and/or behavior
- While controversial, some experts argue that dissociative experiences are universal, comprising a spectrum from normal to pathological. Pathology is loosely defined by the timing/frequency, severity, inability to avoid dissociation, and impact on function (Dell et al. 2009;145:170)
- Dissociative experiences can be conceptualized as "partial" (ie, partially excluded from consciousness; perceived as intrusive and ego-alien) vs "full" (ie, fully excluded from consciousness) (Psychiatr Clin North Am. 2006;1:26)

Possible Symptoms of Pathologic Dissociation

Symptom	Description | Whether Experienced as Partial (P) or Full (F)
Depersonalization	Sense of disconnection from one's self, body, actions | P
Derealization	Detachment from one's surroundings, eg, foggy, distorted, "watching a movie" | P
Amnesia; fugue	Inability to recall important biographical information; dissociated, purposeful travel | F
Memory problems	Distressing, nonspecific forgetfulness (less than frank amnesia) | P
Flashbacks	Intrusive experience of prior traumatic situation | P
"Trance," autohypnotic	Examples include staring/unresponsive episodes, spontaneous age regression, or a sudden change in linguistic expression. Easily recognizable by an observer | P
Somatoform and conversion	Alteration of bodily sensation or function without physical or medical explanation, such as loss of ability to move limbs, below the neck anesthesia/analgesia, etc | P
Hallucinations	Voice or full A/V hallucination of a child; conversant or persecutory voices | P
Thought insertion or withdrawal	Ego-alien experience of thoughts being either added or removed from ones consciousness | P
Intrusive feelings, impulses, actions	Ego-alien, feeling overpowered, "taken over," controlled, or possessed, which may frequently be experienced as an intrusion from an alter identity | P
Loss of knowledge, skills	Temporary amnesia for well-rehearsed knowledge or abilities, such as forgetting how to read, play a game, do one's job, etc | P
Identity confusion	Sudden distressing experience of an intrusive change in self, such as seeing another's image in the mirror, feeling one is of wrong height or gender, etc | P
Identity alteration	"Personality switching," with 2+ "alters" that have autonomous ways of thinking, perceiving, and acting, often in conflict with one another. Core symptom of DID | F
Lost time, "coming to"	Realization that time has passed or events occurred with no recollection | F
Finding objects, evidence of recent actions	Common for individuals with DID to discover new objects (eg, clothes, toys) among their possessions or find evidence of acts that only they could have performed (eg, newly painted room, completed tasks at work) | F

- Some experiences (eg, trance/possession) may be a normative cultural-bound experience
- Dissociative disorders are **highly associated with trauma**, with significantly greater reports of childhood physical (71 vs 27%) and sexual abuse (74 vs 29%) compared to controls not meeting criteria for a dissociative disorder (AJP. 2006;623:629)
- **Ddx for all dissociative disorders:** trauma-spectrum disorders, borderline personality, substance use–related (eg, ketamine, GHB, salvia), neurocognitive disorder, transient global amnesia, seizures (eg, TLE), somatization disorder, conversion disorder, intermittent explosive disorder, acute and transient psychotic disorder, malingering
- **DSM-5 recognized diagnoses** include Dissociative Identity Disorder, Dissociative Amnesia (specifier With Dissociative Fugue), Depersonalization/Derealization Disorder, and Other specified and Unspecified Dissociative Disorder

Epidemiology and Pathogenesis

- Poorly understood, in part due to dissociation's historic association with the concept of "hysteria" and subsequent neglect of the study of its physiological underpinnings
- Some evidence implicates limbic structures including the thalamus and hippocampus; dissociative symptoms have been noted in patients with thalamic lesions (Michelson, Ray. 1996;163:190) with severity of dissociation negatively correlated with hippocampal volume (AJP. 2003;924-932)
- NMDA-antagonists (eg, ketamine), produce dissociative symptoms (Arch Gen Psych. 1994;199:214), which may be mediated via receptors in the limbic system
- Ongoing research focuses on imaging (fMRI/MRI), genotype/phenotype variation (saliva studies), neuropsychiatry, and physiology (pain tolerance, fear-potentiated startle)

Evaluation

- Due to the current lack of objective markers of dissociation, evaluation currently relies on clinical interviews and subjective rating scales
- Urine tox and medical workup needed to exclude substance and neuromedical causes
- Assessment tools include Dissociative Experiences Scale (DES), Clinician-Administered PTSD Scale for DSM-5 (CAPS-5), Structured Clinical Interview for DSM-IV Dissociative Disorders (SCID-D), Multidimensional Inventory of Dissociation (MID)

Dissociative Identity Disorder (DID)

- Formerly known as multiple personality disorder (MPD)
- Historically, one of the most controversial diagnoses in psychiatry, due to high prevalence (80%) of childhood traumatic experiences (Can J Psychiatry. 1989;413:418) and frequent symptomatic overlap with trauma-spectrum disorders, borderline personality, and psychosis (J Traumatic Stress. 2012;241:251)
- Criteria since DSM-III have led to high rates of the "unspecified" designation (57–90% of cases), further bringing our diagnostic schema into question (Dell et al. 2009;383:428)

- While "full" dissociative symptoms (amnesia, identity alteration) are most pathognomonic, they may account for only 1% of total dissociative experiences (Dell et al. 2009;225:237)
- Diagnosis: Existence of 2 or more distinct personality states, with associated gaps in the recall of personal information or events in excess of normal forgetfulness
- Epidemiology: prevalence 1.1% nonclinical population, 2.5% outpatient, 3.5% inpatient (Dell et al. 2009;403:428)

Dissociative Amnesia

- Diagnosis: Inability to remember important information about one's self. Memory deficits are usually episodic or semantic, not procedural. Most commonly manifests as retrograde amnesia; isolated anterograde amnesia is rare

    Localized: Memory loss affects specific periods, usually of a traumatic nature

    Generalized: Memory loss affects identity or major life history

    Dissociative fugue specifier: Bewildered wandering with associated amnesia
- Epidemiology: prevalence 0.2–7.8%; typically diagnosed between 20 and 40 years old; equal M:F; likely underdiagnosed in males (Lancet Psych. 2014; 226:241)

Depersonalization/Derealization Disorder

- Diagnosis: Experiences of depersonalization and/or derealization, during which period reality testing remains intact
- Epidemiology: brief experiences of depersonalization/derealization are common, with an estimated 23% annual prevalence in the general population (Social Psych & Psychiatric Epidem. 2001;63:69); 50% adults have ≥1 transient episode in lifetime, with a significant number due to illicit drug use (J Clin Psychiatry. 2009;1358:1364); prevalence 1–2% (F = M), typically onset in late adolescence to 40's (Psych Clin North Am. 1991;503:517)

Nonpharmacologic Treatment

- The first-line treatment for all dissociative disorders is psychotherapy
- General consensus is that the best treatment for chronically traumatized individuals with dissociative disorders is a phase-oriented therapy (J Trauma Dissociation. 2005;11:53)
- While numerous therapies (eg, CBT, DBT, psychoeducation, sensory modalities, grounding techniques, EMDR) have shown a large overall effect size (0.71) in reducing dissociative symptoms and other depressive, anxious, and personality disorder-based symptoms, the supporting research suffers from flaws in methodology (J Nerv Ment Dis. 2009;646-654). Research with better validity and randomization is needed to definitively demonstrate reduced dissociative experiences

Pharmacologic Treatment

- There are no FDA-approved medications for dissociative disorders. No pharmacotherapy has demonstrated clear reduction of dissociation (Innov Clin Neurosci. 2013;22:29)

- Pharmacotherapy is typically used for treatment of symptoms and comorbid conditions, such as prazosin (nightmares), naltrexone (self-injurious behavior), SSRI/SNRI (depression/anxiety), and propranolol or second-generation antipsychotic (hypervigilance, aggressiveness)
- Mixed results reported for chemical-assisted (barbiturates, benzodiazepines) interviews. There are no RCTs so far, and this practice is not the standard of care (Adv Psychiatr Treat. 2009;152:158)

EATING DISORDERS

General Principles
- Eating disorders are characterized by a disturbance of eating-related behaviors that disrupts functioning or physical health
- Commonly comorbid with depression, anxiety, OCD, body dysmorphic disorder, PTSD, personality disorders (OCPD, avoidant, paranoid, borderline) and substance use
- Treatment approach is interdisciplinary (psychiatrist, therapist, dietician, PCP) with focus on psychotherapy

ANOREXIA NERVOSA
Definition and Clinical Features
- Intense fear of weight gain or persistent behavior interfering with weight gain (eg, restricting, bingeing/purging, excessive exercise); distorted body image; severe dietary restriction leading to lower-than-normal body weight

Epidemiology and Pathogenesis
- Onset usually occurs during early- to mid-adolescence or young adulthood; 8:1 F:M ratio; lifetime prevalence 1% in F and <0.5% in M (sex distribution is less skewed in children) (Lancet Psychiatry. 2015;10.1016)
- Mortality 5.1 per 1000 person-years; 1 in 5 deaths occur by suicide, otherwise mostly 2/2 medical complications (cardiac, infectious), highest mortality among psychiatric disorders (Arch Gen Psychiatry. 2011;724-731)
- Appx 50% have good outcomes (remission), time to remission is 5–6 y, higher rates of full recovery, and lower mortality in adolescents vs adults
- Genome studies suggest AN is strongly famillal; emerging literature suggesting genetic correlations between AN and schizoaffective disorder as well as OCD
- Neuroimaging suggests AN has global reductions in gray/white matter, increased CSF, regional gray matter decrease in L hypothalamus and reward-related regions of basal ganglia and somatosensory cortex; abnls can recover w/ weight regain

Evaluation
- Psychiatric history w/ in-depth interview and consideration of attitude toward food, attitude to self and weight, suicidality, behaviors around food such as meal pattern, restricting, bingeing, purging, eating

rituals, food restrictions, frequency of weighing; note that patients tend to hide symptoms, or present somatic complaints; can use scales such as SCOFF, EDE, EDQ, EDE-Q

- Medical history with full exam and ROS, height, weight, menstrual status; vital signs, exam of hair and nails, blood counts, biochemical profile, EKG; in cases of low BMI or starvation and dehydration, monitor cardiac, muscular, and electrolyte complications; in cases of long-term illness course, consider DEXA scan
- Collateral history: involve family, partners, and significant others if possible
- Risk factors: female gender; body dissatisfaction; personality traits: perfectionism, compulsivity, obsessional, narcissism, anxiety, depression; adverse perinatal and neonatal events, feeding and sleeping difficulty during infancy; globalization and industrialization in lower-income countries
- Differential diagnosis: MDD, other ED, hyperthyroid, malabsorption syndromes, IBD, diabetes, chronic infection, neoplasm
- Comorbidities: 75% of pts w/ AN report lifetime mood disorder (usually MDD); 25–75% report an anxiety disorder (usually precedes AN); 15–29% report OCD; 9–25% report alcohol misuse (lower in restricting subtype); 21% pts have osteoporosis; 54% pts have osteopenia of the lumbar spine

Treatment: Goal to Improve Nutrition Status

- Hospitalize if vitals unstable, abnormal electrolytes, BMI < 14%, rapid weight loss, severe bingeing and purging, safety concern, failure to respond to outpatient treatment; medically manage nutrition to prevent refeeding syndrome morbidity of hypokalemia and hypophosphatemia (complications 2/2 electrolyte and fluid shifts, eg, rhabdomyolysis, szs, hemolysis)
- **Nonpharmacological treatment:** psychotherapy is first line: family-based therapy (especially with younger pts), CBT, IPT, exposure therapy, focused psychodynamic therapy; nutrition: careful weight gain schedule
- **Pharmacological treatment:** No FDA-approved meds; antidepressants for mood (fluoxetine, citalopram, sertraline); some evidence that fluoxetine may reduce risk of relapse after weight restoration *(Bio Psych. 2011;644-652; JAMA. 2006;2605-2612)*; atypical antipsychotics (olanzapine) or mirtazapine for weight gain and to reduce obsessional thinking and distorted cognition *(Am J Psych. 2008;1281:88; Ment Health Clin. 2018;127-137)*, evidence for D-cycloserine adjunct to CBT *(J Clin Psychiatry. 2015:787-793)*; bupropion contraindicated (sz risk)

BULIMIA NERVOSA

Definition and Clinical Features

- Recurrent binge eating (eating a larger-than-normal amount of food in a discrete time period, feeling out of control); recurrent compensatory behaviors to prevent weight gain (eg, purging, laxatives, restricting, exercise); self-worth unduly affected by weight and shape

Epidemiology and Pathogenesis
- Usually begins during adolescence or young adulthood; 10:1 F:M ratio; prevalence 2.5% in F; mortality 2% per decade. Comorbidity also specific phobia and social anxiety disorder. Association with impulsivity, BPD, substance use

Evaluation
- Similar to AN (above). Consider history of arranging schedules to accommodate bingeing and purging, use of laxatives or diuretics; monitor for medical complications of self-induced purging including dental enamel erosions and gum disease, parotid gland enlargement, Russell sign (knuckle callouses from purging), GI complications (Mallory–Weiss), renal or electrolyte instability, endocrine dysfunction, cardiac sequelae; can use scales, bulimia-specific scale BULIT-R
- Differential diagnosis: other ED, gastric outlet obstruction
- Risk factors: Similar to AN (above), weight dissatisfaction

Treatment
- **Nonpharmacological treatment:** therapy: CBT, IPT (focuses on interpersonal deficits, role disputes, role transitions, grief, in order to adjust interaction and communication styles, modify expectations, explore feelings, enable emotional processing, takes longer to have effect vs CBT), DBT (mindfulness, interpersonal effectiveness, emotion regulation, distress tolerance) (*Int J Eat Disord.* 2007;95-101); nutrition: education, reduce frequency of binge-purge cycle; no weight gain goals; light therapy has been shown to reduce binge frequency (*Compr Psychiatry.* 1999;442:48); case reports have suggested efficacy for TMS (*Med Hypotheses.* 2005;1176:8)
- **Pharmacological treatment:** fluoxetine (1st line, the only FDA-approved med for BN, use higher average doses than for treating depression); citalopram, sertraline, fluvoxamine (2nd line), tricyclic (3rd line); topiramate may reduce binge days (*J Clin Psychiatry.* 2003;1335:41); ongoing research on opiate antagonists given the interaction between feeding and endogenous opioid system; bupropion contraindicated (sz risk)

BINGE EATING DISORDER
Definition and Clinical Features
- Recurrent binge eating episodes (eating too rapidly, eating until uncomfortably full, eating large amounts when not hungry, eating alone due to embarrassment, feeling guilty or depressed or disgusted with self afterward); no compensatory behaviors

Epidemiology and Pathogenesis
- Onset usually during late adolescence or young adulthood; prevalence ranges from 0.7 to 6.6% from various studies and 1.75× higher for F; persistence appx 6.5 y (*Biol Psychiatry.* 2013;904:14); higher rates of spontaneous remission compared to AN/BN, a longitudinal study suggested only 18% subjects still had BED after 5 y

Evaluation
- Similar to AN (above). Monitor for complications of metabolic syndrome if overweight/obese

- Differential diagnosis: obesity, DM, genetic syndromes: Kluver–Bucy, Kleine–Levin, Prader–Willi
- Risk factors: depressive symptoms, weight dissatisfaction

Treatment

- **Nonpharmacological treatment:** primary goal to reduce bingeing behavior (secondary goal to reduce weight); therapy is 1st line: meta-analysis showed CBT (individual or group) led to most treatment success for reduction as well as remission of binge eating behavior (though does not directly reduce body weight); evidence for other therapies including IPT, DBT, structured self-help, psychoanalytic, psychoeducation, mindfulness; behavioral weight loss most effective for weight loss and less effective for reducing binge eating compared to psychotherapy; nutrition: education with focus on health over weight status, break binge-purge cycle; no weight gain or loss goals *(Int J Eat Disord.* 2010;205:17)
- **Pharmacological treatment:** no FDA-approved meds; less effective than psychotherapy; can use SSRIs for depressive sx and reducing binge eating; antiepileptics such as topiramate for reducing binge eating and weight loss *(Biol Psych.* 2007;1039:48); ADHD meds (lisdexamfetamine, atomoxetine, armodafinil), naltrexone; other antiobesity meds not recommended

---

OTHER EATING DISORDERS

Avoidant/Restrictive Food Intake Disorder (Previously Feeding Disorder of Infancy)

- Eating disturbance (eg, lack of interest in food, avoidance based on food characteristics) leading to significant weight loss, nutritional deficiency, or disrupted functioning, without distorted body image; usually in infants or children

Rumination Disorder

- Recurrent regurgitation of food for at least 1 mo not attributable to other medical condition or eating disorder; often comorbid with intellectual disability

Pica

- Persistent eating of nonnutritious nonfood substances for at least 1 mo, inappropriate to developmental level, not culturally normative; often comorbid with intellectual disability

FACTITIOUS DISORDER

Clinical Features *(Gen Hosp Psychiatry.* 2003;25(5):358; *Ann Clin Biochem.* 2013;50:194; *Lancet.* 2002;359:346; *Child Abuse Neglect.* 2003;27(4):431; *Child Abuse Neglect.* 2017;72:45; *Am J Psychiatry.* 1983;140:420; *Current Psychiatry.* 2005;13)

- Defined by intentional falsification of medical or psychological signs and/or sx in oneself (**factitious disorder imposed on self**) or another (**factitious disorder imposed on another**) in the absence of external reward (ie, though the patient is intentionally falsifying signs/sx, he/she has no tangible motivation for doing so—distinguishes from malingering)

- Patients with feigned illness can be seen across any medical speciality. The spectrum of presentations is broad (see table below)
- Presentation may include fabricated history, falsified clinical/laboratory/imaging findings and/or induced illness. Pts may present known benign abnormality as pathologic
- **Munchausen syndrome**—subset of pts (10% of those with factitious d/o) with severe and chronic form of factitious d/o marked by 3 components: (1) recurrent simulated or feigned illness, (2) travel from hospital to hospital (**peregrination**), (3) **pseudologia fantastica** (production of detailed, colorful stories associated with presentation)

  Outcomes generally worse than typical factitious disorder
- **Factitious disorder imposed on another**—typically presents as either (1) caregiver intentionally causing injury/illness on another while deceiving treating providers with false/exaggerated info or (2) caregiver fabricating sx to cause overly aggressive medical eval/interventions

  Victims typically ≤4 y/o though can be adults with intellectual or other disabilities, equal in males/females; avg 22 mo between onset of sx and diagnosis

  Sx usually physical rather than psychological: apnea, anorexia, feeding issues, diarrhea, sz

Common Presentations of Factitious Disorder	
Gastrointestinal	Abdominal pain Vomiting 2/2 Ipecac use (can see elevated CK and transaminases) Hematemesis Diarrhea 2/2 laxative use or watering down stool samples
Pulmonary	Hemoptysis Dyspnea
Cardiac	Chest pain Palpitations
Neurologic	Pseudoseizures TIAs Unexplained weakness
Endocrine	Hypoglycemia 2/2 exogenous insulin (low C-peptide and proinsulin) Hyperthyroidism 2/2 exogenous thyroid hormone (inc serum total/free thyroid hormone, undetectable thyrotropin, low thyroglobulin, suppressed RAIU, no goiter, no antithyroid antibodies)

Common Presentations of Factitious Disorder (continued)	
Genitourinary	Renal colic Hematuria due to tampering with urine specimen (suspect if hematuria varies significantly between samples and other aspects of UA are normal; can also obtain 3-tube urine collection to exclude urethral trauma) Hypernatremia 2/2 salt overload, typically seen in infants and young children (FeNa > 2% in volume replete pts with salt overload; Na concentration in gastric aspirate can be checked in infants, >200 mmol/L suggestive of salt overload)
Infectious	Bacteremia 2/2 self-injected feces Urinary tract infection due to placement of feces in urine sample
Musculoskeletal	Self-induced injuries/wounds
Hematologic	Anemia 2/2 bloodletting Easy bleeding 2/2 exogenous anticoagulants
Psychiatric	Depression Bereavement—often see multiple reports of death of same or similar family member in record, often by dramatic/violent death, often accompanied by thoughts of self-harm for pt Psychosis—often see low-yield/uncommon sx (black and white VH, pt conduct inconsistent with delusions) Suicidal ideation and behavior

Epidemiology and Pathogenesis (Psychol Res Behav Manag. 2017;10:387; Lancet. 2014;383:1422; Lancet. 2014;383:1412; Am J Psychiatry. 2003;160:1163-1168; Gen Hosp Psychiatry. 2016;41:20)

- **Epidemiology:** Difficult to determine prevalence due to deceptive nature of disorder, estimated that 0.5–2% of individuals presenting in hospital settings meet criteria for factitious disorder; more common in women, unmarried, often with health care experience, commonly presents in 30s
  - Munchausen syndrome typically men, have lower SES, are isolated
  - Perpetrators of factitious disorder imposed on another most commonly women, often mother of the victim, usually have some medical training or exposure to illness affecting victim
- **Pathogenesis:** Etiology and pathogenesis are unknown. There are thought to be contributing developmental factors, such as childhood illness/loss/adversity and insecure attachment

Evaluation (Lancet. 2014;383:1422; Gen Hosp Psychiatry. 2003;25(5):358; Am J Psychiatry. 1983;140:420)

- Early suspicion (see table below) is important to avoid colluding with patient in ordering unnecessary tests and subjecting pts to further iatrogenic injury. See table below for characteristics that may raise suspicion
- Collateral information from medical records, family, friends and other/prior providers should be obtained
- Observing the patient may provide useful information
- Certain lab tests (described in table above) may provide useful

- **Differential diagnosis:** somatic symptom d/o, malingering, conversion d/o, delusional d/o, medical illness
- Distinction malingering from factitious disorder is often challenging as evidence of a clear secondary gain may be lacking, and there can be tangible benefits of primary gain (sick role can come with disability benefits, increased family support etc). Some view malingering and factitious disorder as being on the same continuum of motivation and symptom exaggeration
- Clues to Munchausen's subtype: histrionic/dramatic style, borderline traits/personality, medical training/knowledge, vague or inconsistent histories, demanding, often don't allow providers to obtain records, often use multiple aliases/MRNs confounding ability to obtain collateral
- Clues to factitious disorder imposed on another: pt doesn't respond to appropriate tx, sx improve when caregiver doesn't have access, unexplained illness in other kids in family, caregiver becomes anxious when pt improves, caregiver encourages invasive tests

Clinical Characteristics That May Raise Suspicion for Factitious Disorder
Treatment at multiple different facilities
Inconsistencies in patient history
Discrepancies between signs and symptoms
Patient reluctant to allow provider to obtain collateral information/obtain records
Evidence in lab results or other tests not consistent with info provided by pt
Atypical course or presentation of illness
Patient requests invasive medical procedures or surgeries
While requesting of medical/surgical interventions, pt refuses psychiatric assessment

Nonpharmacologic Treatment (Gen Hosp Psychiatry. 2003;25(5):358; Lancet. 2014;383:1422; Gen Hosp Psychiatry. 2017;46:74)

- Once diagnosis is established, only perform diagnostic procedures that are needed based on objective signs/data. Do not rely on pt's symptoms/reported diagnosis
- Consistency in communication and treatment planning among all team members is essential to reduce splitting
- Supportive confrontations (and if in the hospital setting, consideration of a therapeutic discharge) should be decided on a case-by-case basis and are best done after some rapport has been built and there is firm evidence of self injury
- Tips on discharging pt from hospital with feigned illness (note that discharge is contraindicated if pt still requires inpatient care despite deception): physician must have confidence pt is engaging in deceptive behavior → safety assessment should be performed prior to d/c (can neutralize provocative statements made at time of confrontation) → prepare for d/c (prepare Rx, d/c paperwork, alert all in-hospital providers to ensure no further w/u or tx warranted, alert security) → discharge pt (use neutral tone and direct

language with emphasis on pt safety, acknowledge distress, offer f/u and referrals, if pt gets dysregulated allow pt to take time to cool off and return to complete d/c → debrief, document event, alert ED to potential pt will return, add malingering/factitious d/o to pt's chart
- Tips on documentation in case of therapeutic discharge: document justification for discharge, document awareness of risk factors, include subjective risk assessment based on pt's report and objective risk assessment based on objective data, articulate why risk not acutely elevated, document evidence of factitious d/o (or if unsure if primary/secondary gain, can use terms such as "deception syndrome" or "feigning")

Pharmacologic Treatment

While there is no pharmacologic treatment for factitious disorder, co-occurring disorders warrant treatment

FUNCTIONAL AND SOMATOFORM DISORDERS

Overview (Am J Psychiatry. 2010;167:6; J Neurol Neurosurg Psychiatry. 2012;83(8):842-850; Clin Neurol Neurosurg. 2010;112(9):747-751; Psychosomatics. 2018;59(4):358-368)

- Generally functional and somatoform disorders refer to a group of disorders which have manifestation of true (not feigned) physical or neurological symptoms which cannot be explained fully by a general medical or neurological condition/injury and are not attributable to another psychiatric d/o

CHRONIC FATIGUE SYNDROME

Definition and Clinical Features (IOM. Beyond ME/CFS. Report Brief, February 2015)

- AKA systemic exertional intolerance disease (SEID) myalgic encephalomyelitis (ME) or chronic fatigue syndrome (CFS)
- Clinical syndrome including disabling fatigue and other symptoms, such as musculoskeletal pain, sleep disturbance, impaired concentration and headaches
- There is controversy about the validity of the disease, given unclear pathophysiology, broad differential, and strong overlap seen with other disorders, including IBS, fibromyalgia, and multiple chemical sensitivity

Diagnostic Criteria (2015 Institute of Medicine)
Patient must have ALL of the following 3 symptoms and at least 1 of the following 2 manifestations.
Symptoms and manifestations should be present at least half of the time with moderate, substantial, or severe intensity.

(continued)

Diagnostic Criteria (2015 Institute of Medicine) *(continued)*

Symptoms (must have all):

1. Substantial reduction or impairment in the ability to engage in pre-illness levels of occupational, educational, social, or personal activities for > 6 mo; accompanied by fatigue of new or definite onset (not lifelong) not the result of ongoing excessive exertion, not alleviated by rest
2. Postexertional malaise
3. Unrefreshing sleep

Manifestations (must have at least one):

1. Cognitive impairment
2. Orthostatic intolerance

Adapted from *Institute of Medicine of the National Academies. Beyond Myalgic Encephalomyelitis/Chronic Fatigue Syndrome: Redefining an illness. Report Brief*, February 2015.

Epidemiology and Pathogenesis *(Psychosomatics. 2017;58:533-543)*

- CDC estimates 4–10 people/100,000 in the US; CFIDS Foundation estimates 0.3% of US population; women > men (4:1 ratio), ages 25–40
- Low employment rates w/ only ~14–27% employed
- Pathophysiology is not well understood. Possible endocrine/immuno-logical abnormalities
  - Infectious illness (EBV, Q fever, viral meningitis) have also been postulated as a cause, but largely debunked
- Up to 80% of patients have comorbid illness, commonly including fibromyalgia, myofascial pain, multiple chemical hypersensitivity, thyroiditis, hypovitaminosis D, endometriosis
- In a study of 124 patients, 45.2% with psychiatric comorbidity, predominantly mood disorders and anxiety

Evaluation

- **Risk factors** *(Arch Gen Psychiatry. 2009;66(1):72-80; Psychol Med. 2008;38(7):933-940)*

  Childhood trauma: Higher levels of childhood trauma and psychopathological symptoms, patients with childhood trauma have up to a 6-fold increase risk, highest correlation with sexual abuse, emotional abuse, and emotional neglect

  Psychiatric illness: People ages 15–36 with psychiatric illness shown to be more likely to experience later in life (OR 2.65); depression and anxiety most common co-morbid psychiatric disorders. Correlation between severity of psychiatric symptoms and likelihood of developing

- **Differential diagnosis:** Broad, infection (EBV, HIV, Hepatitis, Lyme), neurologic (MS, CVA), rheumatic (SLE, RA, Sjogrens), psychiatric (anxiety, MDD), endocrine (thyroid dysfunction, adrenal insufficiency), metabolic disturbance, sleep apnea, anemia, fibromyalgia, dehydration/orthostasis

- **Screening:** CBC, ESR, LFTs, CMP, TSH, urinalysis

Nonpharmacologic Treatment *(Chronic fatigue syndrome. BMJ Clin Evid. 2015;2015:1101; Psychol Med. 2013;43(10):2227-2235; Cochrane Database Syst Rev. 2016;(6):CD003200)*

- PACE trial found graded exercise therapy (GET) and CBT to have up to 22% recovery rate; however, these success rates have recently

been called into question. Adaptive pacing therapy has not been found to be effective
- GET and CBT have also been shown to decrease fatigue, improve sleep, and improve perceived general health among patients
- Treatments without good evidence: dietary supplements, primrose oil, galantamine, immunotherapy, intramuscular magnesium, and prolonged rest

Pharmacologic Treatment (Chronic fatigue syndrome. *BMJ Clin Evid.* 2015;2015:1101)
- Antidepressants can be considered in patients with comorbid depression
- TCAs can be considered in patients with comorbid chronic pain

FUNCTIONAL NEUROLOGICAL DISORDER/CONVERSION DISORDER

Diagnosis
Conversion disorder (functional neurological disorder): Sx of altered voluntary motor/sensory fxn; clinical findings are *incompatible* w/ recognized neurologic/medical condition; causes distress or functional impairment

Definition and Clinical Features (*Am J Psychiatry.* 2010;167:6; *J Neurol Neurosurg Psychiatry.* 2012;83(8):842-850; *Clin Neurol Neurosurg.* 2010;112(9):747-751; *Psychosomatics.* 2018;59(4):358-368)
- **Definition:** Characterized by real (not feigned) neurologic sx (eg, weakness, nonepileptic sz, abnl movements) that cause distress and/or psychosocial impairment, but are inconsistent w/ structural neurologic dz
- **Subtypes:** altered awareness—PNES (see separate section 2-66), dissociation; motor—weakness/paralysis, abnl movement, dystonia, functional speech change (dysphonia, slurred); sensory—pain/touch/visual/auditory/olfactory disturbance, sensation of lump in throat ("globus sensation" or "globus pharyngeus"); mixed (2+ other subtypes)
- **History:** The term "Conversion d/o" is based on the psychoanalytic hypothesis that psychological conflict is "converted" into neurologic sx, implying often unverifiable etiologic assumptions. In contrast, the term "functional" implies that sx arise from abnl *functioning* of nervous system rather than structural pathology. DSM-5 does not require identification of psychological factors or proof that sx are not feigned

Epidemiology and Pathogenesis
Epidemiologic study is challenging, but functional neurologic sx are the 2nd most common complaint to neurology clinics and dxed in 16% of neurology outpts. **Predisposing/risk factors:** female sex, comorbid medically unexplained sx, other nervous system dz, preexisting psychiatric d/o, insecure attachment, hx trauma, psychosocial stressors.

Evaluation (*J Neurol Neurosurg Psychiatry.* 2005; *Psychosomatics.* 2018;59(4):358-368; *Pract Neurol.* 2013; 13(2):104-113)

- **History:** Comprehensive medical and psychiatric interview w/ full ROS. Compile list of all current sx

  Predisposing factors: comorbid medically unexplained sx, other nervous system dz, preexisting psychiatric d/o, hx trauma, family hx
  Precipitating factors: physical injury/head trauma, acute anxiety/panic, dissociative event, recent psychological stressors
  Perpetuating factors: course of illness, deconditioning, illness beliefs, avoidance of sx exacerbation, social benefits of being ill, disability
  Note: (*Br J Psychiatry.* 2006;188:204) *la belle indifférence* has no validity in discriminating conversion d/o from neurologic dz

- **Exam:** Perform complete mental status, physical, and neuro exams. Physical/neuro exam can help to validate pt concerns and reveal undiagnosed medical/neurologic problem(s). **Specific exam signs to support dx (demonstrate inconsistency or incompatibility w/ recognized conditions):** hoover sign -- w/ pt supine place a hand under each heel and ask pt to attempt to lift each leg individually. When pt lifts unaffected leg, + if downward pressure felt from "weak" leg *or* + if ↓ strength in unaffected leg when pt attempts to lift "weak" leg; collapsing/give-way weakness; motor inconsistency (pt unable to perform particular movement but able to perform different movement using same muscle); variability; entrainment; dragging monoplegic gait; splitting of vibration; nonanatomical deficits

- **DDx:** Neurologic dz (MS, myasthenia gravis, movement d/o, stroke, sz [especially frontal lobe], spinal d/o [eg, lumbar nerve root entrapment, cervical myelopathy], autoimmune limbic encephalitis, laryngeal dystonia, stiff person syndrome); somatic symptom d/o; depersonalization d/o; factitious d/o; malingering

- **Workup:** Collaborate w/ other treaters, obtain prior dx and tx records, and collect indicated laboratory and radiologic tests

Treatment (*Am J Psychiatry.* 2006;163(9):1510-1507; *Epilepsia.* 2010;51:70-78; *Pract Neurol.* 2018;0:1-8)

Treatment Approach	
First line	• **Share the dx:** Share which medical/neurologic conditions have been ruled out while emphasizing that pt's sx are *real*, and provide dx name (eg, "functional neurologic d/o"). Explain how the dx was made by demonstrating relevant exam signs, eg, Hoover sign • **Education:** Provide written materials. Refer pt to www. neurosymptoms.org • **CBT** (*Neurology.* 2011;77(6):564-572): Target dysfxnal thoughts (eg, illness beliefs) and maladaptive or perpetuating behaviors • **Physical therapy:** (*J Psychosom Res.* 2013;75(2):93-102) Esp helpful for motor sx/deficits

Treatment Approach *(continued)*	
Other tx consid-erations	• **Medication:** *(J Clin Psychiatry. 2005;66:1529-1534; Neurology. 2010;75(13):1166-1173)* Antidepressants may be beneficial, particularly in the presence of comorbid anxiety or depressive d/o • **Hypnosis:** *(Int J Clin Exp Hypn. 2003;51(1):29)* Relaxation techniques may be helpful for sensory sx or speech disturbance • **Psychodynamic psychotherapy:** *(Int J Clin Exp Hypn. 2003;51(1):29)* Examine relationship patterns to reduce use of sx as defense against conflict • **Family therapy:** *(Am J Psychiatry. 2006;163(9):1510-1517)* Identify and address perpetuating family factors • **Group therapy:** *(Am J Psychiatry. 2006;163(9):1510-1517)* Peer education and support about sx

FIBROMYALGIA

Clinical Features *(JAMA. 2014;311(15):1547-1555)*

• Current diagnostic criteria, per American College of Rheumatology, consists of assessment with Widespread Pain Index and Symptom Severity Scale

Diagnostic Criteria for Fibromyalgia			
A score ≥ 13 points is consistent with fibromyalgia			
Widespread Pain Index (0–19 points): Widespread pain (in axial skeleton, above and below the waist, on both sides of body) **Tenderness in 11 or more of 18 "tender points"**			
Symptom Severity Scale (0–12 points)			
Symptom survey filled out by patients (score 0–12) For each symptom listed below, use the following score to indicate the severity of the symptom **during the past 7 d**			
	No Problem	Slight or Mild Problem	Moderate Problem	Severe Problem
Fatigue	0	1	2	3
Trouble thinking/ remembering	0	1	2	3
Waking up tired (unrefreshed)	0	1	2	3
During the past 6 mo have you had any of the following symptoms?			
Points	0	1	
Pain or cramps in lower abdomen	No	Yes	

(continued)

Diagnostic Criteria for Fibromyalgia (continued)		
Depression	No	Yes
Headache	No	Yes

Adapted from *Clauw DJ. Fibromyalgia: a clinical review. JAMA. 2014;311(15):1547-1555.*

- Individuals with Fibromyalgia are more likely to have anxiety, depression, OCD, and PTSD
- Other common comorbidities: chronic headaches, dysmenorrhea, temporomandibular joint d/o, SEID, IBS, OA, RA, SLE; 10–30% patients with OA/RA/SLE meet diagnostic criteria for fibromyalgia

Epidemiology and Pathogenesis (*JAMA. 2014;311(15):1547-1555*)

- Prevalence: 2–8%, similar across different countries, cultures, ethnic groups
- With new symptom-based diagnostic criteria, F:M ratio 2:1, predominantly affects women aged 40–50 y (*Pain Pract. 2010;10:520-529*)
- Pathophysiology may be related to augmentation of sensory and pain processing, but exact mechanisms are unknown. One hypothesis is a centralized pain state where there is amplification of pain caused by dysfunction of CNS in ascending and descending neural pathways (*Expert Opin Pharmacother. 2014;15(12);1671-1683*)

Evaluation (*Pain Research and Treatment. 2012;2012:15. Article ID 140832*)

- **Risk factors:** Family members with chronic pain or depression, childhood trauma (including physical, emotional, and sexual abuse), early life adversity (premature birth, stressor exposure)
- **Differential diagnosis:** Broad, including rheumatic (RA, OA, Sjogren's, SLE, spondyloarthritis, PMR), muscle (dermatomyositis, polymyositis, metabolic myopathy), infection (HIV, EBV, Lyme, dengue fever, hepatitis), endocrine (thyroid, adrenal insufficiency), neurologic (MS, myasthenia gravis), iatrogenic (statin myopathies, glucocorticoid-induced myopathy), psychiatric (somatic manifestations), SEID

Nonpharmacologic Treatment (*Curr Pain Headache Rep. 2016;20:25; Rheumatol Int. 2016;36:1379*)

- Multicomponent treatments are more effective than single method treatments
- Nonpharmacologic are often considered more effective than pharmacologic and include CBT, education, exercise
- Complementary/alternative treatments: trigger point injections, chiropractic manipulation, tai chi, yoga, acupuncture, myofascial release therapy have some evidence of efficacy
- Other important factors: good sleep hygiene, stress reduction

Pharmacologic Treatment (*Curr Pain Headache Rep. 2016;20:25; Rheumatol Int. 2016;36 1379*)

- Opiates and other peripheral pain meds (NSAIDs) are ineffective
  - 4 classes are generally used for treatment, **bold drugs have FDA approval for fibromyalgia**, other drugs off-label
  - TCAs

- Amitriptyline (10–50 mg daily)—improves pain and sleep disturbances vs placebo (performed well in combination with SSRI, ex, fluoxetine)
- SNRIs
  - **Duloxetine** (60 mg daily)—improves pain and depressive sx, no effect on fatigue or sleep disturbance
  - **Milnacipran** (100–200 mg daily)—improves pain and fatigue
- SSRIs
  - Multiple SSRIs have been studied, but limited evidence for improvement in pain, may be helpful for depressive symptoms
- AEDs
  - **Pregabalin**—improvement for pain and sleep
  - Gabapentin (1200–2400 mg daily)—pain improvement

ILLNESS ANXIETY DISORDER

Diagnosis
Illness anxiety disorder: mild or **nonexistent** somatic sx paired w/ preoccupation of having a serious, undiagnosed illness; anxiety about health and low threshold for alarm about health; excessive health behaviors or avoidance of activities thought to threaten health. Duration 6+ mo.

Definition and Clinical Features (Anxiety Stress Coping. 2016;29(2):219; Am J Psychiatry. 2005;162:847-855; Br J Psychiatry. 2013;202(1):56-61; NEJM. 2001;345:1395)
- **Definition:** Characterized by excessive concern about having or developing a serious general medical dz, generated by *fear* rather than *presence* of physical sx
- **History:** (Anxiety Stress Coping. 2016;29(2):219; J Psychosom Res. 2017;101:31-37) Dx was introduced in DSM-5. Pts previously dxed with "hypochondriasis" are now dxed with somatic symptom d/o (56–74%) or illness anxiety d/o (26–36%). Key difference is presence (somatic symptom d/o) or absence (illness anxiety d/o) of physical sx

Epidemiology and Pathogenesis (Curr Psychiatry Rev. 2014;10:14; J Psychosom Res. 2004;56(4):391)
Largely unknown due to limited study since publication of DSM-5 in 2013. More commonly presents in general medical settings. Estimated prevalence is 0.4–0.75%. Thought to occur equally between men and women; may be associated with fewer years of education and other anxiety + depressive d/o

Evaluation (Cogn Behav Ther. 2016;45(4):259; Am J Psychiatry. 2015;172(8):798-802)
- **Clues to dx:** Dissatisfaction w/ extensive medical care; multiple clinicians/specialists; reassurance unhelpful
- **History:** Comprehensive medical and psychiatric interview w/ full ROS. Consider Health Preoccupation Diagnostic Interview for structured but more time-intensive approach. Include thorough evaluation of following:
  - **Illness fears/beliefs:** Which sensations trigger anxiety; response to anxiety; insight about potential excessiveness of concerns

- **Psychiatric hx:** anxiety d/o, depressive d/o, other somatic symptom d/o
- **Medical hx:** Current and past serious illness or medical evaluation(s); quality of relationships with other clinicians
- **Family hx:** Family members w/ pattern of health anxiety, psychiatric illness, or medical dz
- **Social hx:** Psychosocial stress (relationships, work, housing, finances, etc) and fxning
- **Exam:** Perform complete mental status and physical exam
- **Workup:** Obtain prior dx and tx records, speak to prior and current treaters, pursue judicious laboratory testing and avoid repeat testing

Nonpharmacologic Treatment (*JAMA.* 2004;291(12):1464; *Psychosom Med.* 2007;69(9):881; *Cochrane Database Syst Rev.* 2007)
- **Approach:** Largely based on studies of pts with hypochondriasis and thus overlaps w/ tx of somatic symptom d/o. PCP often plays central role. Main goal is to improve pt's coping and fxnal status, rather than eliminate sx. Initial tx includes regularly scheduling visits; acknowledging health fears; limiting unnecessary tests/referrals; reassuring; assessing for comorbid psychiatric d/o; educating about coping rather than curing; focusing on fxnal improvement
- **Therapy:** (*Lancet.* 2014;383(9913):219-225; *Behav Res Ther.* 2014;58:65-74) CBT is first-line tx and involves cognitive restructuring of dysfxnal beliefs and modification of maladaptive behaviors. Other forms of therapy include (*J Consult Clin Psychol.* 2012;80(5):817-828; *Psychol Med.* 2016;46(1):103; *Behav Res Ther.* 2007;45(5)887-899; *J Gen Intern Med.* 2013;28(11):1396-1404; *Br J Psychiatry.* 1998;173:218): mindfulness-based cognitive therapy; acceptance and commitment therapy; problem-solving therapy, relaxation training, behavioral stress management

Pharmacologic Treatment (*J Clin Psychopharmacol.* 2008;28(6):638)
- **Medications:** Evidence suggests SSRIs may be effective even in the absence of comorbid psychiatric sx. When comorbid psychiatric sx are present, antidepressants should be strongly considered. Start low, go slow given somatic sensitivity to SEs

---

IRRITABLE BOWEL SYNDROME

Definition and Clinical Features (*JAMA.* 2015;313(9):949-958)
- Abdominal pain or discomfort with altered bowel habits without any other identifiable physical, radiologic, or laboratory indications of organic disease
- **Typical features:** Loose/frequent stools, constipation, bloating, abdominal cramping, discomfort or pain, symptoms brought on by specific food, symptoms change over time (pain location, stool pattern)
- 3 types, equally distributed in the US: IBS with diarrhea (IBS-D), IBS with constipation (IBS-C), and IBS with a mixed bowel pattern (IBS-M)
- **Rome IV Criteria for Irritable Bowel Syndrome** (*J Clin Med.* 2017;6(11):99)

- Recurrent abdominal pain on average at least 1 d/wk in the last 3 mo, associated with 2 or more of the following criteria:
  1. Related to defecation
  2. Associated with a change in frequency of stool
  3. Associated with a change in form (appearance) of stool
- Subtypes by predominant stool pattern
  1. IBS with constipation—hard or lumpy stools ≥ 25% and loose or watery stools <25% of bowel movements
  2. IBS with diarrhea—loose or watery stools ≥ 25% and hard or lumpy stools <25% of bowel movements
  3. Mixed IBS—hard or lumpy stools ≥ 25% and loose or watery stools ≥ 25% of bowel movements
- **Poor prognostic indicators:** comorbid anxiety and depression, previous surgery, longer duration of disease

Epidemiology and Pathogenesis (JAMA. 2015;313(9):949-958)
- Most commonly diagnosed GI condition, 12% prevalence in North America
- In the US, M:F = 1:1.5–2

Pathophysiology of Irritable Bowel syndrome	
Environmental	**Host Factors**
Early life stressors (abuse, psychosocial stressors) Food intolerance Antibiotics Enteric infection	Altered pain perception Altered brain–gut interaction Dysbiosis (imbalance in gut microbiome) Increased gut permeability Increased gut mucosal immune activation Visceral hypersensitivity

Adapted from Chey WD, Kurlander J, Eswaran S. Irritable bowel syndrome: a clinical review. JAMA. 2015;313(9):949-958.

Evaluation (JAMA. 2015;313(9):949-958; J Neurogastroenterol Motil. 2010;16(1):47-51; Nat Rev Gastroenterol Hepatol. 13.2 (Feb. 2016):64)
- **Risk factors:** F, current smoking, previous gastroenteritis, anxiety and depression, number of life stressors
- **DDx:** Broad, including other causes of chronic diarrhea (celiac dz, microscopic colitis, SIBO, Crohns dz, UC) and other chronic causes of constipation (neurologic dysfunction, colorectal cancer, diabetes, anorexia, dyssynergic defecation)
- **Features concerning for other GI illness:**
  - Onset after 50 y/o
  - Severe or progressively worsening symptoms
  - Unexplained weight loss
  - Nocturnal diarrhea
  - Family history of organic GI disease
  - Rectal bleeding/melena
- **Common comorbidities:** Depression, anxiety, somatic pain syndromes (fibromyalgia, SEID and chronic pelvic pain), other gastrointestinal disorders (GERD, dyspepsia)

- All IBS subtypes have a high level of association with depression, anxiety, and somatization, up to 60% prevalence of psychiatric disorders

Nonpharmacologic Treatment (*JAMA.* 2015;313(9):949-958)
- **Principles of treatment:** Importance of good therapeutic alliance with provider, focus on lifestyle goals vs GI symptoms
  Exercise—increased physical activity increases colon transit
  Diet—remove gas-producing foods (beans, pork, cabbage, broccoli, brussels sprouts, wheat germ, high carbohydrate), avoid lactose, possible evidence for a gluten-free diet. Consider referral to nutrition
  Psychological therapies—CBT, hypnotherapy, multicomponent psychotherapy, and dynamic psychotherapy have all been proven effective (NNT 4)

Pharmacologic Treatment (*JAMA.* 2015;313(9):949-958)
- Of note, laxatives (such as polyethylene glycol) and antidiarrheals (such as loperamide) have very limited evidence in IBS. While they may benefit symptoms of constipation or diarrhea, there is poor evidence for treatment of global symptoms or pain.

Pharmacological Treatment		
Treatment	**Treatment Benefits**	**Comments**
Over-the-counter		
Fiber: psyllium *(not insoluble fiber)*	IBS-C > IBS-D	SE: bloating, gas
Antispasmodics: peppermint oil	Global sx, cramping	SE: GERD, constipation
Prescription		
TCAs/SSRIs/SNRIs	TCAs may be better for IBS-D due to anticholinergic effects; SSRIs may be better for IBS-C due to serotonergic effects	Some evidence for greater efficacy of TCAs (*PLoS One.* 2015;10(8))
Prosecretory agents: linaclotide, lubiprostone	Improves global sx in IBS-C	SE: diarrhea, nausea
Antibiotic: rifaximin	Improves global sx, pain and bloating in IBS-D	None
5-HT$_3$ receptor antagonists: ondansetron	Improves globa sx in women with severe IBS-D	SE: constipation, rare ischemic colitis
Mu-opioid receptor agonist: eluxadoline	IBS-D	Pancreatitis risk in patients w/o gallbladder

Adapted from Chey WD, Kurlander J, Eswaran S. Irritable bowel syndrome: a clinical review. *JAMA.* 2015;313(9):949-958

Treatment of Comorbid Psychiatric Conditions (Eur Arch Psychiatry Clin Neurosci. 2014;264:651-660)

- Abdominal symptoms can cause/worsen anxiety and depression (hypothetically through autonomic nervous system dysfunction, stress hormone secretion, and immune dysfunction)
- Given this relationship, treating IBS may improve psychiatric symptoms

PSYCHOGENIC NONEPILEPTIC SEIZURE

Definition and Clinical Features (Psychosomatics. 2016;57:1-17)

- Involuntary, paroxysmal episodes of altered movement, sensation or awareness that appear similar to epileptic events but are not associated with epileptiform activity on EEG
- DSM-5: Subtype of conversion disorder (functional neurological symptom disorder)—"with attacks or seizures"
- Presenting symptoms incongruent with physical exam and other tests obtained for further workup
- No identified circumstantial or psychological trigger required for diagnosis

Epidemiology and Pathogenesis (Psychosomatics. 2016;57:1-17)

- Incidence 1.4–4.9 per 100,000 per year
- Prevalence 2–33 per 100,000 per year
- Onset most common between 2nd and 4th decades of life but has been noted in both children and the elderly
- More common in women
- Estimated that 10–30% of patients with PNES also have comorbid, active epileptic seizures or a history of epilepsy
- Model for pathogenesis with multiple, interacting psychological, neuromedical, and social etiological factors that predispose, precipitate, and perpetuate illness
- Limited neuroimaging studies suggestive of changes in brain areas related to emotion processing, perceptual awareness, cognitive control, and motor behavior

Evaluation (Psychosomatics. 2016;57:1-17; Epilepsia. 2012;53:1679-1689; Psychosomatics. 2011;52:501-506; Neurology. 2004;62:834)

- Diagnosis is challenging, often delayed 5–7 y from seizure onset
- Rapid diagnosis associated with improved outcomes, prevents unnecessary use of AEDs, and prevents excessive health care costs
- **Differential:** Epilepsy (particularly frontal lobe), autoimmune encephalitis, transient ischemic attacks, paroxysmal dyskinesias, convulsive syncope, migraine with aura, parasomnias, narcolepsy with cataplexy
- **Semiological factors suggestive of PNES:** eye closure during event, resistance to eye opening during event, partial responsiveness during event, undulating motor activity, side-to-side head shaking, prolonged event (>2 min)
- **Historical factors suggestive of PNES:** treatment resistance to >2 AEDs, AEDs not impacting seizures, events consistently associated with specific environmental or emotional triggers, presence of

witnesses at time of the events, repeatedly normal EEGs in the presence of recurrent seizures

- **Associated psychological risk factors:** trauma (particularly hx of physical or sexual abuse), hx of family dysfunction, alexithymia, fear sensitivity, avoidance behaviors, impaired attention regulation
- **Associated neuromedical risk factors:** coexisting epileptic seizures, hx of mild TBI, fibromyalgia, chronic pain, opioid medication use, intellectual disability
- **Risk factors perpetuating illness:** Social isolation, chronic stress, sick role/illness behavior, and misdiagnosis/mistreatment
- **Common comorbid psychiatric dx:** Depressive disorders, anxiety disorders, PTSD, other somatic symptom disorders, and personality disorders
- **Gold -standard diagnosis:** Video EEG with ictal recording in which clinical seizure lacks accompanying EEG abnormalities

Nonpharmacologic Treatments (*Psychosomatics.* 2016;57:1-17; *Neurology.* 2010;74:64-69)

- See also conversion disorder treatment approach p. 2-59
- **First step:** communicate diagnosis, ideally utilizing a multidisciplinary team consisting of a neurologist and mental health professionals
- **Emphasize:** Presence of genuine symptoms, how diagnosis was made, no diagnosis of epilepsy and no need for medication, effective treatments available
- Patient awareness that events are psychogenic can be therapeutic with one study reporting remission rate close to 40% at 6–12 mo in a subset of patients
- **Psychotherapy:** CBT most supported by evidence to significantly reduce monthly event frequency. Psychodynamic psychotherapy, mindfulness techniques, and group therapy studies also report favorable results
- **Challenges in treatment—patient factors:** Lack of acceptance of diagnosis, avoidance tendencies, external locus of control, social isolation, disability benefits
- **Challenges in Treatment—provider factors:** Mental health professionals lack knowledge, suspicion of malingering, liability concerns

Pharmacologic Treatment (*Psychosomatics.* 2016;57:1-17)

- No specific PNES treatments
- Treat comorbid psychiatric illness as appropriate

Prognosis (*Psychosomatics.* 2016;57:1-17)

- Long-term outcomes not well defined
- Limited studies report varied findings from 26% with continuing symptoms at 5–10 y to 71% with continuing symptoms at 1–10 y
- **Predictors of better outcomes:** Higher education, younger at age of onset/diagnosis, acceptance of diagnosis, antecedent bullying, shorter duration of illness, good social support, employment at baseline, lower somatization and depersonalization scores
- **Predictors of poorer outcomes:** Comorbid epilepsy, various psychiatric diagnosis, violent motor semiology, high emergency department use, receiving social security benefits

Somatic Symptom Disorder

Diagnosis
Somatic symptom disorder: Sx cause distress and/or functional impairment; excessive thoughts, feelings, and behaviors related to and time devoted to sx and health. Typical duration 6+ mos.

Definition and Clinical Features (*J Psychosom Res.* 2004;56(4):391; *Am J Psychiatry.* 2005;162:847-855; *JAMA.* 2009;302(5):550; *J Psychosom Res.* 2013;75(3):223)
- **Definition:** Characterized by 1+ somatic sx associated w/ excessive thoughts, feelings, and/or behaviors that cause significant distress and/ or dysfxn
- **History:** Dx was introduced in DSM-5 and largely replaced "somatoform disorders" including dxes of "hypochondriasis," "somatization disorder," "undifferentiated somatoform disorder," and "pain disorder" to improve predictive validity and interrater and test–retest reliability

Epidemiology and pathogenesis
Thought to be common and to present most often to PCPs; associated w/ ↑ use of medical services. Risk factors may include female sex, lower SES, fewer years of education, hx childhood chronic illness or trauma, other psychiatric or medical illness, or family hx of chronic illness.

Evaluation (*J Psychosom Res.* 2013;74(6):459; *JAMA Intern Med.* 2014;174(3):399-407; *Lancet.* 2006;367:452; *Med Clin North Am.* 2014;98(5):1079; *Cogn Behav Ther.* 2016;45(4):259)
- **Screening:** Self-report measures such as the Patient Health Questionnaire-15 item (PHQ-15), Somatic Symptom Scale-8, Symptom Checklist-90 somatization scale, Whiteley Index, 12-item Somatic Symptom Disorder-B Criteria Scale, 14-item Somatic Symptoms Experiences Questionnaire, 14- and 18-item versions of Short Health Anxiety Inventory, and 29-item Illness Attitude Scale
- **History:** Comprehensive medical and psychiatric interview w/ full ROS. Consider Health Preoccupation Diagnostic Interview for structured but more time-intensive approach. Include thorough evaluation of following:
  - **Sx:** Types of somatic sx triggering health anxiety; pt's beliefs about cause of sx; associated thoughts, behaviors, emotions; impact on fxn; duration of sx (acute or chronic); mitigating and exacerbating factors; prior pattern of similar presentations; prior and concurrent workups; relationships w/ previous treaters; insight re: thoughts/emotions/behaviors
  - **Psychiatric hx:** anxiety d/o, depressive d/o, substance use d/o, personality d/o, other somatic symptom d/o, trauma hx (physical/sexual/emotional abuse)
  - **Medical hx:** Past serious illness or medical evaluation(s)

- **Family hx:** Pattern of somatization or disability, psychiatric illness, medical illnesses w/ similar sx
- **Social hx:** Psychosocial stress (relationships, work, housing, finances, etc)
- **Exam:** Perform complete mental status and physical exam. Physical exam can help to validate pt concerns and reveal undiagnosed medical problem(s)
- **Workup:** Obtain prior dx and tx records, speak to prior treaters, pursue judicious laboratory testing and avoid repeat testing

Nonpharmacologic Treatment (Med Clin North Am. 2014;98(5):1079; BMJ. 2017;356:J268; Lancet. 2007;369(9565):946)
- **Approach:** PCP often plays central role although collaboration w/ mental health clinicians is key for refractory pts. Main goal is improving pt's coping and fxnal status, rather than eliminating sx
- **Initial tx:** Regularly scheduled visits with PCP, not contingent on the presence of active sx or complaints
- **Visit structure:** (BMJ. 2017;356:J268) Inquire about different aspects/ dimensions of sx including somatic (location, severity, duration), cognitive (thoughts about sx), emotional (feelings about sx), behavioral (impact of sx)
  - **Share dx and educate:** Identify which medical conditions, including ones that are life-threatening, have been ruled out and offer evidence. Educate that real sx can be present even in the absence of other dz
  - **Validate:** Empathically acknowledge complaints and clarify sx are *real* (not feigned)
  - **Alliance and common goals:** Collaborative, therapeutic alliance, ensure pt feels heard. Explicitly set goal of fxnl improvement. Caring/coping rather than curing
    - **Collaborate:** Communicate with any specialists also treating pt. Limit additional specialist referrals and unnecessary, potentially harmful dx tests
    - **Cognitive and Behavioral Therapies:** (J Gen Intern Med. 2013;28(11):1396-1404; Lancet. 2007;369(9565):946) *Relaxation training:* diaphragmatic breathing, progressive muscle relaxation; *Behavioral activation:* ↑ pt participation in activities despite physical or emotional barriers; *CBT:* identify and alter ⊖ thinking, cognitive distortions, and misattributions of sx

Pharmacologic Treatment (J Psychosom Res. 2004;56:455; Cochrane Database Sys Rev. 2014;356; BMJ. 2017;356:J268)
- **Medications:** Limited/weak evidence to support use of SSRIs in the absence of comorbid psychiatric sx, but conversely, SSRIs should be strongly considered when comorbid psychiatric sx are present. Low-quality evidence suggests combined tx w/ SSRIs +antipsychotics may be more effective. Start low, go slow given somatic sensitivity to SEs

IMPULSE CONTROL DISORDERS

Overview
- Conditions involving problems in the self-control of emotions and behaviors, manifested in behaviors that violate the rights of others and/or that bring the individual into significant conflict with societal norms or authority figures
- These disorders include oppositional defiant disorder, intermittent explosive disorder, conduct disorder, antisocial personality disorder, pyromania, kleptomania, and other related disorders
- Harsh, neglectful, and abusive practices by the family are implicated in all of them
- Dysfunction of corticolimbic, serotonergic, and dopaminergic systems have been implicated
- Treatment strategies include psychotherapy in conjunction with pharmacotherapy

OPPOSITIONAL DEFIANT DISORDER (ODD)

Clinical Features and Diagnosis
- Essential features include frequent and persistent pattern of angry and irritable mood, argumentative/defiant behavior toward authority figures, and vindictiveness. Differential diagnoses include mood disorders, ADHD, intellectual disability, social anxiety disorder, and other impulse control disorders

Pathophysiology and Risk Factors
- The cause of ODD is unknown. It tends to occur in families with a history of ADHD, substance use disorders, or mood disorders. Malnutrition, lead poisoning, and mother's use of alcohol or other substances during pregnancy may increase the risk of developing ODD. Harsh, neglectful, and inconsistent child-rearing practices are common in families of children with ODD.

Treatment
- Approaches to the treatment of ODD include parent management training, individual psychotherapy, family therapy, cognitive behavioral therapy, and social skills training

INTERMITTENT EXPLOSIVE DISORDER (IED)

Clinical Features and Diagnosis
- It is characterized by impulsive outbursts of anger and aggression, typically with little or no prodrome, and out of proportion to the provocation or precipitating stressor. Differential diagnoses include mood and psychotic disorders, substance use, and other impulse control disorders. Clinically, numerous other diagnoses must be ruled out before it can be diagnosed.

Pathophysiology and Risk Factors
- Imaging studies suggest a dysfunction in the corticolimbic system. Some studies implicate serotonin neurotransmission, high testosterone levels, or low oxytocin levels in the CSF

Treatment
- CBT and pharmacotherapy (anticonvulsants, lithium, beta-blockers, anxiolytics, neuroleptics, antidepressants) can be used. Pharmacotherapy alone has a limited success.

CONDUCT DISORDER
Clinical Features and Diagnosis
- A repetitive and persistent pattern of behavior in which the basic rights of others or age-appropriate societal norms or rules are violated and is associated with a lower level of fear. The onset is often in childhood and adolescence and is seen as the precursor to antisocial personality disorder

Pathophysiology and Risk Factors
- Dysfunction in corticolimbic system and amygdala is implicated. Slower resting heart rate has been reliably noted in individuals with conduct disorder. It is more prevalent with biological parents having severe alcohol use, ADHD, mood disorders, and schizophrenia. Parental neglect, abuse, and harsh disciple are among the family-level risk factors.

Treatment
- Psychotherapy that aims to integrate individual, school, and family settings, including parent management training (PMT)

PYROMANIA
Clinical Features and Diagnosis
- Multiple episodes of deliberate and purposeful fire setting. It involves experience of tension or affective arousal before setting a fire, and fascination with, interest in, curiosity about, or attraction to fire and its situational contexts. It is a diagnosis of exclusion with a broad differential diagnosis, including delusions and hallucinations, manic episodes, conduct disorder, etc.

Pathophysiology and Risk Factors
- Knowledge of the pathophysiology of pyromania is very limited. Deficit in serotonergic functioning have been suggested. Environmental factors include neglect from parents and physical or sexual abuse in earlier life.

Treatment
- CBT treatments, including chain analysis or graphing of the behavior, relaxation training, and social skills training, have been used successfully. Topiramate, SSRIs, and lithium have helped some patients.

KLEPTOMANIA
Clinical Features and Diagnosis
- A recurrent failure to resist impulses to steal items even though they are not needed for personal use or for their monetary value. It associates with increased sense of tension before the act of stealing that is relieved by the act of stealing. Malingering, manic and psychotic episodes, and other impulse control disorders are among the differential diagnoses.

Pathophysiology
- Cause of kleptomania is still ambiguous. A complex interplay of neurotransmitters including serotonin, dopamine, and opiates; hormones; and genetic expression are implicated. Positive reinforcement of the act of stealing, as well as a lack of negative reinforcement (punishment) may play a role.

Treatment
- Antidepressants, anticonvulsants (such as topiramate), or anxiolytics, or combinations of these medications, have been tried with some benefit. Psychotherapy (including insight-oriented psychotherapy and CBT) may be helpful.

OTHER RELATED IMPULSE CONTROL DISORDERS
- Historically, pathological gambling has been classified within the category of impulse control disorders, but DSM-5 classifies it as an addictive disorder
- Antisocial personality disorder is discussed in cluster B personality disorders, even though it has several features in common with impulse control disorders
- Other disorders exist that involve disruptive, impulse-control, and conduct disorder but are not fully consistent with any of the above disorders (such as trichotillomania, ie, the repeated urge of pulling hair)

INTELLECTUAL DISABILITY

Definition
- Intellectual disability (ID) is a neurodevelopmental disorder characterized by impairments in **both** adaptive and intellectual functioning that **present before age 18** (vs "neurocognitive impairment", which develops >18 y) (AAIDD, 2018)
- ID replaces the older term "mental retardation"
- ID can have syndromic and nonsyndromic etiologies
- Global developmental delay (GDD) describes those who have adaptive and intellectual difficulties before age 5. Not all of these children develop ID
- Some studies have shown increased risk of developing dementia later in life (*J Policy Pract Intellect Disabil.* 2013;10(3):245-251)

Clinical Features
1. **Adaptive function impairment**
   - Conceptual domain: literacy (reading, writing), mathematics, memory, self-direction, judgment in novel situations
   - Social domain: interpersonal social communication, empathy, ability to relate to peers as friends, social problem-solving
   - Practical domain: activities of daily living (eating, dressing, mobility, toileting), following a schedule/routine, occupational skills
2. **Intellectual function impairment**
   - IQ<70 (or 2+ standard deviations below mean)

Classification of Severity of ID	
Class	IQ
Mild	Between 50–55 and 70
Moderate	Between 35–40 and 50–55
Severe	Between 20–25 and 35–40
Profound	Less than 20–25

Epidemiology and Pathogenesis

Prevalence (*J Am Acad Child Adolesc Psychiatry.* 1999;38(12 suppl):5S-31S)
- GDD affects 1–3% of the US population
- ID affects approximately 1% of the US population
- ID is mild in approximately 85% of those affected
- More common in boys (partially explained by X-linked causes of ID)

Risk factors (*Am J Ment Retard.* 2002;107(1):46-59)
- Low level of maternal education
- Advanced maternal age
- Poverty

Common causes of ID
- Genetic causes (eg, chromosomal abnormalities, mitochondrial disorders) (*Semin Pediatr Neurol.* 2008;15(1):27-31)
- Environmental causes (eg, prenatal infection, intracranial hemorrhage, birth trauma, hypoxia, psychosocial deprivation, CNS malignancy, accidental or nonaccidental trauma, acquired hypothyroidism) (*Ment Retard Dev Disabil Res Rev.* 2002;8(3):117-134)

Evaluation (*Neurology.* 2003;60(3):367-380; *Pediatrics.* 2014;134(3):749-757)
- Focused history and comprehensive physical exam
- Referral to a developmental pediatrician, pediatric neurologist, or psychologist for neurodevelopmental testing
- School-based assessment
- Genetic evaluation for those with unexplained GDD or ID
- Speech, language, and communication evaluation
- Vision and hearing screening
- Occupational and physical therapy assessment
- Psychiatry for complex psychiatric needs

Associated conditions
- Medical/physical: cerebral palsy, congenital heart disease, constipation, dental caries, endocrine abnormalities, gastroesophageal reflux disease, hearing loss, leading poisoning, obesity, seizures, sleep disorders, undescended testes, vision impairment
- Psychiatric: anxiety, autism spectrum disorders, ADHD, behavioral problems, depression, dementia (early-onset), feeding/eating disorders, injury/neglect/abuse, learning disabilities, movement disorders, PTSD, self-injurious behaviors

Issues of particular concern
- Legal issues: clarify issues of guardianship early on
- Sexuality: address issues of birth control, sexual abuse, and sexually transmitted infections

- Victims of violence: individuals with ID are at 60% increased risk for experiencing abuse and violence (*Lancet.* 2012;379(9826):1621-1629)

Treatment
Goals of treatment
1. Decrease effects of the disability
2. Prevent or slow deterioration
3. Improve and optimize functioning (in home, school, community, vocational settings)

General principles (*Am J Med Genet C Semin Med Genet.* 2015;169(2):135-149)
- Communicate effectively (clear, concise, concrete)
- Encourage independent functioning
- Support families
- Advocate for the child
- Collaborate with others

Components of treatment
- Speech and language therapy
- Occupational therapy
- Physical therapy
- Family counseling and support, respite care
- Behavioral interventions
- Educational assistance
- Case management
- Assistive technology (for communication, mobility, etc)

Services
- The Individuals with Disabilities Act (IDEA) provides early intervention and special education for children with disabilities from birth to age 21
- Referrals should be made *as soon as possible* if a child has or is at risk for developing ID

  Early intervention (age 0 to 3): includes a comprehensive evaluation and individualized multidisciplinary services, usually in the child's home

  Special education (age 3 to 21): provides school-based services; focus is on the *least restrictive environment*; here, individualized education plans (IEPs) are generated annually

MAJOR NEUROCOGNITIVE DISORDERS

Clinical Features (*Nat Rev Neurol.* 2014;10(11):634-642)
- **Major neurocognitive disorder (MND):** evidence of **significant decline in one or more cognitive domains** (eg, complex attention, executive function, learning and memory, language, perceptual-motor or social cognition); preferably documented via standardized neuropsychological testing

  For diagnosis, deficits must interfere with (at minimum) instrumental activities of daily living (iADLs—examples include shopping, cooking, managing medications, managing finances, etc) and cannot occur solely in setting of delirium or another medical/psychiatric disorder

- **Mild neurocognitive disorder:** less severe symptoms; no impairment in daily activities

Major Etiologies*		
	Symptoms	Types
Subcortical (basal ganglia, thalamus, mesen- cephalon)	Dysmnesia (forgetting to remember—difficulty retrieving learned memory can be achieved with cuing) Depletion (impaired manipulation of acquired knowledge) Dysexecutive (apathy/abulia) Delay (slow thought) Comorbid neurologic findings	Wilson disease Parkinson disease Huntington disease HIV dementia Alcohol-related dementia Subcortical vascular dementia
Cortical	Amnesia (cannot learn new material) Aphasia (loss of language usage; temporal) Apraxia (loss of learned motor skills) Agnostic (loss of naming and recognizing deficits) Normal process time Neurological findings less common	Alzheimer dementia Frontotemporal dementia Cortical vascular dementia Lewy body dementia Prion disease
Mixed		Dementia of depression (often has subcortical profile) TBI/dementia pugilistica Huffing (inhalant abuse) Heavy metal exposure Lupus Multiple sclerosis

*Note: Often etiology is multifactorial.
Neurologist. 2008;14(2):100-107

- **Most patients with MND have neuropsychiatric symptoms**; symptoms are often more distressing to patient and family than memory loss
- Common neuropsychiatric symptoms: apathy (most common behavioral symptom in Alzheimer dementia), depression, anxiety, agitation, disinhibition (often seen in frontotemporal dementia), hallucinations, delusions, paranoia, wandering, sleep disturbance

Epidemiology and Pathogenesis (Clin Geriatr Med. 2014;30(3):421-442; Neuroepidemiology. 2007;29:125-132)

- **Prevalence** (varies by cause): increases exponentially with age; Alzheimer dementia by far most common cause of MND in elderly;

prevalence rates highly variable based on methodology used, with sample estimates being 5.0% of those aged 71–79 y to 37.4% of those aged 90 and older

- **Risk factors** (vary by cause): age is strongest predictor; female gender (presumably because women live longer); genetic factors; association with certain psychiatric disorders (depression, late-life anxiety, PTSD, substance abuse)
  - 35% of dementia cases thought to be attributable to 9 potentially modifiable risk factors: smoking; social isolation; physical inactivity; diabetes; late-life depression; hearing loss; morbid obesity; hypertension; low educational attainment (*Lancet. 2017;390:2673*)
- **Pathogenesis:** Dependent on etiology (see below sub-chapters for details), typically involves macroscopic, microscopic, and neurochemical changes

Evaluation (*Continuum (Minneap Minn). 2013;19:397-410; Clin Geriatr Med. 2014;30(3):421-442*)

- **Interview:** Evaluate onset and course of memory loss and associated symptoms (eg, inattention, anomia, poor executive functioning, behavioral changes, impaired ADLs and/or iADLs); mental status exam; review of symptoms; PMH (look for history of head trauma, TIA/stroke, seizure, hallucinations, gait disturbance, falls); past psychiatric history; social history (substance usage, including alcohol and cigarettes; education and previous occupation); FH of memory loss; physical exam (look for tremor, rigidity, gait disorder, abnormal eye movements, any focal neurological signs)

  Collateral is key: best if both patient and caregiver complete questionnaires (eg, patient: MOCA; caregiver: AD8 Dementia Screening Interview) (*Neurology. 2005;65(4):559-564*)

- **Labwork:**

  Standard: CMP, CBC, glucose, calcium, Cr/BUN, B_{12}, vitamin D, thyroid panel, LFTs

  Depending on clinical context: Lyme titer, RPR, HIV screening, heavy metals panel; EKG; urinalysis; ESR

  Apolipoprotein E (APOE) testing not routinely recommended (*Neurol Int. 2011;3(1):e1*)

- **Neuroimaging:** Noncontrast MRI (or noncontrast CT) (can evaluate for strokes, lesions, cortical atrophy); SPECT or PET if atypical presentation or younger patient; LP for CSF analysis not typically used clinically

- **Cognitive testing:** Assess neurocognitive domains: complex attention; executive functioning; learning/memory; language; perceptual-motor; social cognition (recognition of emotions, etc)

  Bedside tests include **abstractions** (similarities, proverbs); **perseveration** (go/no-go, pattern copying, Luria sequence); **executive functioning** (find maze exit, digit span forward/backwards, serial 7s); **primitive reflexes** (grasp, glabellar, palmomental, snout); **praxis** (salute, comb hair, brush teeth); **language** (listing words starting with letter F or animals in 1 min); **judgment** (ask what patient would do in an emergency) (*Arch Neurol. 1998;55(3):349-355*)

- **Differential diagnosis:** Delirium, depression, normal cognition (normal decline in elderly includes slower speed, decreased recall of names/faces, increased trials needed for learning, decline in divided attention, decreased abstract thought)

    Also, evaluate for intracranial pathology (eg, tumors, stroke, multiple sclerosis); systemic disease (eg, porphyria, paraneoplastic syndrome); vitamin deficiencies or toxins; endocrine diseases (eg, recurrent hypoglycemia, Addison disease, Cushing disease); autoimmune diseases (eg, lupus, sarcoidosis); **drugs or medication side effects**

- **Goals of assessment:** clarify diagnosis and establish cognitive baseline for further assessment; help to guide clinical decision-making and treatment options

Nonpharmacologic Treatment (*JAMA.* 2002;288(12):1475; *JAMA.* 2012;308(19):2020)

- Nonpharmacological treatment goals: educate caregivers on disease progression and potential safety issues; use nonpharmacological interventions/environmental aides to support functioning and address behavioral issues; improve quality of life; reduce caregiver stress; delay entry into nursing homes
- **Strategies for cognitive symptoms:** Use **external memory aids** (eg, calendars, lists); focus on creating habits (ie, enhancing procedural memory); encourage **participation in social and cognitively stimulating activities**; introduce activities that tap into preserved capabilities; allow patient sufficient time to respond to questions; simplify environment and tasks; **encourage aerobic exercise**; limit smoking and alcohol usage; oral nutritional supplements (inadequate nutrition is a common problem; note supplementation will help with weight gain but not other outcomes) (*J Am Geriatr Soc.* 2011;59(3):463)
- **Strategies for neuropsychiatric symptoms:** For new/worsening symptoms search for underlying cause (eg, pain, delirium, medication side effects, sensory deficits); **redirection** (eg, change conversation topic, avoid direct confrontation of delusions, participate in safe and familiar activities such as listening to old music or looking at photo albums); **manage environment** (eg, consistent routines, nightlights); **establish safety** (eg, Medic alert bracelet; GPS tracking for phone/car; lock doors, gates; disconnect stove; remove potentially dangerous objects)
- Care for caregivers: support groups, counseling/therapy, respite care

Pharmacologic Treatment (*JAMA.* 2003;289(2):210-216; *Ann Intern Med.* 2008;148(5):379; *N Engl J Med.* 2004;351(1):56-67; *JAMA.* 2004;292(23):2901)

- Combination therapy (cholinesterase inhibitor + memantine) gives best outcomes in patients with Alzheimer dementia; current treatments can help improve memory to where it was 6–12 mo prior but are **not curative**
- Unproven benefit for estrogen replacement, anti-inflammatory drugs, gingko biloba, statins, dietary supplementation, fish oil
- Future goal: more specific disease-modifying treatments

Pharmacological Treatments for MND (Cognitive Symptoms)			
Medication	**Mechanism of Action**	**Side Effects**	
Cholinesterase inhibitors: **Donepezil Rivastigmine Galantamine**	Reversibly **inhibits acetylcholinesterase** > increases acetylcholine > increases functioning of remaining cholinergic neurons > increases cognition	Well tolerated; most common GI (nausea, poor appetite)—typically subsides in days; vivid dreams; dehydration; bradycardia (check EKG first); peptic ulcer disease	CYP2D6 substrate; CYP3A4 substrate; can decrease seizure threshold; can worsen behavioral symptoms in FTD
Memantine Memantine XR	**Regulates NMDA receptor**; also, presumed to be a **dopamine agonist**	Well tolerated; most common dizziness, confusion, drowsiness	CYP450 substrate

Note: Memantine only FDA approved for moderate to severe AD, but can be helpful in mild AD, vascular dementia, and dementia with Lewy bodies; cholinesterase inhibitors often used in mixed etiologies, vascular dementia, dementia with Lewy bodies as well

Pharmacological Treatments for MND (Neuropsychiatric Symptoms)		
Depression	SSRIs first-line Also, bupropion, mirtazapine, SNRIs	Fluoxetine takes longer to become effective and may interact with warfarin; paroxetine has rapid-onset withdrawal if dosage forgotten
Anxiety	SSRIs first-line	Atypical antipsychotics can be added *with caution*
Pseudobulbar affect	dextromethorphan/quinidine (Nuedexta)	
Insomnia	Stimulants (eg, methylphenidate ER; modafinil) can increase daytime wakefulness Low-dose sedatives (eg, trazodone, zolpidem, quetiapine if underlying psychotic symptoms) can be used WITH CAUTION (may contribute to falls)	Maximize sleep hygiene and treat underlying sleep disorders first

(continued)

Pharmacological Treatments for MND (Neuropsychiatric Symptoms) (continued)		
Agitation	Low-dose atypical anti-psychotics (eg, risperidone—less sedating but can cause prolactinemia/exacerbate osteoporosis; quetiapine—sedating, less likely to worsen parkinsonism symptoms; aripiprazole—very little sedation; ziprasidone; olanzapine—most metabolic side effects)	
Failure to thrive	Can use appetite stimulants (eg, megestrol acetate or dronabinol) with caution	Enteral feeding does NOT improve survival

*Note: In general, if urinary incontinence and on a cholinesterase inhibitor, only keep incontinence medications (eg, oxybutynin) if controlling symptoms enough that patient can avoid wearing incontinence undergarments.

From: *Am J Psychiatry.* 2016;173(5):543-546; *N Engl J Med.* 2004;351(1):56-67.

ALZHEIMER DEMENTIA

Clinical Features (*Alzheimer's Dement.* 2016;12(4):459-509; *N Engl J Med.* 2004;351(1):56-67; *Learn Mem.* 2004;11(1):43-49)

- **Overview:** Alzheimer dementia (AD) = **progressive, irreversible neurodegenerative brain disease.** Clinical symptoms: dementia with prominent memory impairment. Microscopic pathology findings: **senile/neuritic plaques** (extracellular β-amyloid deposits) and **neurofibrillary tangles** (intracellular deposits of tau protein). Macroscopic pathology findings: **prominent cortical atrophy** in temporal (**esp. hippocampus**), parietal and frontal lobes. Neurochemical deficits: **prominent acetylcholine deficiency;** imbalances in dopamine, norepinephrine, glutamate, serotonin
- **Cardinal cognitive symptoms:** Impairments in **memory** (eg, recall of recent events; episodic memory; semantic memory); **language** and communication (eg, anomia; word-finding difficulties; decreased fluency); **reasoning** (eg, difficulty with judgment, executive functioning, problem-solving, insight); **visuospatial functioning**; attention
- **Cardinal behavioral symptoms:** Apathy and irritability very common; agitation, anxiety, depression, exacerbation of premorbid personality traits also common
- **Additional signs and symptoms:** Dyspraxia (occurs after memory loss); sleep disturbance; olfactory dysfunction; severe AD: difficulty with speaking, swallowing, walking (basic ADLs); seizures
- **Clinical course:** Continuous decline (often measured via repeat MMSE or MoCA). Early neuropsychiatric symptoms (eg, agitation) may signify more rapid decline. Average life expectancy after

diagnosis 3–9 y (highly variable depending on multiple factors, including age of onset and level of impairment when diagnosed) (*Neurology.* 2008;71(19):1489)

Epidemiology and Pathogenesis (*Alzheimer's Dement.* 2016;12(4):459-509)

- **Prevalence:** Most common form of dementia; 60–80% of cases (1/2 AD alone; others mixed pathology). Incidence roughly doubles every 5 y from ages 65 (2.5–3% incidence) to 85 (32–50% incidence). Estimated 5–6 million Americans currently with AD, projected to increase to 13.8 million by mid-century
- **Risk Factors (RF):** Greatest RF: older age (but AD not considered a normal part of aging)
  Nonmodifiable RF: family history of AD (2–4× increased risk if 1st-degree relative); APOE-e4 gene; Down syndrome; genetic mutations (~1%, often cause of early-onset AD; mutation in amyloid precursor gene (APP); presenilin 1 protein or presenilin 2 protein); small head size/brain volume
  Modifiable RF: traumatic brain injury; low educational attainment; low lifelong occupational attainment; lack of social/cognitive engagement; cardiovascular disease; many other presumed RF exist: smoking; substance abuse; exposure to certain metals; cerebrovascular disease; diabetes; thyroid disease; obesity, etc
- **Pathogenesis:** Exact etiology of AD unknown. Amyloid cascade hypothesis is an example causation hypothesis, although many exist (eg, oxidative stress hypothesis, cholinergic hypothesis, tau hypothesis) (*J Neurosci.* 2005;25(34):7709-7717)

Evaluation (*Alzheimer's Dement.* 2016;12(4):459-509; *Neurol Ther.* 2017;6(suppl 1):15-24)

- **General evaluation** of patient with memory loss: Please see "Major Neurocognitive Disorder" section, p. 2-79 for more information
- **National Institute on Aging—Alzheimer's Association (NIA-AA) working group** revised criteria in 2011 to include biomarker evidence (levels of beta-amyloid in the brain and biomarkers showing injured/degenerating neurons in the brain); clinical criteria similar to criteria in *Diagnostic and Statistical Manual of Mental Disorders 5* (DSM-5)—both include presence of dementia, gradual onset and steady progression of impairment, evidence of decline in memory, learning and other cognitive domains, and rule-out of other causes (*Alzheimer's Dement.* 2011;7(3):253-256)
- Can use multiple different rating scales (eg, Clinical Dementia Rating scale) to further categorize **preclinical** (eg, very mild cognitive decline, memory lapses, decline in ability to plan and organize); **mild** (eg, memory loss, confusion about location of familiar places, difficulty with iADLs), **moderate** (eg, increasing memory loss and confusion, problems recognizing friends and family, restlessness, agitation, anxiety), or **severe/late stage** (eg, inability to recognize family or communicate, lost sense of self, lack of bladder and bowel control, aspiration pneumonia, weight loss) (*Br J Psychiatry.* 1982;140:566-572)

- **Differential diagnosis:** Normal aging, dementia with Lewy bodies, vascular dementia, frontotemporal dementia, depression, nondementia causes of cognitive impairment (eg, medication side effects; B_{12} deficiency; syphilis)
- **Screening guidelines:** USPSTF concludes current evidence is insufficient to assess the balance of benefits and harms of screening for cognitive impairment. Common clinical practice for is discretionary screening between ages 65–74; every 2 y between ages 75 and 84; and annually after age 85 (*Geriatrics.* 2005;60(11):26-31)
- **Neuroimaging:** MRI sometimes obtained as part of evaluation; often see generalized and focal atrophy and white matter lesions (all nonspecific). Atrophy of temporal and medial parietal cortex (esp. hippocampus) slightly more specific (*Neurology.* 2001;56(9):1143). Other neuroimaging used: decreased metabolism in temporal/parietal cortex on FDG-PET; positive PET amyloid imaging; SPECT or fMRI imaging (*JAMA.* 2001;286(17):2120)
- **Biomarkers:** Not yet routinely used in clinical practice; core CSF biomarkers for AD include total tau (T-tau), phosphorylated tau (P-tau) and β-amyloid 42 (Aβ42)

Nonpharmacologic Treatment (*Ageing Res Rev.* 2016;25:13-23; *Ageing Res Rev.* 2013;12(1):253-262)

- No curative treatment exists for AD. Goal of treatment is to improve quality of life and slow progression of memory loss and impaired functioning
- Meta-analyses have shown cognitive stimulation and exercise (particularly aerobic) are beneficial to patients with AD

Pharmacologic Treatment (*Cochrane Database Syst Rev.* 2006;(1):CD005593; *J Alzheimer's Dis.* 2014;41(2):615-631)

- **Medications: cholinesterase inhibitors** (donepezil, rivastigmine, galantamine) and **memantine** are FDA approved for treatment of AD
- SSRIs and atypical antipsychotics are not FDA approved but are often used for management of neuropsychiatric symptoms. Note these symptoms are often more distressing to caregivers than memory impairment

---

FRONTOTEMPORAL DEMENTIA (FTD)

Definition
FTD is cluster of neurocognitive syndromes d/t degeneration of frontal and temporal lobe, characterized by progressive dysfunction in executive functioning, social behavior, and language

Clinical Features (*Ther Adv Psychopharmacol.* 2018;8(1):33-48)
- 2 subtypes of FTD: behavioral variant and primary progressive aphasia
Behavioral variant (bvFTD)
- The International Behavioral Variant FTD Criteria Consortium (FTDC) established criteria for diagnosis of bvFTD
  - Possible bvFTD can be diagnosed in the patient with 3 of 6 clinical features (disinhibition, apathy/inertia, loss of sympathy/empathy, perseverative/compulsive behaviors, hyperorality, dysexecutive neuropsychologic profile)

- Probable bvFTD can be diagnosed in the patient who meets criteria for possible FTD plus functional decline and imaging that shows frontal and/or temporal lobe atrophy, hypometabolism, or hypoperfusion

Primary progressive aphasia (PPA): deficits in word finding, comprehension, or sentence construction. There are three subtypes:
- Nonfluent: difficulty with articulation, effortful speech
- Semantic: difficulty with comprehension (both spoken and written, especially single words), naming objects; preservation of fluency, repetition, grammar
- Logopenic: impairment in sentence repetition and word retrieval

Epidemiology and Pathogenesis *(Ther Adv Psychopharmacol. 2018;8(1):33-48)*
- FTD is the 3rd most common degenerative dementia after AD and LBD
- 2nd most common dementia in <65 y/o population
- bvFTD is the most common subtype (50% cases)
- FTD has earlier onset than other dementias, typically occurs in 6th decade
- Highly heritable; family history of dementia or psych illness in 40% of pts with FTD
- Pathogenesis of FTD is heterogeneous. Syndromes often correlate with brain atrophy patterns (frontal and temporal lobe atrophy) and protein inclusions found in neuronal cell bodies, including tau and TDP-43

Evaluation *(Am J Geriatr Psychiatry. 2012;20(9):789-797)*
- Clinical evaluation to rule out neuromedical causes and identify pattern of deficits. **General evaluation** of patient with memory loss: Please see "Major Neurocognitive Disorder" section, p. 2-79 for more info
- Due to frontal lobe atrophy, have significant difficulty with executive functioning
- Neuroimaging: MRI will often show frontal or anterior atrophy; is supportive data, not diagnostic
- PET or SPECT: typically shows hypoperfusion in frontal or anterior temporal regions
- Neuropsychological testing: focus on tests of executive functioning (Luria sequence, trail making, clock drawing)

Pharmacologic Treatment *(Ther Adv Psychopharmacol. 2018;8(1):33-48)*
- SSRIs: target irritability, depression, apathy, disinhibition, improvement in NPI score
- Trazodone: targets overeating, irritability, dysphoria, depression
- Stimulants: decreased risk-taking behavior, improved cognitive functioning
- Gabapentin: insomnia, restless legs
- SGAs: target agitation; increased risk of mortality in dementia associated agitation, so not used first-line with these patients; increased risk of EPS, confusion, sedation
- No significant evidence for use of AEDs, memantine, cholinesterase inhibitors
- Avoid use of benzodiazepines—negative cognitive effects, paradoxical agitation

DEMENTIA WITH LEWY BODIES

Clinical Features

- Dementia with Lewy bodies (DLB) is a neuropsychiatric disease characterized by dementia, parkinsonism, sleep disturbances, and behavioral and perceptual distortions
- DLB appears to be the 2nd most common degenerative dementia after AD. DLB accounts for ~ 4% of new dementia cases by clinical diagnosis (*Psychol Med.* 2014:44;673), but pathologically diagnosed DLB was present in 26% of dementia autopsies in an American brain bank (*Alzheimer Dis Assoc Discord.* 2002:16;203)
- DLB is defined pathologically by the presence of Lewy bodies (intra-cytoplasmic inclusions with aggregations of alpha-synuclein) in the deep cortical layers of the brain

Presentation and Diagnosis

The DLB Consortium Consensus Criteria, 4th revision (*Neurology.* 2017;89:88):

- **Probable** DLB can be diagnosed in the patient with dementia plus 2 or more core clinical features, with or without indicative biomarkers; *or* dementia plus one core clinical feature who has one or more indicative biomarkers
- **Possible** DLB can be diagnosed in the patient with dementia plus one clinical feature and no biomarker evidence; *or* when one or more biomarkers is present but there are no core clinical features besides dementia

Core Clinical Features in Addition to Dementia:	Indicative Biomarkers:
Fluctuating cognition with pro-nounced variations in attention and alertness	Reduced dopamine transporter uptake in basal ganglia on SPECT or PET
Recurrent visual hallucinations	Low uptake ^{123}iodine-MIBG myocardial scintigraphy
REM sleep behavior disorder (commonly precedes cognitive symptoms by many years)	PSG-confirmed REM behavior disorder (REM sleep without atonia)
Bradykinesia, resting tremor, and/or rigidity	

See full criteria for additional supportive clinical features and biomarkers.

Evaluation

- There is **considerable overlap between the degenerative dementias**, and diagnosis is imprecise. In addition, patients may have multiple comorbid dementias (eg, DLB and vascular dementia). Pathological features of multiple dementias are often seen concurrently on autopsy

- **The most discriminating clinical features are those that appear *early* in the course of illness**, as the major dementias tend to increasingly resemble each other as the illness progresses
- DLB may be suspected in patients who:
  - Experience the **onset of dementia before, or concurrently with, features of parkinsonism.** If movement features are present long before cognitive decline, consider Parkinson Disease dementia, a discrete disease process
  - Suffer **early deficits in attentional, executive, and visuospatial domains.** Unlike in AD, memory and naming are usually preserved in early DLB
  - Experience **visual hallucinations.** Although not all DLB patients report hallucinations, they are highly unusual in other dementias
  - Had a **severe extrapyramidal reaction to dopamine antagonists**, especially typical (first-generation) antipsychotics. Because these can be irreversible or even fatal, neuroleptic sensitivity is no longer a core clinical feature and should not be used for diagnosis

Treatment

- **Cholinesterase inhibitors** (eg, rivastigmine and donepezil) have been shown to improve or sustain cognition and functional ability (*Lancet.* 2000;356:2031; *Ann Neurol.* 2012;72:41)
- **Memantine** may also be effective and is well-tolerated (*Lancet Neurol.* 2009;8:613; *Lancet Neurol.* 2010;9:969)
- **Antipsychotics should be avoided**, especially 1st-generation due to risk of EPS
- **SSRIs, SNRIs, and mirtazapine** are frequently used to control mood symptoms, but systematic data are lacking
- Motor symptoms tend to be less responsive to dopamine agonists in DLB than in PD (*Neurology.* 2004;63:376), and dopaminergic treatment can provoke psychosis. **DA agents, if used, should be carefully titrated from low starting doses.** Levodopa may be better tolerated and less likely to produce psychosis compared to dopamine agonists, but data are not specific to DLB (*JAMA.* 2000;284:1931; *NEJM.* 2000;342:1484)

Prognosis

- The median survival from the onset of cognitive symptoms is 7–8 y (*Neurology.* 1998:51;351; *Neurology.* 2006:67;1935)

VASCULAR DEMENTIA

Clinical Features (*DSM.* 5th ed.; *APA.* 2013)

- Mixed cortical and subcortical dementia characterized by executive dysfunction, mood disturbance, apathy/abulia, and motor sx that classically worsen in "stepwise" fashion
- Emerging cognitive deficits assoc temporally w/ cerebrovascular events or prominent decline in complex attention and frontal-executive fxn
- **Motor sx:** gait disorder, incontinence, parkinsonism, slowing
- **Psychiatric sx:** personality and mood change, abulia, emotional lability, depression

MND 2-87

"Vascular depression": depressed mood and cognitive impairment 2/2 vascular dementia (BMC Med. 2016;14(161):1-16)
- VaD and AD have similar sxs + cerebrovascular risk factors ↑ risk for both → difficult to differentiate VaD from AD (Alzheimers Dement. 2015;11(6):718-726)

Epidemiology and Pathogenesis
- 2nd most common cause of dementia (Lancet. 2015;386(10004):1698-1706)
- Linked to deep small vessel arteriolar disease
- Higher prevalence among males, African Americans
- Develops following major stroke or collection of small strokes, lacunes, or chronic subcortical hypoxia (Circ Res. 2017;120(3):573-591)
- Risk factors include cerebrovascular disease, diabetes, HTN, a. fib, and heart disease
- Pure genetic forms: CADASIL, MELAS

Evaluation
- **Screening:** MOCA > MMSE b/c of emphasis on exec fxn (J Am Geriatr Soc. 2005;53(4):695-699)
- **Neuropsych testing:** Emphasis on tests of exec fxn such as Luria sequencing, go/no-go, trail making; NINDS-CSN Vascular Cognitive Impairment Battery has been validated in several countries (BMC Neurol. 2015;15(20):1-6)
- **Imaging:** MRI w/ cortical and subcortical infarcts, WM lesions
- **Vascular disease workup:** carotid ultrasound, echo, screening for HTN, DM, HLD, smoking

Treatment
- Goal of reducing neuropsychiatric sxs, maximizing independence, supporting pt and caregivers
- **Risk factor reduction:** Area in need of further study; evidence suggests benefit of ↓ vascular risk factors: smoking cessation; ↑ physical activity; HTN tx; glycemic control in DM (Circ Res. 2017;120(3):573-591)
- **Cholinesterase inhibitors:** Donepezil may improve cognition/ADLs (Stroke. 2011;42(9):2672-2713)
- **Memantine:** NMDA-R antagonist; well-tolerated; some improvement in cognition but not in global fxn (Stroke. 2002;33(7):1834-1839)

MALINGERING

Definition and Clinical Features (Current Psych. 2005;4(11):12-25)
- **Malingering:** Intentional production of false or grossly exaggerated physical or psychological symptoms, motivated by external incentives (Current Psych. 2005;4(11):14)
- Distinct from factitious disorder, when motivation is internal (to assume sick role)
- Lying exists on broad spectrum, including creating fictional details in a narrative, minimizing or maximizing symptoms, exaggerating frequency, omitting details or events, distorting timelines, editing narratives, or manufacturing symptoms

- 3 categories: **pure malingering** (feigning nonexistent disorder), **partial malingering** (consciously exaggerating real symptoms), **false imputation** (ascribing real symptoms to cause known to be unrelated to patient's symptoms)
- Motivation for deception generally about (1) avoiding pain or other negative consequences, and/or (2) seeking pleasure. Examples include:
  - Fear that treatment will not be obtained, immediate needs will not be met
  - Aim to obtain shelter, food
  - Aim to avoid legal action
  - Aim to obtain certain medications
- **Epidemiology:** In a study of 40 patients admitted to the hospital for suicidal ideation or attempt, 10% self-reported malingering. Mental health providers were no better than chance in detecting malingerers (*Crisis.* 1998;19(2):62-66)

Evaluation (*Psychiatr Clin North Am.* 2007;30(4):645-662; *Current Psych.* 2005;4(11):12-25; *Gen Hosp Psych.* 2017;46:74-78)

- Detection of lying in others is difficult. The average person is able to differentiate lies from truth 54% of the time (*Pers Soc Psychol Rev.* 2006;10(3):214-234)
- Always consider malingering when there is a medicolegal context to presentation
- Do not initially confront patient to avoid putting patient on defensive
- **Obtain as much information as possible** from EMR, medical records from outside hospitals, collateral information from other staff and family/friends/coworkers, if possible
  - May find pattern of deceptive behavior in other care settings
- **Take detailed history of symptoms,** compare to what is known about phenomenology of psychiatric illness
  - That is, schizophrenia unlikely to present with only visual hallucinations
- Monitor for **rare or improbable symptoms**
  - That is, ask if when severely depressed, does patient find his/her thoughts speed up?
- Monitor for **internal inconsistencies** (ie, gives clear explanation of being confused or gives conflicting account of story) or **external inconsistencies** (ie, reports AH/VH but shows no evidence of responding to internal stimuli, behaves differently around psychiatrist than around other patients)

  In certain cases, may be helpful to **confront the patient** and **discharge** from emergency or inpatient setting, to minimize further harm to the patient and medical system (*Gen Hosp Psychiatry.* 2017;46:74-78; *Gen Hosp Psychiatry.* 2018;51:30-35)

- Must be relatively certain of deception
- Complete safety assessment prior to confronting patient
- Prepare for discharge by packing patient belongings, preparing prescriptions and discharge paperwork, alerting all treaters, utilizing security personnel
- Inform patient of discharge with direct, neutral language. Offer outpatient follow-up. Acknowledge patient's distress and avoid confrontation
- Postdischarge, debrief with staff. Document rationale clearly

OBSESSIVE–COMPULSIVE DISORDER

Clinical Features (JAMA. 2017;317(13):1358-1367)
- Hallmark of obsessive-compulsive disorder (OCD) is the presence of obsessions, compulsions, or both
- **Obsessions:** Recurrent, unwanted, illogical, intrusive thoughts (eg, fear of contamination, violent/sexual thoughts to harm someone, morality, symmetry, religion), urges (eg, to stab someone), or images (violent scenes) that cause distress. Beyond excessive worry about life problems. Not related to another mental d/o (eg, autism, GAD, depression)
- **Compulsions:** Repetitive activities (eg, hand-washing, ordering, checking) or mental acts (eg, counting). Usually recognized as excessive (ego-dystonic). Usually in response to obsessions, but not required for diagnosis. Compulsions are aimed at preventing or reducing anxiety/distress
- Obsessions and compulsions are time-consuming, cause distress and interfere w/ functioning

Epidemiology and Pathogenesis (Mol Psychiatry. 2010;15(1):53-63; Psychol Med. 2014;44(1):185-194; J Clin Psychiatry. 2013;74(3):233-239; J Clin Psychiatry. 2007;68(11):1741-1750; Arch Gen Psychiatry. 1999;56(2):121-127; Mol Psychiatry. 2017;22(11):1626-1632)
- **Epidemiology:** Prevalence 1–2% in the general population. Bimodal age of onset during early adolescence (11–14 y) and early adulthood (~20–29 y). Mean age of onset: ~20 y. M:F1:1. Same incidence across cultural boundaries, monozygotic > dizygotic twins
- **Pathogenesis:** brain imaging and neurosurgical tx support hypothesis of neuronal dysfunction in caudate nucleus, putamen, thalamus, globus pallidus, and orbital frontal cortex loop. Past research shows serotonin, glutamate, and dopamine involvement
- **Prognosis**:
  - If untreated, course is usually chronic and remission rate among adults is ~20%
  - One study showed ~22% achieved partial remission and ~17% achieved full remission within 5 y
  - After adjusting for psychiatric comorbidities, the risk of dying by suicide was ~10 times higher in those with OCD than that of the general population

Evaluation
- **Screening w/ YBOCS:** gold standard for baseline OCD sx, severity, and response to treatment (see Commonly Used Rating Scales, p. 1-9)
- **Evaluate** for safety of pt and others
  - Does it affect home life and lead to danger (ie, parenting, physical illness).
  - Does the person have insight?
- **Differential diagnosis:**
  - **Bipolar:** Unlike in OCD, bipolar has egosyntonic grandiose delusions
  - **Body dysmorphic disorder:** in BDD, preoccupation is circumscribed to perceived body imperfections

- **Depressive disorder:** in depressive disorders, depressive ruminations around self-image, including self-criticism, guilt, regret, failures, pessimism may be present in the context of an episode. No compulsive rituals
- **Eating disorder:** in eating disorders, the behaviors and thoughts are restricted to weight and eating alone
- **Generalized anxiety disorder:** in GAD, there are no rituals associated with worries. Worries usually focus on real-life problems without irrationality
- **Hypochondriasis:** in hypochondriasis, fear of illness arises from misinterpretation of regular body symptoms, unlike in OCD where fear stems from external stimuli (ie, contamination)
- **Obsessive-compulsive personality disorder:** in OCPD, global traits of perfectionism and rule preoccupation are egosyntonic, not specific to a worry or fear; obsessions not typically present
- **Paraphilias:** in paraphilic disorders, have sexual arousal with images/thoughts, whereas pts with OCD have ego-dystonic anxiety with images/thoughts
- **PTSD:** in PTSD, intrusive thoughts/images are a result of actual events, unlike in OCD where future consequences are anticipated
- **Schizophrenia:** in schizophrenia, there are usually IOR and/or grandiose, bizarre, persecutory delusions
- **Tourette's syndrome:** in Tourette, tics are not in response to thoughts; may be comorbid with OCD

Goals of Treatment
- Decrease of sx frequency/severity
- Improved functioning and QOL
- Quantifiable goals: ie, <1 h QD obsessing and/or doing behaviors
- Preventing relapse: Medication tx for 1–2 y before slow taper then stopping. If CBT completed, periodic sessions can be helpful to reinforce skills

Nonpharmacologic Treatment (N Engl J Med. 2014;371:646-653; J Consult Clin Psychol. 1997;65:44; Am J Psych. 2002;159:269)
Psychotherapy
1st line: Exposure and response prevention therapy (ERP)
- Repeated and prolonged exposures to fear-eliciting situations or stimuli; focus on anxiety reduction (vs CBT)
- RCT showed improvement in 60–85% patients; improvement was maintained after treatment finished
- Weekly sessions totaling 20–30 h with daily homework
  Other: CBT
- Challenge automatic unrealistic thoughts and patient's interpretations
- RCT showed improvement in 60–80% patients, similar effect size as exposure therapy
    Surgical: Anterior cingulotomy, capsulotomy deep brain stimulation can be effective in refractory cases

Pharmacologic Treatment (N Engl J Med. 2014;371:646-653; J Consult Clin Psychol. 1997;65:44)
- SSRIs or clomipramine lead to improvement in 40–60% pts
- On average, pts experience 20–40% reduction in sx w/ meds alone, but best in combination w/ CBT

First Line
- SSRIs: No difference in efficacy w/in class, choice is determined by which SSRI pt will tolerate best; 4–6 wk for initial response, 10–12 wk for max benefit; first-line over clomipramine due to better adverse effect profile
  - Higher doses are often required as compared to tx for MDD and above standard treatment guidelines (eg, sertraline >200 mg)

Second Line
- TCAs: clomipramine 50–250 mg; monitor for anticholinergic s/e
- Antipsychotics: Consider if partial response w/ SSRI/clomipramine (risperidone has the most data)
- Venlafaxine

Third Line
- SSRI + clomipramine, buspirone, memantine, pindolol, *or* riluzole
- Residential treatment

PERSONALITY DISORDERS

Definition
- Personality: enduring patterns of emotions, cognitions, behaviors in response to one's environment
- Personality disorder: combination of maladaptive personality traits that lead to distress and poor social fx and (1) is stable across time/situation, (2) originates in adolescence, and (3) is not better explained by sociocultural environment, medical or substance use
- Estimated that 4.4–13.4% of general population meets criteria for a PD (Br J Psychiatry. 2006;188:423-431; Arch Gen Psychiatry. 2001;58(6):590-596)

CLUSTER A

Clinical Features
- **Shared features:** "odd" behaviors in interpersonal context, generally characterized by withdrawal from social relationships
  Historically grouped on the hypothesis that cluster A PDs exist on a spectrum with SCZ (see relationship to SCZ below)
  - **(1) Paranoid PD:** pervasive mistrust of others and their intentions, eg, that others are exploiting, harming, or deceiving; can be hostile and litigious
  - **(2) Schizoid PD:** pervasive withdrawal from social relationships and reduced range of affect; appear aloof and detached
  - **(3) Schizotypal PD:** pervasive withdrawal from social relationships AND odd beliefs and behaviors, eg, magical thinking

Epidemiology and Pathogenesis
- **Prevalence:** rare; in general population paranoid (~2%), schizoid (~1%), schizotypal (~1%) (Br J Psychiatry. 2006;188:423-431); in psychiatric outpatients, paranoid (4.2%), schizoid (1.4%), schizotypal (0.6%) (Am J Psychiatry. 2005;162(10):1911-1918)
- Relationship to SCZ:

Schizotypal PD has a strong familial and genetic overlap with SCZ (*Arch Gen Psychiatry. 1993;50(10):781-788*) and shares many of the same neurophysiologic deficits (*Am J Psychiatry. 2004;161:398-413*)

10–20% of children dx with schizotypal PD go on to develop full-blown SCZ (*J Child Adolesc Psychopharmacol. 2005;15(3):395-402*)

Paranoid and schizoid PD thought to have some familial overlap with SCZ, though < schizotypal (*Arch Gen Psychiatry. 1993;50(10):781-788*)

- **Pathogenesis:** as with all PDs, dominant theory postulates that PDs arise out of a mix environmental factors and genetic vulnerabilities

Genetic vulnerabilities for schizotypal PD overlap with risk alleles for SCZ, while paranoid and schizoid PD genetics are less well defined

Environmental factors which increase risk include trauma (Correlates with paranoid PD. *CNS Spectr. 2003;8(10):737-754*), maternal intrapartum nutritional deficiency (correlates with schizoid and schizotypal PD) (*Soc Psychiatry Psychiatr Epidemiol. 1998;33:373-379*)

Parenting style also postulated to be important: overly critical and/or anxious parents can foster a view of the world as dangerous, leading to paranoid PD; overly dismissive or overbearing parents foster defensive self-sufficiency leading to social withdrawal in schizoid/schizotypal PD (McWilliams. *Psychoanalytic Diagnosis.* 2nd ed.; 2011)

Evaluation

- PD diagnosis is mired by poor interrater reliability esp in a single cross-sectional encounter; can improve reliability by (1) evaluating longitudinal hx to establish chronicity and (2) obtaining collateral (*Arch Gen Psychiatry. 1985;42(6):591-596*)
- **Diagnostic clues:** should prompt consideration of the dx

Schizoid PD: absence of meaningful relationships, elaboration of rich fantasy lives (eg, hours spent playing fantasy games); preference for jobs that require minimal human interaction (eg, graveyard shift)

Schizotypal PD: magical thinking or odd beliefs (eg, in a sixth sense, telepathy); identification with community that shares similar beliefs

- Distinguishing schizotypal PD from SCZ: schizotypal cognitive/perceptual disturbances are less well-formed, systematic than positive symptoms in SCZ, and schizotypal pts will oscillate spontaneously between skepticism and endorsement (eg, "this probably sounds crazy but…"); schizotypal pts can have brief psychotic episodes, but these are self-limited with a return to normal functioning following the episode
- Distinguishing schizoid and schizotypal PD from autism: challenging to distinguish; autistic pts have stereotyped behaviors and interests which are not present in cluster A PDs

Nonpharmacologic Treatment

- Evidence limited to case series: psychodynamic and CBT could be helpful, though rate of improvement is slow (*J Nerv Ment Dis. 1992;180(4):238-243; J Am Acad Psychoanal. 1983;11(1):87-111; Psychother Theor Res Pract Train. 1988;25(4):570-575*)

Pharmacologic Treatment

- Two small trials (n = 11 and n = 25) found olanzapine and risperidone moderated psychotic symptoms and increased functionality in schizotypal PD (*Schizophr Res. 2004;71(1):97; J Clin Psychiatry. 2003;64(6):628*)

- No Rx trials exist for paranoid or schizoid PD; small case series (n = 15) demonstrated modest improvement in fx in patients w/ paranoid PD admitted to an inpt unit started on antipsychotics (*Int Clin Psychopharm.* 2013;28:283-285)

CLUSTER B

Clinical Features
- **Shared features:** characterized by dramatic, emotional or erratic relationship styles
- **Antisocial PD (ASPD):** Manipulating or antagonizing others without remorse
- **Histrionic PD:** Extreme emotionality, attention seeking behavior
- **Narcissistic PD (NPD):** Grandiosity, desire for admiration/attention, limited empathy
  Borderline PD: Instability in affective, behavioral and interpersonal functioning; see p. 2-95

Epidemiology and Pathogenesis
- **Prevalence:** estimates vary; in general population, antisocial (0.2–4%, M > F), histrionic (0.3–2% M > F), narcissistic (0.9–9.3% M > F) (*J Clin Psychiatry.* 2004;65(7):948-958; *Br J Psychiatry.* 2006;188:423-431)
- **Pathogenesis:** as with all PDs, the dominant theory postulates that PDs develop from a combo of genetic vulnerability + environmental stressors
  Genetics: cluster B PDs likely moderately heritable; twin studies estimate heritability for NPD at 45% and ASPD at 67% (*Acta Psychiatr Scand Suppl.* 1993;370:19; *Compr Psychiatry.* 2000;41(6):416); low MAO-A activities correlated with antisocial behavior in children (*Science.* 2002;297(5582):851)
  Trauma: early childhood trauma associated with all PDs; some evidence to suggest physical abuse esp predisposes to ASPD (as opposed to sexual or neglect). Less well-defined relationship between trauma and histrionic/NPD (*Psychiatr Res.* 2011;45(6):814-822; *J Pers Disord.* 2010;24(3):285-295; *Psychiatry Res.* 2014;215(1):192-201)
  Parenting style: excessive parental rigidity surrounding rules is associated with antisocial traits in adulthood (*Acta Psychiatr Scand.* 2002;106(2):126); overly-evaluative parents (eg, "you made me proud/I'm disappointed") may → NPD; familial environments in which sexuality is perceived as threatening may → histrionic PD (McWilliams. *Psychoanalytic Diagnosis.* 2nd ed.; 2011)

Evaluation
- **Evaluation of ASPD:** consider the dx in pts who malinger, have a hx of arrests/incarcerations (present in 80% of pts) and SUD (present in 75%) (*Robins Deviant Children Grown Up.* 1966)
- **Evaluation of histrionic PD:** consider the dx in pts who use impressionistic language (colorful but devoid of content) or are seductive in interview
- **Evaluation of NPD:** "They talk in the interview as if addressing a large audience" (Gabbard. *Psychodynamic Psych in Clin Practice.* 2014)
  NPD subtypes: DSM-5 criteria correspond to the **grandiose** subtype; growing evidence suggests existence of a **vulnerable**

subtype, in which pts appear shy and hypersensitive, which cloaks a deeper hidden grandiosity and sense of entitlement (*Personal Disord.* 2016;7(4):363)

Risk of suicide: NPD is associated with low-impulsivity high-lethality suicide attempts, esp when suffering *narcissistc injury* (ie, a loss of status, such as divorce, being fired, etc.) (*J Clin Psychiatry.* 2009;70(11):1583-1587)

Nonpharmacologic Treatment

- Antisocial PD: 2 trials of CBT for ASPD have been negative (*Psychol Med.* 2009;39(4):569; *Br J Psychiatry.* 2007;190:307); no trials of other modalities exist. Evolving psychoanalytic conceptions of ASPD place it on a spectrum of severity with NPD (ie, NPD → malignant narcissism → ASPD → psychopathy) and the presence of more narcissistic features is hypothesized to make therapy more viable, though not empirically validated (*Meloy. Antisocial Personality Disorder.* 1995)
- Histrionic PD: generally a positive prognosis in psychodynamic psychotherapy and CBT (*Am J Psych.* 2003;160:1223). Erotic transference is a common therapeutic pitfall
- Narcissistic PD: no clinical trials of psychotherapies for NPD; expert clinicians modify modalities for borderline PD for use with NPD eg, dialectical behavioral therapy, mentalization-based therapy, transference-focused therapy

Pharmacologic Treatment

- No trials demonstrate efficacy of any medication for ASPD, histrionic, or NPD
- Case studies suggest that ASPD aggression could be treated with second-generation antipsychotics (quetiapine, risperidone) (*Int J Offender Ther Comp Criminol.* 2003;47(5):556)
- Experts' guidelines recommend treatment of comorbid psychiatric conditions first rather than targeting specific cluster B PDs given lack of demonstrated efficacy

BORDERLINE PERSONALITY DISORDER (BPD)

Clinical Features

BPD is a syndrome characterized by a pervasive pattern of instability in affective, behavioral, and interpersonal functioning:

- Emotions: intense, reactive, and quickly changing moods including dysphoria, anxiety, irritability, and anger, usually in response to a stressful interpersonal event, lasting only hours up to a few days; intense anger and difficulty controlling anger that often leads to interpersonally or self destructive behaviors
- Behaviors: recurrent impulsive tendencies toward suicide and self-injurious behaviors (eg, cutting); impulsive risky behaviors (eg, excessive spending, sexual behaviors, reckless driving, substance use)
- Relationships: intense relationships with impulsive shifting between idealizing or devaluing the other person leading to behavioral dysregulation and frantic efforts to avoid perceived abandonment
- Sense of identity: feeling detached, like one does not know oneself; chronic feelings of emptiness or boredom
- Distorted perceptions: transient psychotic or dissociative episodes usually in response to acute stressor

Epidemiology and Pathogenesis

- **Prevalence:** estimates vary from 0.5 to 6% (median 1.4%) of the general US population; most common PD in clinical population; 10% of psychiatric outpatients, 15–25% of psychiatric inpatients; prevalence is 4× greater among primary care patients compared to general population (*Lancet. 2011;377:74-84*)
- **Risk factors:** family history of BPD, antisocial personality, substance use disorder; childhood trauma; young adult age
- **Comorbidities:** comorbid with axis I and II disorders; most frequently associated with mood disorders, anxiety disorders, and substance use disorders; 39% borderline pts meet criteria for PTSD; eating disorders more common in F, substance use disorders more common in M
- **Course:** higher rate of functional and vocational impairment, high use of treatment services; high risk of suicidal behavior (69–80% of BPD pts), mortality 8–10% from suicide (50× higher than general population); however, despite the myth that BPD pts are refractory to treatment, most BPD pts go into remission even without stable long-term treatment (10% remit in 6 mo, 25% in 1 y, 45% in 2 y); recent study of 175 BPD pts showed 85% remission within 10 y although slower than other PDs (*Arch Gen Psychiatry. 2011;68(8):827-837; Compr Psychiatry. 2001;42(6):482-487*)
- **Pathogenesis:** similar to all PDs, BPD emerges from a combination of hereditary and environmental contributions:

  Genetics: BPD is more heritable than other PDs (65–75% per twin studies compared to 40–60%) (*Psychiatr Clin North Am. 2008;31(3):441-461*); ongoing gene studies examining targeted polymorphisms (serotonin promoter region, COMT allele, MOA tandem repeats) though no specific genes have been demonstrated as causative

  Biological correlates: Research demonstrates increased cortisol and HPA reactivity among BPD pts; also suggests several neuropeptide abnormalities correlating with dysregulated traits including increased sensitivity to rejection and abandonment (low opioids), increased social sensitivity and distrust (low oxytocin), impulsive aggression (reduced serotonergic responsiveness), increased anger (high vasopressin) (*J Clin Psychiatry. 1989;50(6):217-225; Harv Rev Psychiatry. 2009;17(3):167-183*)

  Neuroimaging: MRI studies demonstrate that BPD pts have increased amygdala activation when viewing aversive images and faces, and reduced activation of cognitive control structures (*Psych Res. 2009;172(3):192-199*); PET studies also suggest prefrontal and frontolimbic dysfunction correlating with poor emotion control (*J Psychiatry Neurosci. 2009;34(4):289-295*)

  Trauma: BPD pts report many more childhood adverse events (eg, trauma, neglect) compared to other PDs; childhood trauma can distort development of self-image, emotion regulation, and interpersonal skills, as well as disrupt capacity to examine one's identity or relationships, resulting in hypersensitive insecure attachments

Evaluation

- Assess for pervasive patterns of instability in affective and behavioral regulation, interpersonal functioning, impulse control, and cognitive distortions in the patient's history and presentation
- Present the definition and clinical features of BPD to the patient for nonstigmatizing collaborative discussion about likelihood of diagnosis, accompanied by psychoeducation regarding effective treatment options available with good prognosis. Evidence that even a single psychoeducation session can reduce anxiety about a highly stigmatized diagnosis and improve awareness of treatment options (*CMAJ.* 2012;184(16):1789-1794). Develop safety plan for pts w/ chronic suicidality to enable learning of coping strategies in the outpatient setting and prevent maladaptive patterns of high utilization of health care services (eg, repeated hospitalizations)
- Diagnostic pearls: history of self-injury, chronic suicidal ideation (vs MDD when suicidality is episodic), mood–affect incongruity (pts can look neutral or even cheerful when discussing morbid content); pts often self-present, classically when in crisis triggered by interpersonal conflict (eg, fight or breakup with partner)
- Several scales and structured interviews to assess BPD are available though rarely used within clinical practice; of note, mood disorder questionnaires frequently misdiagnose BPD as BPAD (*J Clin Psychiatry.* 2010;71(9):1212-1217)

Nonpharmacologic Treatment

- First-line treatment of BPD is via psychotherapy with pharmacotherapy as adjunct for periods of acute decompensation and comorbidities (*Am J Psychiatry.* 2001;158(1):1-3)
- Multiple specialized treatments for BPD exist:

  Dialectical behavioral therapy (DBT): shown to be effective in BPD to reduce several key outcome measures including suicidality and self-injurious behaviors compared to nonmanualized therapies in the community; evidence for impact on substance use and mood symptoms is mixed (*Arch Gen Psychiatry.* 2006;63(7):757-766; *Behav Res Ther.* 2009;47(5):353-358; *Br J Psychiatry.* 2003;182(2):135-140)

  Mentalization-based therapy and transference-focused therapy: have been shown to be more effective than treatment as usual for BPD and esp effective for affect regulation, impulsivity, and attachment (*Am J Psychiatry.* 2007;164(6):922-928; *Am J Psychiatry.* 2009;166(12):1355-1364)

  Good psychiatric management (GPM): focus on case management, psychoeducation, and integration of multimodal interventions, that have been shown to be as effective as DBT, but do not require specialized provider training or intensive therapy schedule (*J Pers Disord.* 2016;30(4):567-576; *Am J Psychiatry.* 2012;169(6):650-651)

- Improvements in behavior and interpersonal functioning are often followed by improvements in depressive sx; therefore in pts with BPD comorbid with MDD, it is important to focus on treating BPD first (*J Clin Psychiatry.* 2004;65(8):1049-1056)

Pharmacologic Treatment (Br J Psychiatry. 2010;196(1):4-12)

- Pharmacotherapy has modest effect and use should be adjunctive; provide early psychoeducation about this to pt to avoid externalization and medication iatrogenesis; taper unhelpful medications and minimize polypharmacy; minimize lethal medications when concerned for impulsive suicidal behaviors (eg, MAOIs, lithium)
- Antidepressants (targeting affective sx): no clear agent superior to others; evidence that SSRIs (eg, fluoxetine, escitalopram) as well as TCAs (eg, amitriptyline, imipramine) can be helpful to treat depressive symptoms, limited evidence that MAOIs are superior to placebo
- Antipsychotics (targeting cognitive and perceptual symptoms as well as mood stabilization): no clear agent superior to others; evidence that olanzapine and haloperidol were effective with or without accompanying antidepressant treatment; quetiapine can be used as adjunct for antidepressant with sedating properties for insomnia
- Mood stabilizers (targeting impulsive and behavioral dysfunction): lamotrigine shown to improve affective instability and impulsivity (Int Clin Psychopharmacol. 2009;24(5):270-275) though more suitable for treatment reliable pts given risk of SJS with inconsistent use; some evidence of VPA being helpful for aggression and interpersonal sensitivity (J Clin Psychiatry. 2002;63(5):442-446); carbamazepine does not appear to be superior to placebo

---

CLUSTER C

Clinical Features
- **Shared Features:** characterized by anxiety, fearfulness
- **Avoidant PD:** social inhibition, feelings of inadequacy, rejection sensitivity
- **Dependent PD:** excessive need to be taken care of, fear of abandonment/rejection
- **Obsessive–compulsive PD (OCPD):** preoccupation with perfectionism and control, rigidity

Epidemiology and Pathogenesis
- **Prevalence:** estimates vary; in gen pop avoidant (0.4–5%), dependent (0.4-1.6%), OCPD (0.9–9.3%) (Br J Psychiatry. 2006;188:423-431)
- **Pathogenesis:** like all PDs, dominant theory postulates a combo of genetic vulnerability + environmental factors

  Genetics: twin studies demonstrate that cluster C PDs are moderately heritable (~30%), avoidant and dependent PD likely share common genetic factors; OCPD is possibly genetically unrelated to other cluster C PDs (Psychol Med. 2007;37(5):645-653; Arch Gen Psychiatry. 2008;65(12):1438-1446)

  Parenting style: pts with avoidant PD perceived their parents to be shaming in childhood (Acta Psychiatr Scand. 1989;80:415-420); pts with dependent PD had early family environments, which were rule-oriented and discouraged self-sufficiency (J Pers Disord. 1991;5(3):256-263)

Evaluation

- Avoidant PD:
  - vs schizoid PD: pts with schizoid and avoidant PD both avoid social connection; unlike schizoid PD, avoidant PD pts desperately crave social connection
  - vs social anxiety disorder: significant overlap in criteria for both disorders; controversy exists around whether these two disorders should be merged as they are not distinguishable genetically or epidemiologically (*Depress Anxiety.* 2010;27(2):168-189)
- Dependent PD clinical pearls: frequent intersession contact is common; may frantically seek new relationships when a key relationship is threatened
- OCPD:
  - vs OCD: in pure OCPD, there are no actual obsessions or compulsions; however, comorbid OCD and OCPD are common
  - Screen for eating d/os in pts with OCPD; estimated that OCPD increases odds of eating d/o 7-fold (*Am J Psychiatry.* 2003;160(2):242-247)

Nonpharmacologic Treatment

- CBT efficacious for cluster C PDs, with enduring effects 2 y after termination (*Am J Psychiatry.* 2004;161(5):810-817)
- Efficacy of psychodynamic psychotherapy for cluster C disorders is mixed (*Br J Psychiatry.* 2006;189:60-64); possibly more effective when self-compassion is targeted as an explicit goal of treatment (*Psychotherapy (Chic).* Sep;48(3):293-303)

Pharmacologic Treatment

- No RCTs of any Rx for any cluster C PD
- As with all PD care, consider Rx for comorbid axis I conditions

POSTTRAUMATIC STRESS DISORDER

Clinical Features (*Nat Rev Dis Primers.* 2015;1:15057; *PLoS One.* 2013;8(4):e59236)

- Disorder following **exposure to trauma (inc threatened/witnessed):** death/injury, violence (sexual, physical, emotional), inc exposure to details of traumatic incidents (eg, first responders). Symptom spectrum > 1 mo:
  - **Re-experiencing:** recurrent and intrusive distressing memories, dreams, flashbacks, or reactions to triggers associated w/ trauma
  - **Avoidance of triggers:** internal (eg, memories) or external (eg, locations)
  - **Cognitive/emotional disturbance:** inability to remember traumatic details; negative self-beliefs/emotional state; distorted self-blaming; anhedonia
  - **Hyperarousal:** angry outbursts; self-destructive behavior; hypervigilance; exaggerated startle response; poor sleep or concentration

- **Dissociative symptoms:** derealization/depersonalization
- Most experience PTSD within 3 mo of traumatic event; ~4% symptomatic 3 mo after; 40% of PTSD patients develop chronic PTSD (>3 mo duration)
- Course related to nature of trauma; *unintentional* (eg, accidents, natural disasters) → likely to resolve, 30% exposed w/ PTSD sx at 1 mo → 14% at 12 mo; *intentional* (eg, abuse, rape) ↑ prevalence 12% at 1 mo → 23% at 1 y
- Severity of sx may ↑ w/ chronic course related to *kindling* (stimulation of fear circuit in amygdala leading to hyperexcitability) and *sensitization* (autonomic hypersensitivity to intense, novel, or fear cues) (*World Psychiatry.* 2010;9:3-10)
- Independent predictor of suicidality/suicide attempts (*Psychosom Med.* 2007;69:242-248)
- **Acute stress disorder:** above sx for <1 mo; stressor-related disorders: reactive attachment disorder, disinhibited social engagement disorder, adjustment disorder

Epidemiology and Pathogenesis (*Euro J Psychotrauma.* 2017;8:suppl 5:1353383; *Nat Rev Dis Primers.* 2015;1:15057; *Depress Anxiety.* 2014;31:130-142).
- **Prevalence:** 70% respondents to WMH surveys in 2000s reported a prior traumatic event, 4% w/ dx PTSD. 2013 US study → 12 mo prevalence 2.5%
- F>M, highest risk = rape (19% WMH survey) >> other sexual assault (10%) >> >> witnessing atrocities + refugee status each (5%)>>Combat (4%)>> man-made disasters (2.9%) >>> natural disasters (0.3%)
- Comorbid conditions: 40–60% w/ MDD/persistent depressive disorder; 46–86% w/ anxiety disorders; 8–14% w/ SUD, overlaps with BPD/personality disorders; see *Complex PTSD*
- **Neurobiology:** incompletely understood; dysregulation of HPA-axis w/ poor attenuation by 5-HT circuits, predisposed by low cortisol during trauma → dysregulated attenuation of amygdala by ACC and vmPFC, default mode network (MPFC and PCC) → self-referential processing → may mediate guilt/shame

Evaluation (*Nat Rev Dis Primers.* 2015;1:15057; *SAMHSA Trauma-Informed Care in Behavioral Health Services.* 2014; *Chapter 4: Screening and Assessment*)
- **Interview:** Ask about each symptom cluster. Potential limitations: pt minimization/avoidance; appreciation of culture-bound experiences of stress (eg, *ataque de nervios, taijin kyofusho*); memory deficits, preoccupation; exaggeration for secondary gain
- Sample questions include the following:
  - Have you or someone you know experienced an event or events in which you (or they) feared for your (or their) life? Do you have a trauma history?
  - Do you have intrusive thoughts or memories about the event? Do you ever have flashbacks or nightmares? What are they like for you?
  - Do you avoid people, places, things, and thoughts associated with the event?
  - Do you ever blame yourself? Are you depressed?
  - Do you often find yourself on edge? Do you startle easily?

- **Trauma-informed interview:** SAMHSA 6 principles if suspected/ known prior trauma: (1) safety, (2) trustworthiness + transparency, (3) peer support, (4) collaboration + mutuality, (5) empowerment, voice, + choice, (6) cultural, historical, + gender issues (https://www.samhsa.gov/nctic/trauma-interventions)
  - Clarify expectations at the outset of the interview, including benefits for the patient
  - Be supportive, kind, and matter-of-fact in your statements
  - Respect personal space
  - Match tone and volume of the patient, paying attention to verbal and nonverbal cues of discomfort
  - Provide symbols of safety in the physical environment
  - Monitor your own emotional responses during and after, watching for secondary traumatization
  - Use a qualified medical interpreter
  - Elicit only as much information as necessary + appropriate to your clinical setting (eg, unlikely that details of trauma are necessary in the ED)
  - Allow the patient options for timing and gender of the interviewer as able
  - Avoid phrases that pass judgement
  - Provide feedback about clinical impressions
- **Differential diagnosis: psychiatric:** (1) mood + anxiety d/o (inc. hyperarousal → mania); (2) psychotic d/o (hypervigilance→ paranoia, dissociation→ behavioral disorganization); (3) ADHD (impulsivity); (4) antisocial and BPD co-occur or result from PTSD. **Neuromedical:** (1) somatic features vs medical diagnoses (eg, stomach ulcer, angina, tachycardia, arthritis, HTN); (2) medical causes of depression may result in negative PTSD symptoms; (3) sympathomimetic conditions (eg, hypercortisolism, pheochromo-cytoma, stimulant intoxication); (4) seizure disorders (eg, TLE) vs dissociation

Nonpharmacologic Treatment (Cochrane Rev. 2013;12:CD003388; Cochrane Rev. 2016;4:CD010204; Am J Psych. 2017;174:943-953; Couns Psychother Res. 2018;18:237-250)

- **Trauma-focused CBT:** TF-CBT more effective than usual care. Exposure therapy → disrupt link between trauma-cues and emotional disturbance; cognitive processing→ understand/change distorted beliefs (eg, "I am a helpless person" or "I am responsible for what happened")
- In co-occurring SUD, TF-CBT + SUD tx more effective than either alone
- CBT most effective for children and adolescents (Cochrane Rev. 2012;12:CD006726)
- **Eye-movement desensitization and reprocessing (EMDR):** mindfully ↓ threat-responses w/ directed eye movements
- **Psychodynamic psychotherapy:** demonstrated to be useful, disputed efficacy as compared to TF-CBT, goal to explore the meaning of the event

Pharmacologic Treatment (*Psych Med. 2018;48:1975-1984; Cochrane Rev. 2006;1:CD002795; Neuropsychobiology. 2014;69:235-242*).

- **First-line:** SSRIs, typically high doses, best efficacy and tolerability; SNRIs also effective and well-tolerated, primary = venlafaxine
- **Second-line:** TCAs (desipramine + imipramine > amitriptyline) + MAOIs (phenelzine) effective + well-tolerated, 2nd line 2/2 SE profile
- **Third-line:** Mirtazapine (particularly if insomnia); data less robust
- **Symptom targets:** *Nightmares:* evidence for hydroxyzine or prazosin; however: double-blinded RCT of prazosin in veterans w/out efficacy in ↓ nightmares or improving sleep (*N Eng J Med. 2018;378:507-517*). *Anxiety:* propranolol → hyperarousal; however, meta-analysis did not establish efficacy (*J Psychopharmacol. 2016;30:128-139*). *Intrusive thoughts:* atypical antipsychotics adjunct (*Psychiatry MMC. 2005;2:43-87*)
- **Prevention:** moderate evidence for administering hydrocortisone s/p event may prevent the onset of sx (*Cochrane Rev. 2014;7:CD006239*)

COMPLEX PTSD

Overview
- Has been described as "the syphilis of psychiatry" as it "at one time or another mimics every personality disorder" as well as other psychiatric syndromes (*J Traum Stress. 1992;377:391*)
- Was called Disorders of Extreme Stress Not Otherwise Specified (DESNOS) in DSM-IV
- Neurobiology: Likely involves changes in HPA and SAM stress axes, conditioned by prolonged exposure to severe stress; evidence suggesting higher T-cell counts associated with autoimmune diseases; brain regions involved include reduced volumes of hippocampus, anterior cingulate, and orbital prefrontal cortex, with resulting functional deficits in memory encoding bias toward negative stimuli and increased but failed attenuation of fear signaling in the amygdala by the prefrontal cortex (as compared with overall reduced inhibition in borderline personality disorder) (*BPD and Emotion Dysreg. 2014;1:9*)

Clinical Features
- Exposure to *prolonged, repeated* interpersonal trauma whereby the patient was under another person's coercive control and unable to escape due to physical, psychological, maturational, environmental, or social constraints (eg, child abuse, domestic violence, repeated sexual assault, imprisonment, refugees, religious cults, trafficking, slavery)
- Negative self-concept (low self-esteem, self-hatred, guilt, shame)
- Emotional dysregulation (mood lability, chronic suicidality, self injury, poor distress tolerance, dissociation, rage outbursts, irritability, anhedonia, numbness)
- Unstable interpersonal relationships (difficulty developing and maintaining close relationships)
- Somatization (eg, headaches, GI sx, chronic pain, fatigue, tremors)
- Pervasive vulnerability and fear of recurrent trauma and high risk of re-traumatization (either self-inflicted or by others) even in the absence of traumatic reminders

Differential

- Whereas PTSD usually follows a circumscribed traumatic event, complex PTSD typically emerges from exposure to chronic repeated interpersonal trauma from which a person cannot flee ("subordination to coercive control") (*J Traum Stress.* 1992;377:391)
- Symptoms in complex PTSD have more characterological features than in simple PTSD (suggesting that repeated trauma affects development of personality and identity)
- Significant overlap with borderline personality features. Complex PTSD has more fear of recurrent trauma, whereas borderline personality has more fear of abandonment and unstable sense of self (*Eur J Psychotraumatol.* 2014; 10.3402); notably, DSM-5 diagnosis of PTSD strongly overlaps with diagnostic features of BPD

Epidemiology

- Limited evidence; suggested prevalence 0.6% in the US, 13% of veterans, and 32% of psychiatric inpatients (*Clin Psychol Sci.* 2015;215-229)
- After child abuse, risk of developing complex PTSD is double the risk of developing simple PTSD (*Eur J Psychotraumatol.* 2013; 10.3402)
- Highly associated with mood and anxiety disorders, PTSD, borderline personality (some argue complex PTSD is concomitant PTSD and borderline personality)

Treatment

- Limited yet growing body of literature. Survey of trauma experts emphasize phase-based treatment program that initially focuses on safety, stabilization, psychoeducation, basic life competencies; later focuses on therapeutic exploration of trauma memories to recreate trauma narrative into a coherent positive identity. Targeted interventions: emotional regulation strategies, anxiety management, interpersonal effectiveness, reinforcing adaptive narrative (*J Traum Stress.* 2011;615-627)
- Traditional therapy strategies for PTSD (exposure therapy, CBT, psychoeducation, trauma-informed care) remain important for treating complex PTSD. Traditional therapy strategies for borderline personality (DBT, mindfulness, ACT) are also effective
- Unclear evidence regarding medication strategy in complex PTSD. Treat similarly to PTSD and address comorbidities (SSRIs, BZDs, prazosin, target symptom management)
- Risk for relapse include life stressors and poor social supports warranting extension of treatment program

PSYCHOTIC DISORDERS

Clinical Features *DSM-5®. American Psychiatric Pub; May 22, 2013*
- Brief psychotic disorder
  Must have 1 of (1) delusions, (2) hallucinations, (3) disorganized speech
  Can also have (4) disorganized behavior
  Duration: ≥1 d, <1 mo

- Schizophreniform disorder

  Must have 2+ of the following for a significant portion of a **1 mo period**: (1) delusions, (2) hallucinations, (3) disorganized speech, (4) grossly disorganized or catatonic behavior, (5) negative symptoms

  Duration = ≥1 mo, <6 mo

  Is NOT schizoaffective disorder, depression, or bipolar disorder w/ psychotic features because no major depressive or manic episodes have occurred w/ active sx and mood sx present for minority of total duration of active sx

- **Schizophrenia**

  Same criteria as schizophreniform, but duration = **>6 mo**

  For significant portion of time since onset of sx, level of functioning is markedly impaired

- **Schizoaffective disorder**

  An uninterrupted period of illness during which there is a major mood episode along with criteria for schizophrenia

  Delusions or hallucinations for 2+ wk in the absence of a major mood episode

  Sx that meet criteria for major mood episode present for majority of illness

- **Delusional disorder**

  Presence of 1 or more delusions >1 mo, has NOT met criteria for schizophrenia

  Aside from the delusion, functioning NOT impaired

  Types of delusions: Erotomanic, grandiose, jealous, persecutory, somatic, mixed, unspecified if with bizarre content

- **Substance/medication-induced psychotic disorder**

  Presence of one or both: (1) delusions, (2) hallucinations

  Symptoms thought to develop during or soon after substance intoxication or withdrawal or after exposure to medication

  Consider: EtOH (as part of delirium tremens or alcoholic hallucinosis), cannabis (especially synthetic cannabinoids), PCP, hallucinogens, inhalants, sedatives, hypnotics, anxiolytics, amphetamines, cocaine

- **Psychotic disorder due to another medical condition**

  Evidence from history, physical, or labs that disturbance is direct pathophysiological consequence of another medical condition; not explained by another mental disorder, not occurring exclusively during delirium

- **Other specified schizophrenia spectrum and other psychotic disorder**

  Does not meet full criteria for above disorders, but sx causing significant distress or impairment

  Examples:

  Persistent auditory hallucinations (in absence of other features)

  Delusions with significant overlapping mood episodes

  Attenuated psychosis syndrome

  Delusional sx in partner of individual with delusional disorder

- **Unspecified schizophrenia spectrum and other psychotic disorder**

  Used in situations where clinician chooses *not* to specify the reason that the criteria are not met for a specific disorder

Used if insufficient information to make more specific diagnosis (ie, an ED evaluation)

- **Symptoms of anomalous experience** *(Scz Bulletin. 2009;35(1):5-8)*
—ask patient about these often subtle, self-experienced changes to better understand/encapsulate their reality

  Thought interference: intrusive insignificant thoughts

  Thought perseveration: obsessive repetition of insignificant thoughts or mental images

  Thought pressure: chaos of thoughts

  Thought blocking: sudden loss of thread

  Disturbance of receptive language: difficulty understanding

  Expressive speech: finding appropriate words; often abnormal pronoun use

  Disturbance in abstraction

  Inability to multitask/switch attention

- **Six symptom clusters—schizophrenia** *Current Psych 8.6 (2009);74*
a concise yet comprehensive, cross-sectional diagnostic framework, helpful to target specific problem areas within SCZ aside from pos and neg sx

  Motor Symptoms (restlessness, tremor, bradykinesia, TD, catatonia)

  Disorganization (speech, thinking, appearance)

  Delusions/hallucinations

  Negative symptoms—blunted affect, alogia

  Cognitive symptoms—executive dysfunction, verbal memory impairment

  Affective symptoms—depression, anxiety, demoralization, suicidality, mania

Epidemiology and Pathogenesis *(Epidemiol Rev. 2008;30:67; Int Rev Psychiatry. 2010;22:417. DSM-5®. American Psychiatric Pub. May 22, 2003; Schizophr Bull. 2011;37(5):1039-1047; Schizophr Bull. 2006;32(1):3; Nature. 2014;511(7510):421; J Clin Psychiatry. 2014;75:e184-e190)*

Schizophrenia

Prevalence ~1%, incidence ~1.5 per 10,000, M:F 1.4:1

  Age of onset 18–25 for males, 25–35 for females with second peak perimenopause

  Risk factors: obstetrical complications, late winter/early spring birth, advanced paternal age

  Genetic: ~108 single nucleotide polymorphisms associated

  Pathogenesis not completely known, though likely represents multiple diseases that present with similar signs/sx; complex interplay btw gene/environment

  Higher rates than general population of: depressive disorders, anxiety disorders, EtOH and substance use d/o, 20× higher risk for suicide compared to general population (240 per 100,000 annually compared to general population 12 per 100,000 annually)

Evaluation *(Harvard Rev Psych. 15.5 (2007):189-211)*

History/Intake

- Clarify onset/duration of symptoms
- History of prodromal period (school/work/social difficulties, poor self care, depression)

- Substance use
- Mood sx
- Medical and family history
- Carefully document episodes—can evolve into different dx (70% of 1st episode can achieve full remission and can remain stable)
- Consider rating scale—PANSS, SAPS, SANS, BPRS
- **Risk** assessment for suicide and aggression

First Episode Workup (*Early Intervent Psych* 3.1(2009):10-18)
- Thorough physical and neuro exam
- Labs: CBC, CMP, LFTs, TSH, U tox, vit B_{12}, folate, FTA-ABS, pregnancy test, metabolic screen, lipid panel, A1C, ESR, ANA, HIV, MRI (preferred over CT)
- Nonroutine but consider by history: EEG, neuropsychiatric testing, heavy metal screen, copper/ceruloplasmin screen, prolactin level, genetic testing

Nonpharmacologic Treatment (*Psych Serv* 65.7 (2014):874-880; *Schizophr Bul* 44.3 (2017):475-491)
- Address stress, family needs, supportive employment, social skills training, assertive community treatment (ACT)
- Monitor weight, height, BMI, waist circumference, DM2 (fasting blood glucose), lipids, prolactin, EPS, EKG
- CBT (for positive symptoms)
- Family involvement and education
- Increase community connection
- Minimize exposure to MJ, stimulants

Pharmacologic Treatment (*Acta Psychiatr Scand.* 2012;125(1):15-24; *Arch Gen Psych.* 2003;60(1):82-91; *Cochrane Database Syst Rev.* 2005;2; *Am J Psych.* 2004;161(2 suppl))
First Line
- Positive symptoms: All antipsychotics w/ similar efficacy aside from clozapine. Base on degree of sx, past results, or SE, available formulation (SL, injection). 2nd-generation antipsychotics have lower risk of EPS/TD but greater metabolic effects. **Consider long-acting injectables right away**
- Negative symptoms: treat depression if present, consider parkinsonism from meds, treat anxiety (note: some antidepressants inhibit catecholamine reuptake, which may worsen/sustain positive sx)
- Agitation/aggression: BZD in acute phase, mood stabilizers or beta-blockers helpful long term

Second Line
- Clozapine (should also be considered if persistent thoughts of suicide or suicide attempts, or persistent aggressive behavior)
- ECT: for persistent psychosis or SI after clozapine has failed, or for catatonic features (if no response to Ativan)

Third Line
- Augment clozapine with lamotrigine, 2nd antipsychotic, ECT, or TMS

Background (Neuropsych Dis Treat. 2010;6:297-308; MMWR. 2017;66(31):821-825)
- ~1.2% of US population (2015 estimate)
- 60–75% of epilepsy is focal, **Temporal lobe epilepsy (TLE) is most common**
- Causes → neurodevelopmental d/o (eg, autism), substance withdrawal, metabolic disturbance, TBI, vascular dx, infectious dx, degenerative dx, tumor

Classification (Epilepsia. 2017;58(4):522-530)
- **Seizure:** transient disturbance of brain function d/2 abnormal neuronal discharge
- **Epilepsy:** recurrent, unprovoked seizures
- *Focal (formerly partial):* localized onset, generally related to cerebral insult or congenital malformations: +/− alteration in consciousness (formerly simple/complex); +/− motor onset; +/− evolving to bilateral convulsive status (formerly secondarily generalized)
- **Generalized:** generalized onset, can be genetic, origin typically in subcortical tract that immediately spreads to cerebral cortex

Clinical features (Neuropsych Dis Treat. 2010;6:297-308; Semin Neur. 1991;11(2):167-174; Epilepsia. 2017;58(4):522-530)
- Focal
  - *Temporal focus:* most common, attributed to cognitive/behavioral alteration
    - *Medial temporal lobe:* oral automatisms (lip smacking, kissing, swallowing), manual automatisms (fidgeting, scratching, undressing), expressions suggesting extreme emotion (fear, crying), language dysfunction, AH, déjà-vu/jamais vu, dissociation, psychosis
    - *Uncus:* olfactory hallucination
  - *Frontal focus:* Less common, associated w/ cognitive/behavioral alteration, p/w disinhibition, motor phenomena, vocalizations, language dysfunction, catatonia, often develop during sleep, *typically no aura or postictal confusion*
  - *Parietal focus:* paresthesia/sensory changes, apraxia
  - *Occipital focus:* VH
- **Generalized:** Tonic-clonic, other motor, Absence (children > adults)
- **Nonconvulsive status epilepticus:** can be mistaken for psychotic or affective d/o, particularly status of absence (eg, prolonged state of altered consciousness w/ preserved alertness and some responsiveness)

Evaluation (Neuropsych Dis and Treat. 2010;6:297-308; Acta Neurol Belg. 1990;90(1):11-19; J Clin Neurophys. 2008;25(3):170-180; Am J Neuroradiol. 2018;39:1791-1798)
- **EEG findings:** Interictal spike/sharp wave, or localized slowing. Only 30–55% w/ known epilepsy have abnormalities on rEEG, repeated exams ↑ yield to 80–90%. LTM w/ video EEG, can characterize "spells" and ↑ identification/localization
  - *Focal seizures w/out alteration in consciousness→* only 20–60% w/ EEG changes

- *Focal seizures w/ alteration in consciousness* generally = EEG changes; *frontotemporal seizures* may require foramen ovale electrode placement
- **Imaging:** MRI (eg, 3T epilepsy protocol) used to ID focal lesions for dx and surgical planning. PET useful if MRI does not show structural lesions, particularly TLE

Psychiatric Symptoms Associated With Seizures (*Epil Beh.* 2010;18:13-23; *Epil Beh.* 2016;54:58-64; *Epilep Disord.* 1999;1(2):81-91; *Neurology.* 2002;58(8 suppl 5):S27-S39; *Seizure.* 2015;24:70-76; *CNS Spect.* 2016;21:247-257; *Epil Res.* 2002;49:11-22; *Neuropsych Dis Treat.* 2010;6:297-308; *Semin Neurol.* 1991;11(2):167-174; *Neuropsychiatr Dis Treat.* 2008;4(2):365-370)

- **Psychiatric comorbidity:** Depression ~ 20–50% >> psychosis 5–10%, 6–12× than in gen pop. Seizures 2× more common in psychotic d/o pts than gen pop
- **Medication-related:** Some AEDs used to tx psychiatric sx, others cause irritability/mood changes. See AED chapter for details

Depression	
Preictal	Dysphoria, irritability hrs-3 d leading up to seizure
Ictal	Generally brief, stereotyped mood changes + anhedonia/guilt/SI. Can be primary symptom of focal seizure or a/w other ictal symptoms. *Aura* (early ictal process) can involve mood changes
Postictal	Up to 72 h after last seizure + lasting up to 2 wk, sx similar to MDD, including suicide. A/w postictal cognitive deficits
Inter-ictal	Controversial dx. Can present as major depression, bipolar disorder, dysthymia. Classically described as dysthymic-like disorder, chronic depression punctuated by hours-days w/o symptoms +/– euphoric episodes, irritability, anxiety

Psychosis	
Ictal	Hallucinations, paranoia, grandiosity, unusual behaviors can be clinical manifestation. Hallucinations can be auditory, visual, olfactory, gustatory. *Aura* can involve hallucinations
Postictal	Lucid interval (12 h–7 d) after seizure, followed by 1 d–3 mo of psychotic sx, often heralded by insomnia. More commonly a/w treatment-resistant focal epilepsy + bilateral independent foci
Inter-ictal	Episodes of psychosis independent of seizures, can be acute (days-wks) or chronic (mos-yrs). *Looks similar to primary psychotic d/o* except: later onset, absence of negative symptoms, better premorbid condition, less severe and better treatment response
Forced normalization	*AKA: alternative psychotic episode,* rare, antagonistic relationship between seizure + psychosis; onset of psychosis w/ establishment of seizure control

Other Psychiatric Symptoms	
Anxiety	Panic is the most common emotional experience in focal seizures of the temporal lobe; Preictal/ictal sx may include a rising epigastric sensation (ie, sensation of swelling in abdomen progressing to chest and thorax), which can be mistaken for panic or globus hystericus
Somatization/ conversion symptoms	Todd paralysis (postictal hemiparesis) can be mistaken for conversion disorder or TIA. Transient aphasia after temporal lobe seizure may be mistaken for conversion/ psychosomatic symptoms
Suicidality	Suicide rate much higher than in gen pop; ~11.5% (range in studies 1–33%)
Agitation/ violence	May be part of ictal process or secondary to mood/psy-chotic symptoms
Personality	Temporal lobe seizures classically (now controversial) linked to personality changes (Geschwind syndrome), including increased verbal output, circumstantiality, viscosity (eg, "sticky"), hypergraphia, hyposexuality, inten-sified mental life

Treatment of Psychiatric Disorders in Epilepsy (*Neurology.* 2002;58(8 suppl 5):S27-S39; *Epil Res.* 2002;49:11-22; *Epil Beh.* 2015;51:176-181; *CNS Spect.* 2016;21:247-257)

- **Depression:** Generally equivalent to treatment of depression in patients w/o epilepsy, eg, SSRIs, SNRIs, mood stabilizers, ECT, CBT. ECT ↑ seizure threshold
- **Psychosis:** *Ictal:* Adequate seizure control, *Postictal:* Adequate sei-zure control + antipsychotic, often only days. Early tx can prevent recurrence. *Inter-ictal:* Antipsychotic (preferentially atypicals, ↓ risk to lower seizure threshold). *Forced normalization:* Tx unclear—consider reducing or stopping AED

SEXUAL DYSFUNCTION

Background (*J Sex Med.* 2016;13(2):135-143; *JAMA.* 1999;281(6):537-544)
- **Definition:** clinically significant disturbance in ability to respond sexually or experience sexual pleasure >6 mo
- ~31% of men + 43% of women
- Etiology physiologic (neurological, hormonal, vascular) + nonphysio-logic factors
- **Taking a sexual history:** Facilitates accurate diagnosis. Obstacles: patient/physician embarrassment, time constraints. Screening: *"Is there anything you would like to change about your sex life?", "Are you satisfied with your sex life?", "Are you sexually active? With men, women or both?"*
- **DDx: Endocrine:** hypothyroidism, adrenal dysfunction, hypogonad-ism, DM; **vascular:** HTN, atherosclerosis, stroke, venous insufficiency, sickle cell; **Neurologic:** CNS/PNS damage, MSE; **local genital Dx/**

trauma: priapism, Peyronie disease, urethritis, prostatitis, hydrocele, imperforate hymen, vaginitis, PID, endometriosis, prostatectomy, perineal sx, episiotomy, vaginal trauma

Disorders		
Name	**Criteria**	**Treatment**
Female Dysfunction		
Female sexual interest/ arousal disorder (FSIAD)	• 3+: ↓/absent sexual interest, thoughts, arousal, excitement, genital sensation, activity, w/ reluctant initiation/participation in sex, > 6 mo → significant personal distress • Combined from female arousal d/o + female hypoactive desire disorder	• Flibanserin (5-HT mixed agonist + DA agonist, SE: HoTN, syncope when taken w/ EtOH) • EROS-CTD clitoral suction device • Sildenafil
Female orgasmic disorder	• Delay or ↓ in frequency/intensity of orgasm, normal excitement, >75% encounters • Excluded if orgasm with direct clitoral contact and not intercourse → normal variant	• CBT to promote anxiety reduction, skills training can help • Multiple pharm agents studied w/ out benefit over placebo
Genitopelvic pain/penetration disorder	• Pain w/ fear of during penetration/intercourse +/− pelvic floor tensing, precipitant can be sexual trauma • DDx → poor vaginal lubrication, infection, combined vaginismus/ dyspareunia	• Ospemifene (selective estrogen receptor modulator) →postmenopausal dyspareunia d/2 vulvar/vaginal atrophy • Vaginal dilators • Use of female superior position, lubricant, + Kegel exercises
Male Dysfunction		
Erectile disorder	• Inability to attain/maintain erection in > 75% encounters. 50% of men >60 y/o, 50–85% organic basis • Distinguish if lifelong (present since becoming sexually active) vs acquired + generalized vs situational • *Risk factors:* HTN, DM, AD, vasc. Dx, smoking, EtOH, pelvic trauma/surgery, anxiety/ depression	• PDE-5 inhibitors (contraindicated w/ co-nitrate use) • Yohimbine

Disorders (continued)		
Name	**Criteria**	**Treatment**
Male hypoactive sexual desire d/o:	• Recurrent/persistent absence of sexual thoughts/fantasies/desire for sexual activity > 6 mo	• Behavioral → sensate focus exercises, erotic materials, masturbation training
Premature ejaculation	• Ejaculation w/in 1 min of minimal stimulation/before pt wishes causing distress for 6+ mo, >75% encounters	• SSRIs • Meta-analysis → paroxetine, clomipramine, sertraline + fluoxetine comparable, paroxetine → strongest ejaculation delay
Delayed ejaculation	• Infrequency/delay in ejaculation for 6+ mo, >75% encounters • Rare: 3–10% sex dys. pts • Ddx retrograde ejaculation, secondary (eg, SSRI SE) • Formally male orgasmic disorder	• Investigate and target medical and psychosocial contributor
Other Dysfunction		
SSRI-induced sexual dysfunction	• Significant differences among SSRIs →paroxetine = delay of orgasm/ejaculation; fluvoxamine, fluoxetine, sertraline→impotence • + correlation w/ dose • M> incidence, W > severity	• ↓ dose • Switch SSRI or to non-SSRI • Add bupropion • Add PDE-5 inhibitor • Add high dose buspirone

Reprod Sys Sexual Disorders. 2013;2(2):122; Int J Impot Res. 16(4):369; BJU Int. 2004;93(7):1018-1021; J Sex Med. 2004;1(1):66-68; CNS Drugs. 2015;29(11):915-933; Exp Opin Pharmacother. 2015;16(6):875-887; J Urol. 1998;159(2):433-436; J Urol. 2000;164(2):371-375; J Sex Med. 2007;4:260-268; J Clin Psychiatry;63(4):357-366; Endocr Rev. 2001;22(3):342-388

PARAPHILIC DISORDERS

Clinical Presentation (World J Biol Psychiatry. 2010;11:604; Arch Sex Behav. 2016;45:2173; Aggress Violent Behav. 2012;17:527)

• The concept of acceptable vs unacceptable sexual behavior dates back to biblical era; sexual deviance as a medical condition emerged in the late 19th century. Boundaries for acceptable sexual behavior vary with culture and evolve over time
• Each of the following common paraphilic disorders involve:
  • Recurrent and intense sexual arousal from a particular type of erotic activity or target; can manifest as fantasies, urges, or behaviors, patient may acknowledge or deny these interests

- Symptoms lasting for >6 mo
- Interests cause significant distress or impairment in functioning or has led the patient to act upon these sexual urges
- Paraphilic disorders should be distinguished from paraphilias (see differential diagnosis below); a paraphilia is necessary but not sufficient to be diagnosed with a paraphilic disorder
- DSM-5 provides specifiers for the majority of paraphilic disorders: "in a controlled environment" (primarily one living in a setting in which opportunities to engage in paraphilic behaviors are restricted); "in full remission" (in an uncontrolled setting for at least 5 y, one has not acted on urges with a nonconsenting person and no distress or impairment in that time)

Common Paraphilic Disorders	
Recurrent and intense sexual arousal from urges, fantasies, or behaviors…	
Voyeuristic disorder	…from observing an unsuspecting person who is disrobed or engaged in sexual activities Most common potentially law-breaking sexual behavior Onset usually <15 y/o though minimum age of diagnosis is 18 y/o due to difficulty differentiating from age-appropriate sexual curiosity Lifetime prevalence: 12% in ♂, 4% in ♀
Exhibitionist disorder	…from exposing one's genitals to an unsuspecting person Lifetime prevalence: 2–4% in ♂, less in ♀ Often emerges during adolescence or early adulthood, unclear persistence over time
Frotteuristic disorder	…from touching or rubbing against a nonconsenting person Often emerges in late adolescence or early adulthood but can also appear during childhood (though difficult to differentiate from conduct disorder in children) Comorbidities: Antisocial or conduct disorders Prevalence: 7–30% in ♂, 14% of ♂ seen for paraphilic disorders meet criteria for frotteuristic disorder, low in F ♀
Sexual masochism disorder	…from the act of being humiliated, beaten, bound, or made to suffer in a sexual interaction Practices can involve asphyxiation (risk of accidental death) Patients usually openly acknowledge their preferences Associated with use of masochistic pornography Often emerges in late adolescence or early adulthood
Sexual sadism disorder	…from physical or psychological suffering of another person Prevalence: 2–30%, lower among civilly committed sexual offenders, but higher among sexually motivated homicides Often emerges in late adolescence or early adulthood

Common Paraphilic Disorders (continued)	
Pedophilic disorder	...from sexual activity with prepubescent child or children Patients are over 16 y/o or >5 y older than the child Use of child pornography may be a useful indicator Prevalence: 3–5% in ♂, low in ♀ Often emerges around puberty and is lifelong Men with pedophilia and antisocial personality are more likely to act on their interests Child sexual abuse may be a risk factor
Fetishistic disorder	...from focusing on nonliving objects (eg, female under-garments, footwear, rubber, leather) or nongenital body parts (eg, feet, hair) Fetishes often combine the 2 (eg, dirty socks and feet) Appreciation of culture allows distinguishing between fetish and socially common sexual behaviors Many people with fetishes do not have dysfunction (disorder) Some people prefer solitary sexual activity with fetishes even when in a trusted relationship Fetishes are relatively uncommon among sexual offenders
Transvestic disorder	...from cross-dressing Can occur with fetishism (eg, specific garments or fabrics), gender dysphoria less likely Can occur with autogynephilia, whereby a man is sexually aroused by imagining himself as a woman, gender dys-phoria more likely Purging and acquisition behaviors can be indicators of dis-tress (eg, a man spends significant $ on women's apparel, discards them in an effort to overcome urges, and then begins re-acquiring them again) Individuals usually identify as heterosexual though may have sexual interactions with other men when cross-dressing Often emerges in childhood with fascination of women's attire Prevalence: 3% in ♂, less in ♀

APA. 2013; DSM-5. J Am Acad Psychiatry Law. 2014;42:191-201; J Am Acad Psychiatry Law. 2014; 42:478-483; Am J Forens Psych. 2011;32(2):3-26; World J Biol Psychiatry. 2010;11:604

Epidemiology and Pathogenesis (Psychiatr Clin North Am. 2014;37:149; Aggress Violent Behav. 2012;17:527; Arch Sex Behav. 1997;26(4):343; J Neurol. 2016;263(7):1454; Arch Neurol. 2003;60(3):437; Criminal Behav Ment Health. 2008;18:79-87; J Sex Res. 2017;54(2):161-171)

- Typically interests begin in adolescence, more common in ♂, all eth-nic and socioeconomic groups are represented; people engaging in 1 illegal paraphilic activity commonly engage in multiple
- Prevalence ill-defined
  - Swedish study asked randomly selected men and women about sexual interests: 3.1% reported arousal to exposing one's genitals to a stranger, 7.7% reported arousal spying on others having sex

- Another survey of randomly selected men: 4% reported sexual contact with a child, 9% reported sexual fantasies about children; these surveys don't address intensity, recurrence or persistence, thus likely represent the upper limit of potential prevalence
- Recent Canadian study of 1040 subjects found >50% expressed interest in at least 1 paraphilic category, >30% had experience in at least 1 paraphilic practice, and the most common categories were voyeurism, fetishism, frotteurism, and masochism
- Some categories (eg, masochism) rarely seek professional help thus demographic characteristics are difficult to define
- Pathogenesis unknown
  - Ongoing controversy regarding the validity of paraphilic disorders as medical diagnoses; some nations exclude them as a basis for involuntary commitment
  - Some consider paraphilic disorders to be forms of impulse control disorders, on the obsessional compulsive spectrum, or an intrinsic abnormality of sexual development
  - Multiple biological theories including perturbations in central monoamine neurotransmitter functioning; there have also been case reports involving compression to orbitofrontal cortex
  - No evidence that individuals with paraphilic disorders have higher testosterone or androgen receptor activity

Evaluation (Psychiatr Clin North Am. 2014;37:149; Curr Psychiatry Rep. 2015;17(5):29; J Sex Marital Ther. 2013;39:7; Harv Rev Psychiatry. 2005;13:186)
- **Clinical interview:** Consider demographics, conventional and paraphilic sexual fantasies and activities, substance use prior to sexual behaviors, age of puberty, age of onset of paraphilic behaviors, gender and age of partners, internet use, violence, legal history, impulsivity, relationships, degree of cognitive disability, family history. While interviewing can be informative, some pts are reluctant to discuss interests, particularly if perceived as atypical or potentially resulting in negative consequences. Self-report questionnaires (eg, online survey instead of phone) can improve response rate and detail
- Self-report questionnaires
  - MIDSA: comprehensive, addresses deviant sexual interests/behaviors as well as other domains such as criminal behavior and personality traits
  - MSI/MSI-II: 300-item/560-item true/false questionnaire, assesses comprehensive range of sexual preferences and behaviors
  - SHQ-R: 508-item multiple choice questionnaire, addresses wide range of sexual interests and behaviors
  - BSHI: 81 items, used clinically and in some studies to assess paraphilias
- Psychophysiologic methods
  - Phallometry/penile plethysmography: measures changes in penile circumference/volume in response to stimuli that vary on particular dimensions of interest (eg, age, violence); particularly helpful in assessment of pedophilia; considered the gold standard for objective measurement of sexual arousal in men

- Viewing time: pictures of semiclothed children/adolescents/adults are shown to viewer, and viewing time for each image is covertly recorded. Administered along with a questionnaire. Difficult to assess paraphilias other than pedophilia with this method
- Sex hormone profile screening (free and total testosterone, FSH, LH, estradiol, prolactin, progesterone) should be done to establish a baseline for any pharmacotherapy
- **Differential diagnosis:** normative sexual behavior (line between abnormal and normal sexual behavior is a continuum), OCD (differentiated from paraphilic disorders in that people with paraphilic disorders have sexual arousal with images/thoughts, whereas pts with OCD have ego-dystonic anxiety with images/thoughts), paraphilia (sexual interests outside the usual range of usual sexual interests but do not require psychiatric intervention) vs paraphilic disorder (cause significant distress, impairment, or may cause an individual to harm others)

Nonpharmacologic Treatment (Isr J Psychiatry Relat Sci. 2012;49:291; World J Biol Psychiatry. 2010;11:604; J Marital Fam Ther. 2006;32(3):297; Aggress Violent Behav. 2012;17:527)

- CBT is most widely recognized and most-studied psychotherapeutic tx for paraphilic disorders. Goal is to address distortions in thinking that contribute to rationalization of behaviors (eg, belief that children can consent to sex or victims are responsible for being assaulted). CBT is often combined with empathy training, sexual impulse control training, biofeedback and relapse prevention. Substantial evidence that this tx approach can reduce recidivism among sex offenders, though studies with longer follow-up periods show higher relapse rates suggesting limited durability of effect
- Family/couples therapy can be utilized to restore trust and healthy sexual relationship between partners
- Augmenting therapies targeting contributors to paraphilic behaviors such as anger management or substance use disorders
- Other therapies used include insight-oriented therapy, psychodynamic strategies, supportive psychotherapy, psychosocial programming, though these approaches do not have clear evidence of effect
- Treatment of paraphilic disorders among sex offenders has been ethically controversial throughout history (including psychodynamic psychotherapy, aversion therapy, surgical castration, and antilibido medication) and often negotiate the tensions between public safety, treatment of the individual, and punishment of criminal offenses

Pharmacologic Treatment (Psychiatr Clin North Am. 2014;37:173; Int J Offender Ther Comp Crimnol. 2003;47(4):407; Clin Ther. 2009;31:1; Psychiatr Clin North Am. 2014;37:149)

- Pharmacologic tx should be part of a more comprehensive plan including psychotherapy; goal of pharmacologic tx is to reduce libido, thus helping some pts respond more effectively to psychotherapy
- Choice of pharmacologic tx depends on medical history, compliance, intensity of fantasies, sexual violence risk

- **Antidepressants (SSRIs):** theories include (1) serotonin ↓ sexual arousal and ↓ orgasmic and ejaculatory abilities, (2) paraphilia w/ high comorbidity of anxiety and depressive disorders, (3) similarities in OCD spectrum disorder and paraphilias
  - SSRIs show good efficacy in treating mild symptoms and should be considered in pts w/ comorbid OCD, anxiety, or depression
  - Improvement in sx typically 2–4 wk; doses similar to those used for depression, though can be increased up to doses typically used in OCD
- **Steroidal antiandrogens:** medroxyprogesterone acetate (MPA), ↓ circulating testosterone and DHT
  - Side effects related to hypoandrogenism as well as risk of thromboembolism
  - Contraindicated in pts with abnormal liver fxn, thromboembolic disorder, active pituitary disorder
- **Gonadotropin-releasing hormone analogues or agonists (GnRHa):** triptorelin, leuprolide acetate, goserelin—act on pituitary GnRH receptors to interrupt normal pulsatile stimulation and lead to desensitization of GnRH receptors → ↓ secretion of LH + FSH → ↓ testosterone
  - During initiation, initial ↑ in testosterone, which can lead to ↑ paraphilic behavior, thus other concurrent tx warranted in first weeks of tx
  - Side effects related to hypoandrogenism (hot flashes, ↓ face/body hair growth, gynecomastia, ↓ testicular volume; bone mineral loss) should be monitored and treated
  - Contraindications for tx with GnRHa are osteoporosis and active pituitary disorders

SLEEP DISORDERS

Overview and Initial Approach
- Sleep is a complex process dependent on multiple brain pathways. Dx of the underlying etiology necessary for appropriate tx
- **Contributing factors to sleep dysfunction:** medical illness, psychiatric illness, medication adverse effects, poor sleep hygiene, stress

INSOMNIAS

Condition(s) causing unsatisfactory sleep quality/quantity with difficulty in ≥1 of: sleep initiation, sleep maintenance, early morning awakening (NEJM. 2015;373:1437)

Etiology
Disruption of homeostatic drive and/or circadian rhythm, which jointly control sleep timing and quality (J Biol Rhythms. 2006;21:482):

Homeostatic drive: regulates tiredness + sleep onset; ↑ while awake, ↓ with sleep

Circadian rhythm: timing mechanism separates day into sleep + awakening based on light/dark exposure; opposes homeostatic drive while awake; not affected by previous sleep

- **Medication effect:** stimulants, steroids, bronchodilators, decongestants, antidepressants, dopamine antagonists (akathisia) (*Sleep Med Clin.* 2018;13:147)
- **Psychiatric illness:** mania > schizophrenia > depression and anxiety, 60% = no psychiatric disorder (*JAMA.* 1989;262:1479)
- **Substance use:** intoxication—cocaine, synthetic cannabis, PCP, amphetamines, alcohol (aids sleep onset, disrupts overall sleep), withdrawal—caffeine, BZD, alcohol, opioids
- **Medical illness (*most common cause in geriatric pts*):** cardiac (angina, paroxysmal nocturnal dyspnea), pulmonary (COPD, asthma, cough), GI (reflux), MSK (pain), endocrine (thyroid, diabetes mellitus, menopause), neuro (Parkinson's, CVA, migraine, dementia), GU (nocturia, renal disease) (*Psychiatr Clin North Am.* 2015:38:825)
- **Restless legs syndrome (RLS):** strong urge to move limbs, which worsens at rest and at end of day and which improves with activity, dx supported by ferritin level <50 ng/mL; movements **do not** occur during sleep
- **Primary insomnia:** diagnose if not explained by other medical or psychiatric cause, occurs at least 3×/wk for 3 mo, + no other sleep disorder present

Nonpharmacologic Treatment
- **Address comorbid conditions** (eg, tx of depression > insomnia 2/2 antidepressants)
- **Behavioral interventions**
  - Modify sleep environment: earplugs, sleep mask, bedding/pillow modifications
  - Sleep hygiene (consistent bed time, no naps after 12p, bed only for sleep or sex, no electronics 1 h before bed, ↓ caffeine)
  - CBT for insomnia (CBT-I): different from CBT for psychiatric disorders; available in self-guided apps
  - ↓ sleep anxiety (challenge unrealistic expectations, stop clock watching, relaxation)
- **For RLS:** heating pads, ice packs

Pharmacologic Treatment
- Utilize only after nonpharm intervention or if significant functional impairment. Goal: Short-term use while addressing underlying etiologies or initiating behavioral change
- BZD receptor agonists (those in bold = FDA approved for insomnia): **temazepam**, **triazolam**, clonazepam, lorazepam, **eszopiclone**, **zolpidem**, **zaleplon**; *cautions:* ↓driving performance, anterograde amnesia; avoid in geriatric pts (↑ fall risk, delirium), risk of misuse/dependence
- Melatonin agonists: **melatonin** (0.25–0.5 mg; avoid ↑ doses → vivid dreams, activation, next-day oversedation/fatigue), **ramelteon**
- Orexin antagonists: suvorexant
- Antidepressants + mood stabilizers (target insomnia + comorbid psych disorder): mirtazapine, trazodone, amitriptyline, doxepin, gabapentin

- 2nd-generation antipsychotics (eg, quetiapine) can be utilized short term if other agents ineffective; risk of metabolic disturbance in long-term use
- Alpha blockers: prazosin (tx of nightmares as etiology of insomnia, data evolving)
- **For RLS:** if ferritin low → iron supplementation, dopamine agonists (eg, pramipexole, ropinirole, gabapentin)

HYPERSOMNIAS

Conditions causing excessive daytime sleepiness (regardless of abnormal vs normal sleep)

Etiology
- Obstructive sleep apnea (OSA)
- Narcolepsy: daytime sleepiness, cataplexy (strong emotions → sudden weakness), hypnogogic/hypnopompic hallucinations, sleep paralysis
- Periodic limb movement disorder: Repetitive + rhythmic involuntary movements during sleep, may cause awakening (contrast w/ RLS, which occurs while awake + involves movements to relieve urge)
- Medication: BZDs, antidepressants, neuroleptics, anticonvulsants

Diagnosis
- **OSA scales:** Epworth Sleepiness Scale, STOP-BANG questionnaire, Mallampati score
- **Polysomnography:** Indicated when abnormal behaviors/movements during sleep; repetitive brief awakenings during sleep; suspicion for OSA (snoring/body habitus + ≥1: daytime sleepiness, witnessed apnea, refractory HTN)
- **Multiple sleep latency test:** if narcolepsy suspected

Treatment
- **OSA:** CPAP, weight loss, upper airway surgery, positional devices (prevent moving into positions that exacerbate obstruction)
- **Narcolepsy:** stimulants (modafinil, methylphenidate); sodium oxybate (most effective for cataplexy; venlafaxine second-line for cataplexy)
- **Periodic limb movement disorder:** dopamine agonists (pramipexole, ropinirole), BZDs; avoidance of caffeine and SSRIs

PARASOMNIAS

Conditions characterized by abnormal behaviors (motor or verbal) during sleep

Etiology
Fusion of wakefulness with either REM or non-REM sleep

Differential Dx: Seizures, PTSD, nocturnal panic, dissociative disorders

Diagnosis
Bed partner history often sufficient, polysomnography, expanded workup for RBD (see below)

- **Non-REM sleep behavior disorders:** patients not easily awoken, confusional period after
  Confusional arousals: slow speech, confusion, difficulty responding to questions/commands on awakening, most common in children
  Sleepwalking: walk w/ ↓ consciousness, +/− complex actions (eg, driving); risk: self-injury
  Sleep terrors: express fear (screaming, flailing, diaphoresis); may occur with frightening dreams, commonly no memory of episode
  Sleep-related eating: rapid binge eating (large amounts in <10 min); may be partially/fully conscious but without any control over eating; risk of injury or poisoning (may consume inedible/toxic substances)
- **REM sleep behavior disorders:** do not involve confusion; nonmotor (except RBD)
  Sleep paralysis: inability to use voluntary muscles or speak while fully conscious, at sleep onset or on awakening, often w/ intense fear; onset in teens, most prevalent in 20–30s
  Hypnagogic (sleep onset) or hypnopompic (awakening) hallucinations: commonly visual, can last several minutes
  REM behavior disorder (RBD): vivid dreams + motions corresponding to actions in dream (punching, kicking, jumping); easy to awaken w/ no confusion (pt will often recall details of dream), *expanded assessment:* RBD associated with alpha synucleinopathies (Parkinson's, dementia with Lewy bodies, multiple systems atrophy)

Treatment
- Sleep hygiene + lifestyle modification (stress and sleep deprivation exacerbate all parasomnias); avoid alcohol/caffeine
- **Medication:** short-acting BZDs may have some benefit for sleepwalking or sleep terrors; SSRI or topiramate may reduce sleep-related eating
- **RBD:** bedroom safety precautions to avoid injury to pt or bed partner, discontinuation of serotonergic agents, treatment of underlying neurologic syndrome if present; consider BZDs, melatonin (high-dose 5–10 mg nightly), pramipexole

STROKE

Overview (*JAMA. 2000;284:2901-2906; Circulation. 2017;135:e229-e445; Stroke. 2017;48:1795-1801; J Stroke Cerebrovasc Dis. 2014;23:1837-1842*)
- Acute onset of neurologic symptoms w/ evidence of vascular pathology (infarction = ischemic or rupture = hemorrhagic) on imaging (eg, CT or MRI)
- In contrast to **transient ischemic attacks (TIA)**: neurologic deficits exist 2/2 ischemia w/ absence of imaging evidence, managed similarly given ↑ risk of stroke within days

- **Epidemiology:** In 2017, 795,000 in the US; 140,000 deaths; 87% ischemic + 13% hemorrhagic, ~25% w/ previous stroke
- **Pts w/ psychiatric illness are at risk:** Psychiatric hospitalization associated w/ an ↑ risk of stroke within 1 y, believed to be mediated by stress + immunologic reaction, ↓ medication adherence, ↑ chronic medical illness. ♂ w/ MDD at > risk of dying 2/2 stroke
- **Stroke syndromes mimic psychiatric sx:** ~9% of missed strokes in EDs attributed to psychiatric illness (Neurology. 2015;85:505-511). 39% missed acute strokes initially dx'd as "altered mental status" (J Stroke Cerebrovasc Dis. 2014;23:374-378)
- *Time is brain:* early recognition = better outcomes. Missed strokes → worse neurologic outcomes + > 4× risk of death at 1 y (Neurology. 2015;85:505-511)
- Poststroke neuropsychiatric symptoms are common; treated similarly to primary psychiatric symptoms

---

ISCHEMIC STROKE

Risk Factors and Etiology (Stroke. 2014;45:2160-2236; Drug Alcohol Depend. 2014;142:1-13; Int J Cardiol. 2014;174:669-677)
- **Atherosclerosis** (50% of stroke): ↑ risk w/ DM, HTN, smoking
- **Embolic** (20%): ↑ risk w/ primary cardiac pathology (AFib, cardiomyopathy), hematologic diseases (malignancy, inherited hypercoagulability), + smoking
- **Lacunar** (20%): ↑ risk w/ HTN
- *Other* (10%): eg, arterial dissection, vasospasm, + watershed infarcts
- **Modifiable:** HTN, HLD, DM, smoking, inactivity/obesity, CAD, cardiomyopathy, AFib, PFO, VTE, valvular disease, cocaine or heavy EtOH use, CAD/MI, *mental illness, antipsychotic use*, hypercoagulable state (cancer, antiphospholipid antibody syndrome, factor V leiden), vasculitis, hypoperfusion + anoxia
- **Nonmodifiable:** sex (F>M), race (AA>HA>WA), prior TIA/stroke, prior MI

Diagnosis (Stroke. 2018;49:e46-e99; Stroke. 2018;49:e111-e122)
- Stroke team w/ stroke protocol = ↓ time to tx for alteplase therapy
- **Rapid clinical assessment:** detailed neuro exam w/ localization + triage to imaging + *NIH Stroke Scale* (NIHSS), ≥10 →73% sensitive + 74% specific for large vessel occlusion (https://stroke.nih.gov/documents/NIH_Stroke_Scale.pdf)

Ischemic Stroke Syndromes			
Location	**Vessel**	**Location and Laterality**	**Symptoms (Psychiatric Appearance in Bold)**
Anterior	ICA	N/A	Combinations of other anterior stroke syndromes (see below)
	Ophthalmic	N/A	Ipsilateral amaurosis fugax (transient, painless vision loss) or permanent vision loss
	ACA	Anterior/medial frontal lobe	Contralateral or bilateral leg weakness, urinary incontinence, frontal release, **neuropsych (apathy, disinhibition, depression, perseveration)**
	MCA	Dominant (usually L frontotemporal)	*Superior:* **expressive aphasia**, contra arm and face weakness +/− sensory loss; *Gerstmann syndrome* (1) (acalculia, agraphia, RL confusion, finger agnosia, apraxia) *Inferior:* **receptive aphasia**, sensorimotor loss
		Nondominant (usually R frontotemporal)	*Superior:* **expressive aprosodia**, hemineglect, disability indifference; *Inferior:* **receptive aprosodia**, hemineglect
Posterior	Vert/AICA/PICA	Cerebellum and lateral medulla	Ataxia, dysmetria, nystagmus, nausea, headache, *Wallenberg syndrome* (2), herniation and death
	Vert/ASA/BA	Brainstem	Complex mix of vision and oculomotor deficits, hearing deficits, weakness, numbness, drop attack (which may mimic cataplexy) and *locked-in syndrome* (3)
	PCA (occipital)	N/A	Homonymous hemianopia, cortical blindness, and **Anton syndrome** (4)
	PCA (thalamus)	N/A	Pain syndromes, amnesia, tremor
	PCA (parieto-occipital)	N/A	Loss of voluntary eye movements, optic ataxia, asimultagnosia

(continued)

Ischemic Stroke Syndromes *(continued)*			
Location	**Vessel**	**Location and Laterality**	**Symptoms (Psychiatric Appearance in Bold)**
Lacunar	Subcortical (putamen, caudate, thalamus, internal capsule, pons)	N/A	Pure motor and pure sensory (without aphasia)

1. **Gerstmann syndrome**: dominant parietal lobe stroke resulting from MCA segment stroke characterized by agraphia, acalculia, finger agnosia, left-right confusion, and ideomotor apraxia.
2. **Wallenberg syndrome**: lateral medullary infarction resulting from PICA stroke characterized by vertigo, ipsilateral hemiataxia, dysarthria, ptosis, and miosis (possible etiology of Horner syndrome).
3. **Locked-in syndrome**: pontine infarction resulting from basilar stroke characterized by paralysis of all voluntary movement except extraocular and eyelids.
4. **Anton syndrome**: occipital lobe pathology (eg, infarction of PCA) resulting in visual anosognosia (vision loss without awareness of as much and resulting confabulation).

- **Brain imaging:** preferably < 20 min; *Non-con CT head + neck vessels* → cost-effective + sufficient for most pts, if unclear presentation/ localization, or presentation 6–24 h after last known normal, *MRI head + neck w/ FLAIR and DWI* may change management + improve outcomes
- Routine laboratory tests, ECG, troponin should be considered but should not delay workup, **except blood glucose** to rule out hypoglycemia as etiology
- Etiological workup: EKG +/− telemetry (to r/o atrial fibrillation), TTE (to r/o PFO), PT/INR/PTT (to r/o procoagulant state), risk factor screening (HbA1c, FLP)

Acute Management (Stroke. 2018;49:e46-e99)
- **Supportive care:** O$_2$sat kept >94%; correct hypotension; avoid HTN if thrombolytic therapy (SBP<180, DBP <105 mmHg for ≥24 h); correction of fever; blood glucose goal 140–180 mg/dL
- **Last known normal (LKN) <4.5 h→ IV alteplase:** absolute contraindications: ICH, prior ischemic stroke or head trauma in last 3 mo, coagulopathy, infectious endocarditis, aortic dissection, administration of LMWH or Gp IIb/IIIa inhibitors in last 24 h. Relative contraindications: recent neurosurgery, prior ICH, bleeding
- **LKN 6–24 h → endovascular therapy (EVT)** if: (1) premorbid modified Rankin Score of 0–1, (2) ICA or MCA segment occlusion, (3) age ≥18 y, (4) NIHSS ≥6, (5) MCA severity score (ASPECTS) of ≥6. If eligible, alteplase B4 thrombectomy. *Note:* Pts w/ psychiatric illness significantly less likely to receive EVT (Stroke. 2018;49:738-740)

Postacute Management (Stroke. 2016;47:e1-e72; Cochrane Rev. 2012;11:CD009286; Lancet. 2011;10:123-130)
- Antiplatelet agents + statin within 48 h; delay ASA for 24 h following alteplase
- **Monitor/manage complications:** Edema, seizures (prophylaxis is not recommended), hemorrhagic conversion, delirium (avoid neuroleptics, BZDs, alpha-antagonists)
- **Rehabilitation:** aggressive PT, OT, SLP w/ repeat functional assessment, prevent venous thromboembolism contracture and skin breakdown 2/2 ↓ mobility, Manage incontinence + pain
- SSRI → ↓ psychiatric disturbance + ↑ motor recovery
- **Secondary prevention** (Stroke. 2014;45:2160-2236; J Am Coll Cardiol. 2018;71:e127-e248): Manage HTN, HLD, DM, lifestyle (weight loss, diet, physical activity), OSA

    Carotid artery disease: Stenting in >70% stenosis (>50% by catheter-imaging) vs carotid endarterectomy >70-y, antiplatelet therapy

    A Fib: Following stroke/TIA rhythm monitoring × 30 d → if + anticoagulation (DOACs preferred, no antiplatelet unless is co-occurring CAD)

    Mechanical valve = vit. K antagonist: *aortic* → INR 2-3; *mitral* → INR 2.5-3.5. +/– ASA

    Patent foramen ovale: TTE in-hospital, +/– transcatheter closure if known DVT

HEMORRHAGIC STROKE

Background (Stroke. 2015;46:2032-2060)
- Presentation often any combination of the stroke syndromes +/– headache, nausea, vomiting, meningeal signs, respiratory depression, coma
- May occur as either a subarachnoid hemorrhage (often 2/2 aneurysm) or intracerebral hemorrhage (often 2/2 HTN, amyloid angiopathy)
- **Risk factors:** HTN, amyloid angiopathy, AVMs and aneurysms, tumors, infections, hypocoagulability (clotting disorders, antiplatelet, anticoagulation), vasculitides, cocaine use

Diagnosis
- Noncontrast CT head + angiography
- If high suspicion and negative imaging, LP warranted to identify small bleeds (via xanthochromia or elevated RBC counts)

Management
- Close monitoring of vital signs, preference for SBP<140 mmHg
- Reverse anticoagulation +/– platelets (thrombocytopenia or antiplatelet tx in 24 h)
- AED for seizures (levetiracetam most common → ↓ risk of respiratory depression)
- Neurosurgical consultation, esp. cerebellar hemorrhage → brainstem compression = risk of coma + death

NEUROPSYCHIATRIC SEQUELA

Poststroke Depression (PSD) (Can J Psych. 2010;55:341-349)
- ~20% post stroke, incidence peak 6 mo
- Associated w/ ↑ morbidity (↓ recovery of ADLs, cognitive function) and mortality

- Treat as MDD. May be accompanied by restlessness and mood lability (more commonly L hemisphere)

Psychosis (*J Neuro Neurosurg Psych.* 2018;89:879-885)
- ~ 5%, associated w/ R frontal, R temporal, R parietal, or R caudate
- Associated w/ poor outcomes + high mortality
- Little data on treatment: haloperidol and risperidone common, some data for complete/partial resolution at 3.5 mo

Mania (*Cerebrovasc Dis.* 2011;32:11-21)
- Rare; data of overall prevalence lacking, 2011 systematic analysis → 74 cases in 50 y
- Associated w/ corticobasal injury
- No robust treatment recommendations, differential of seizures + dementia

Vascular Dementia (*Lancet.* 2015;386:1698-1706)
- Subcortical dementia, classically described as progressing in a step-wise fashion 2/2 many "mini-strokes" from small vessel disease of white matter tracts
- Distinguished from "cortical dementias" by motor signs, inattention, slowed processing, and mood symptoms
- **Binswanger disease** is considered a subtype of vascular dementia and is characterized by cognitive impairment co-occurring parkinsonism, upper motor neuron signs, and difficulty with balance (*Expert Rev Neurother.* 2014;14:1203-1213)
- For details see Major Neurocognitive Disorders, p. 2-77

Stroke Symptoms and Their Psychiatric Confounders		
Location	**Symptom**	**May Be Confused With…**
Wernicke's area	Receptive aphasia (pressured speech, clanging, "word salad")	Mania, psychosis, "altered mental status"
Broca's area	Expressive aphasia (poverty of speech)	Depression and catatonia
Orbitofrontal	Disinhibition, excessive joking	Mania
Frontal convexity	Apathy, perseveration	Depression, hypoactive delirium
Thalamus, midbrain	Delirium (extremely rare)	"Altered mental status"
Frontocerebellar circuits	Pseudobulbar affect	Mania, mixed episode, depression, psychosis
Occipital cortex	Visual hallucinations (simple)	Psychosis
Cerebral peduncle, temporal lobe	Auditory hallucinations	Psychosis

Stroke Symptoms and Their Psychiatric Confounders *(continued)*		
Location	**Symptom**	**May Be Confused With…**
R parietal	Paranoia, persecutory delusions	Psychosis
Bi- or R frontal	Delusional misidentification	Capgras syndrome, psychosis, delusional disorder

TRAUMATIC BRAIN INJURY

Backround + Epidemiology *(Vital Health Stat. 2012;10; CDC National Center for Injury. 2010; DoD Defense and Veterans Brain Injury Center. 2017)*

- Result of focal +/− diffuse acceleration/deceleration, leading cause of disability
- Mechanism of injury: falls (28%, highest risk age 0–4 and >75) > MVA (20%, highest risk age 15–24) > head striking object (19%) > assault (11%), >375,000 TBIs reported by DOD 2000–2017, primary d/2 blast injury, EtOH involved in ~50%
- Risk: M > F, blacks > Caucasian > American Indians/Asian/Pacific Islanders, risk is additive: sustaining 1 TBI → 3× ↑ risk of 2nd TBI; 2nd TBI → 10× ↑ risk

Classification *(J Trauma. 2011;70(3):554-559; J Trauma. 2011;70(3):554-559; J Neurotrauma. 2005;22(10):1040-1051; J Neurotrauma. 2004;21(9):1131-1140)*

- LOC is not diagnostic nor reliable severity marker
- Longer posttrauma amnesia→predict future disability
- Use of GCS: **mild:** 13–15; +/− LOC; AKA concussion, **moderate:** 9–12, **severe:** GCS < 8, Utility limited by confounding factors (eg, ETT, EtOH, paralysis, dementia, other neurologic sequelae

Glasgow Coma Scale	
Eye Opening	**Score**
Spontaneous	4
To verbal command	3
To pain	2
No response	1
Best Verbal Response	
Fully oriented	5
Confused	4
Inappropriate words	3

(continued)

Glasgow Coma Scale *(continued)*	
Eye Opening	**Score**
Incomprehensible sounds	2
No response	1
Best Motor Response	
Obeys commands	6
Localizes pain	5
Withdrawal from pain	4
Decorticate (flexor) posturing	3
Decerebrate (extensor) posturing	2
No response	1
Total	

Pathophysiology *(Curr Opin Crit Care. 2002;8(2):101-105)*

- **Primary injury:** at time of trauma; direct mechanical force to head (coup injury) or brain hitting opposite inner surface of skull (countercoup injury) → focal contusions/hematomas, white matter shearing, and cerebral edema
- **Secondary injury:** physiologic response; neurotransmitter-mediated excitotoxicity; inflammation; electrolyte imbalance; apoptosis; vasospasm/vascular injury

Primary Brain Injuries	
Cerebral contusions	Common in basal frontal and temporal areas d/2 acceleration/deceleration injury
Diffuse axonal injury	Axonal shearing primarily affecting corpus callosum + midbrain
Epidural hematoma	A/w torn dural arteries (ie, middle meningeal) + skull fxr
Subdural hematoma	Damage to bridging veins between cortex + venous sinus; ↑ risk w/ anticoagulation and cerebral atrophy (bridging veins stretched)
Subarachnoid hemorrhage	Often 2/2 disruption of pial vessels or ruptured aneurisms w/ bleeding into sylvian fissure/interpeduncular cisterns/between gyri or spinal canal
Intraventricular hemorrhage	Tearing of subependymal veins or extension from adjacent bleed

Evaluation *(J Trauma. 2005;59(4):954)*

- Hx of incident + events leading up to; full neuro eval + GCS; assesst for amnesia
- Signs suggesting severe injury: EDH w/ skull fxr and transient LOC followed by "lucid interval" and MS deterioration; Battle's sign and

raccoon eyes (postauricular and periorbital ecchymoses) w/ basilar skull fxr; *ICP* (dilated pupil(s), HA, vomiting, nuchal rigidity), *Cushing reflex* (HTN, bradycardia, resp depression), hemiparesis can occur w/ SDH 2/2 mass effect of hematoma

- CT w/out contrast → ID bleed, ↑ ICP; NEXUS II criteria, CT indicated for mTBI pts w/ skull fxr, scalp hematoma, neuro deficit, GCS <= 14, persistant vomiting, coagulopathy, or abnormal behavior
- MRI w/out contrast in subacute/chronic setting to eval persistant sxs; may show posttraumatic gliosis, encephalomalacia; patchy WM lesions may be seen in axonal damage (DAI), MRI DTI/DWI = most sensitive for DAI

Clinical Presentation (Brain Inj. 2004;18(2):131-142; Neuropsychiatr Dis Treat. 2017;13:459-465; Arch Phys Med Rehabil. 2004;(85):73-81; Neurology. 2014;83(4):312-319; Prog Neurol Surg. 2014;28:38-49; Brain Pathol. 2015;25(3):350-364)

- **Acute phase:** up to 8d s/p TBI, coma in severe, delirium in up to 70%,↑ w/ ↓ GCS, seizure often occurs 1st 24 h, secondary mania up to 9% of pts, usually R ventral frontal/basotemporal injury (Psychiatr Clin North Am. 2014;37(1):13-29)
- **Subacute + chronic phase:** subacute = 8–89 d, chronic = >90 d s/p TBI, 65% w/ long-term cognitive problems >2 y later (executive fxn, memory, attention, information processing, and language; correlate w/ initial GCS/time in coma); impulsivity, apraxia, 60% ↑ risk of dementia in controlled study of veterans, seizures occurring >1 wk postinjury; indicative of more permanent structural/physiologic brain change
- **Chronic traumatic encephalopathy:** repetitive trauma (ie, football, boxing, combat) → progressive deterioration w/ mood disturbance, cognitive impairment, personality change, +/− sensorimotor impairment incl parkinsonism, characterized by deposition of p-tau protein
- **Frontal lobe syndrome and organic personality disorder:** frontal and temporal lob damage → apathy, poor social judgment, aggression, impulsivity, loss of social graces, lewdness, paranoia; pt may have little insight

Neuropsychiatric Sequela of TBI		
Symptom	**Data**	**Treatment Options**
Depression/MDD	Most common: 14–77%, 15% attempt suicide w/in 5 y iso despair, hopelessness, relationship loss, insomnia, chronic HA, + disinhibition	SSRIs
GAD and PTSD	Most common assoc anxiety d/	SSRIs
Mood lability	Often d/2 frontal + temporal lobe inj and assoc WM tracts → labile affect, disinhibition	SSRIs

(continued)

Neuropsychiatric Sequela of TBI (continued)		
Symptom	**Data**	**Treatment Options**
Aggression		SSRIs, propranolol, neuroleptics; valproate; carbamazepine
Psychosis	Prevalence 0.9–8.5%; delusions +/– AH; disorganized thought process; onset may be delayed up to 5 y postinjury	Neuroleptics
Apathy		Stimulants, SSRI not shown to be effective
Mania	Relatively uncommon w/ rates 2–17%	Valproate, carbamazepine
Cognitive complaints		Stimulants, acetylcholinesterase inhibitors

Am J Psychiatry. 2002;159(8):1315-1321; n J Nerv Ment Dis. 2005;193(10):680-685; Neuropsychiatr Dis Treat. 2015;11:2355-2365; Psychiatr Clin North Am. 2014;37(1):113-124; Am J Psychiatry. 2002;159(8):1315-1321; J Neuropsychiatry Clin Neurosci. 2000;12(3):316-327

Nonpharmacologic Treatment (*Arch Phys Med Rehabil. 2011;92(4):519-530*)

- Cognitive rehab → intervention must be targeted to be effective, environmental modification to ↓ triggers/irritations, supportive therapy, family education/support, PT, OT

Pharmacologic Treatment (*Brain Sci. 2017;7(8):93; Ann Phys Rehabil Med. 2016;59(1):42-57; Neurosci Lett. 2008;448(3):263-267; Brain Inj. 2004;18(1):1-31; J Neuropsychiatry Clin Neurosci. 2009;21(4):362-370*)

- General principles: Start low, go slow; avoid drugs that ↓ sz threshold (ie, bupropion, TCAs); limit anticholinergic + alpha antagonism (risk delirium, HoTN)
- **SSRIs:** Meta-analysis of 37 studies → evidence for depression, emotional lability, aggression, no impact on apathy
- **Beta-blockers:** propranolol ↓ agitation/aggression
- **Mood stabilizers:** VPA, carbamazepine 1st if comorbid sz; improve aggression/agitation
- **Neuroleptics:** can ↓ psychosis, agitation, and aggression; some animal studies suggest chronic neuroleptic use may interfere w/ neuroplasticity and recovery
- **Stimulants:** weak evidence; improvement in apathy, processing speed, attention
- **Acetylcholinesterase inhibitors:** limited evidence w/ mild improvement in memory, attn
- **BZDs:** Risk of worsening cog impairment, ↑ disinhibition; not recommended

ALCOHOL USE DISORDER

Background *(Ann Intern Med. 2016;164: ITC1; Lancet. 1997;349:1897)*
- *At-risk* → >14 drinks/wk in nonelderly M (max 4/d), 7 drinks/wk in F (max 3/d)
- *AUD* → characterized by cravings for EtOH, inability to control intake, + use despite significant consequences
- Chronic use of EtOH and BZD → ↑ signaling GABA and insensitivity → abrupt cessation = CNS overreactivity which is life-threatening, ↑ risk for multiple medical problems

Assessment
- Amount, duration + frequency of use, last drink/use, history of blackouts, withdrawal seizures, DTs, treatment, sobriety, dangerous behaviors (eg, impaired driving), at-risk dependents, legal obligations, other use, psychiatric/medical d/o
- Determine appropriate treatment setting (eg, outpatient, IOP, PHP, inpatient detox, dual dx psychiatric hosp, medical hosp, ICU) (ASAM Criteria)
- **Acute intoxication:** nystagmus, slurred speech, disinhibition, incoordination of movement, depressed level of consciousness. *Exclude ddx:* head trauma, hypoxia, hypoglycemia, hypothermia, encephalopathy, electrolyte abnormality, other intoxication incl. methanol, ethylene glycol, + isopropanol, other causes of AMS
- **Testing:** breathalyzer or BAL; urine/serum tox; LFTs (>2:1 elevated AST:ALT ratio), CBC (macrocytosis, thrombocytopenia, ↑ MCV), BMP (AKI), +/– CK (rhabdo)
- **Long-term/extended daily use:** E/o chronic liver dx (eg, palmar erythema, spider angiomata, caput medusae, ascites/edema, gynecomastia, jaundice)

Clinical Institute Withdrawal Assessment Scale for Alcohol (CIWA-Ar)
- Assign points for each of the 10 criteria; each criterion is scored 0–7, except orientation, which is scored 0–4; add points to calculate score

CIWA-Ar Scale					
Points	**Anxiety**	**Agitation**	**Tremor**	**HA**	**Orientation**
0	None	None	None	None	Oriented
1		Somewhat	Not visible, but felt at fingertips	Very mild	Cannot do serial additions
2				Mild	Disorient. by ≤2 d
3				Moderate	Disorient. by >2 d

(continued)

CIWA-Ar Scale *(continued)*					
Points	**Anxiety**	**Agitation**	**Tremor**	**HA**	**Orientation**
4	Guarded	Restless	Moderate w/ hands extended	Mod severe	Disoriented to person or place
5				Severe	n/a
6				Very severe	n/a
7	Panic	Pacing or thrashing	Severe	Extremely severe	n/a
Points	**N/V**	**Sweats**	**Auditory halluc**	**Visual halluc**	**Tactile disturb**
0	None	None	None	None	None
1		Moist palms	Very mild	Very mild photosens	Very mild paresthesias
2			Mild	Mild photosens	Mild paresth
3			Moderate	Mod photosens	Mod paresth
4	Intermit. w/ dry heaves	Beads	Mod severe	Mod severe visual halluc	Mod severe hallucinations
5			Severe	Severe	Severe
6			Very severe	Very severe	Very severe
7	Constant	Drenching	Cont.	Continuous	Continuous
Score: <8 none to minimal withdrawal; 8–15 mild; 16–20 moderate; >20 severe					

Signs of Withdrawal (*Am Fam Physician.* 2004;69:1443; *Lancet.* 1997;349:1897; *Arch Intern Med.* 2004;164:1405)

- **Uncomplicated:** diaphoresis, anxiety, GI upset, hyperreflexia, HTN, ↑ HR, masked by β-blockers + sedatives
- **Seizure:** 12–48 h s/p last drink, may occur earlier versus much later w/ long-acting BZD
- **Alcoholic hallucinosis:** visual + tactile hallucinations w/ preserved attention and orientation, onset 12–24 h s/p last drink, resolves w/ in 24–48 h
- **Alcohol withdrawal delirium (DTs):** hallucinations, disorientation, agitation, autonomic instability, onset 48–96 h s/p last drink, can last 5+ d, a/w mortality

Treatment (Crit Care Clin. 2017;33:559; Neuroscience. 2002;37:513; World J Crit Care Med. 2014;3:42; Neuroscience. 91:429-438)

- **Withdrawal**
  - For pts able to communicate, symptom-triggered BZD (eg, CIWA-Ar), BZDs used vary (eg, diazepam [5–20 mg], chlordiazepoxide [25–100 mg], or lorazepam [1–4 mg] w/ liver compromise or elderly)
  - Institution-specific protocols may use other GABA-ergic meds (eg, phenobarbital), anticonvulsants (eg, carbamazepine, gabapentin), or α-2 agonists (eg, clonidine) although evidence is variable
  - High-dose thiamine (B1) (eg, 500 mg IV Q8h × 3–5 d) based on Caine criteria (see "WE") w/ volume + electrolyte repletion
  - *Note on BZD withdrawal*: specific BZD withdrawal (eg, alprazolam) may not be completely covered w/ other BZD
- **Addiction/AUD** (APA Practice Guideline; 2017)
  - Determine goals (eg, abstinence vs moderation) incl. any legal obligation
  - Moderate/severe AUD, if pt prefers MAT/failed tx w/o MAT: *1st line*: naltrexone or acamprosate, IM naltrexone if adherence concern, *2nd line*: disulfiram (suggest signing specific contract), gabapentin + topiramate (not FDA-approved)
  - Best practice may incl. random monitoring (breathalyzer, urine ethanol or urine ethyl glucuronide) + other drug screening
  - Psychosocial interventions, CBT, motivational enhancement therapy, marital and family counseling, contingency management, and mutual support orgs (AA, SMART recovery)
  - Family members may benefit from referral to Al-Anon or CRAFT therapist
  - Avoid BZD d/2 risk respiratory depression w/ EtOH + potential for misuse

WERNICKE ENCEPHALOPATHY

- Emergent complication of chronic use (+ other cause Vit. B1 deficiency) (J Neurol Sci. 1989;90:125), can be fatal or → irreversible memory impairment (Korsakoff syndrome)
  - Caine criteria, ≥2 of: Nutritional deficiency, AMS or memory impairment, oculomotor abnormalities, cerebellar dysfunction, w/o hepatic impairment, sensitivity 85% (J Neurol Neurosurg Psychiatry. 1997;62:51)
- **Even if Caine criteria not met but WE on differential, high-dose IV/IM thiamine indicated**, eg, 500 mg TID 3+ d (Eur J Neurol. 2010;17:1408; In Vivo. 2017;31:121), administered before glucose infusion
- Others → prophylactic thiamine PO 100 mg QD, folate 1 mg QD, MVI QD

COCAINE USE

Background (drugabuse.gov, dea.gov, Am J Addict. 2018;(27):477-484)
- **Alternative names:** Powder: coke, blow, dust, yayo, yay. Freebase: crack, rock(s), candy
- **Common forms:** powder, freebase crystal, intravenous, leaf
- **Method of use:** ingestion (leaf), mucus membranes, insufflation (slower onset, ↑ duration), injection (rapid onset, ↓ duration), crack/freebase smoke inhalation (rapid onset, ↓ duration)
- **Method of action:** blocks reuptake of DA, NE, 5-HT, ↑ glutamate/aspartate in CNS, blocks Na^+ channels, ½ **life <60 min, metabolized in liver → benzoylecgonine (detected in urine 36 h after acute use, >7 d if chronic)**
- **Comorbid condition: depression, anxiety**, other psychiatric d/o, other SUD (including nicotine)
- ↑↑ **risk of use:** male, BPAD, BPD, other substance use, family hx SUD, never married/widowed/divorced

Signs of Intoxication (Curr Opin Neurobiol. 2001;11(2):250)
- **Short-term/immediate intoxication:** euphoria, ↑ confidence, ↑ energy/alertness, ↓ appetite, ↑ HR, ↑ BP, vasoconstriction/spasm, ↑ risk of psychosis (hallucinations, paranoia, delusions), ↑ anxiety/panic attacks, tics/tremors, insomnia, mydriasis, diaphoresis
- **Testing:** urine, saliva, hair, blood
- **Longer-term/extended daily use:** risk of viral infection, ↑ suicide, depression, cognitive problems

Signs of Withdrawal (Addiction. 1994;89(11):1477-1481)
- Few physical sx (muscle aches, chills) mostly mood/cognitive, within hours to days after ceasing heavy/prolonged use. Dysphoria +/− SI, fatigue, vivid/unpleasant dreams, insomnia/hypersomnia, ↑ appetite, psychomotor retardation/agitation

Treatment (Addiction. 2016;111(8):1337-1346)
- **Acute intoxication:** Supportive tx (HTN/MI risk), BZD for agitation/aggression, FGA/SGA for psychosis (should resolve within hours to days), avoid β-blockers (c/f unopposed α agonism)
- **Withdrawal:** supportive tx, inpatient hospitalization if SI
- **Addiction (stimulant use disorder, cocaine):** no FDA-approved medication for dependence, topiramate w/ mixed evidence. CBT, support groups

Health-Related Complications (Crit Care Clin. 2012;28(4):517-526)
- **Medical complications:** CP, arrhythmia, AV node block, ↑ QTc, MI (vasospasm), CVA/hemorrhage/coma, seizures, hemoptysis, fever, chest pain, asthma, PNA, resp. depression, nasal septum necrosis (chronic insuffltn), **pregnancy** → fetal hypoxia, placental abruption, ↓ birth weight, LV hypertrophy, urogenital malformation, CNS irritability
- **Adulterants:** levamisole → cutaneous vasculitis/necrosis, agranulocytosis. clenbuterol → hyperglycemia, hypokalemia

MARIJUANA USE

General Facts (drugabuse.gov, dea.gov, *Clin Pharmacokinet*. 2003:327-360)
- Most commonly used illicit, legal for medical use in 31 states (see medical MJ), rec use in 9 states, decriminalized in 22 states
- **Alternative names:** 420, Aunt Mary, Bud, Chronic, Dope, Gangster, Ganja, Grass, Hash, Herb, Kind, Mary Jane, Mota, Pot, Reefer, Sinsemilla, Skunk, Smoke, Swag, Trees, Weed
- **Common forms:** dried leaf/flower, hashish, concentrates (shatter, wax, oil, tincture), edibles (THC lipophilic, partially soluble in EtOH)
- **Method of use:** smoked, vaporized, dab (vaporizing concentrate), or consumed in edible form
- **Method of action:** THC → psychotropic lipophilic metabolite, CBD → nonpsychotropic metabolite, modulate endogenous cannabinoid system. Inhaled → maximum plasma conc. in minutes, psychotrop. effects in sec to min, max effect 15–30 min, last 2–3 h. Oral → effects in 30–90 min, max 2–3 h, last 4–12 h. Hepatic metabolism
- **Comorbid conditions:** high comorbidity with SCZ, SUD, mood/anxiety d/o
- **Risk of use:** male, younger age, less education, less income, other SUD, comorbid psychiatric d/o, ↓ age of 1st use + rate of progression to frequent use

Signs of Intoxication (*JAMA Psychiatry*. 2018;75(6):585)
- **Short-term use:** euphoric, pleasurable feeling, perceptual changes, time perception changes, ↑ appetite, ↑↓ anxiety/tension, paranoia, nausea, tachycardia, ↑ BP, ↑ RR, conjunctival injection, dry mouth, slurred speech. **Mod dose** → impaired motor coordination, attention/concentration, short-term mem., executive functioning. **High dose** → nausea, delirium, anxiety/panic, psychosis in some, can persist past initial high up to 12–24 h. **Children:** may present atypically, more likely to have severe toxicity w/ hyperkinesis or coma
- **Testing:** urine drug screen, UDS+ 10 d after weekly use, up to 25 d after daily use
- **Longer-term/extended daily use:** young adolescent use assoc w/ lower educational achievement + other substance use, frequent adolescent/young adult use assoc w/ small reduction in cognitive functioning, but not after 72 h abstinence. In adults, no neuropsych differences from nonusers after 1 mo abstinence

Signs of Withdrawal (*Subst Abuse Rehabil*. 2017;8:9)
- Within 1 wk of cessation/reduction heavy use: irritability, anger, anxiety, depression, poor sleep. Rare physical symptoms

Treatment (*Curr Pharm Des*. 2016;22(42):6409)
- **Acute intoxication:** mild → dim room, reassurance, can consider BZD. Severe → treat severe anxiety/agitation w/ BZD; consider other substance use/psychiatric d/o
- **Withdrawal:** for severe withdrawal, can use dronabinol, gabapentin, symptomatic support. CBT effective
- **Addiction (cannabis use disorder):** no FDA-approved med, psychosocial interventions, therapy: CBT, MI, mutual help groups

Health-Related Complications

- Chest pain → pneumothorax, exacerbation of underlying pulm dz, case reports of MI. Hyperemesis syndrome in chronic, daily users

---

MEDICAL MARIJUANA

Background

- Although cannabis remains illegal on a federal level, many states have legalized cannabis for recreational and medical use
- As of 2018, Guam, Puerto Rico + 31 states legalized medical MJ: AK, AZ, AR, CA, CO, CT, DE, FL, HI, IL, LA, ME, MA, MD, MI, MN, MT, NV, NH, NJ, NM, NY, ND, OH, OK, OR, PA, RI, VT, WA, WV
- Cannabis comes in different forms (oils, edibles, flowers, topical) and in varying potency

Definitions (Bot Rev. 2015;81:189; Adv Psychol. 2012;2:241)

- **Cannabis:** used broadly, describes organic products derived from plant genus, *Cannabis* (eg, hemp, MJ, cannabinoids), >400 chemical entities
- **Marijuana:** parts of cannabis plant or derivatives w/ considerable level of THC
- **Cannabinoids:** active chemicals in cannabis (eg, CBD, THC), >60 types
- **Hemp:** cannabis plants w/ low THC (<0.3%)
- **K2, Spice:** See "Synthetic Cannabinoids"

Mechanism of Action (Proc Natl Acad Sci USA. 1990;87(5):1932-1936; Ann N Y Acad Sci. 2006;1074:514-536.)

- 2 commonly studied for medicinal use: THC and CBD → Both w/ chemical structure similar to endogenous cannabinoid and act at cannabinoid receptors (CB1, CB2)
- CB1 and CB2 → CNS and CB2 → immune system
- CNS effects primarily through CB1 in basal ganglia, cerebellum, cerebral cortex, substantia nigra, hippocampus
- Linked to the ↓ release of GABA, NE, glutamate, DA, AcH

Cannabinoid-Based Medications

- Pharmaceutical companies created 3 primary drugs that make use of THC:
  - Nabilone—*Cesamet*
  - Dronabinol—*Marinol, Syndros*
  - Cannabidiol—*Epidiolex*

FDA Approved			
Generic Name	**Cannabidiol**	**Nabilone**	**Dronabinol**
Trade Name	*Epidiolex*	*Cesamet*	*Syndros* *Marinol*
Active ingredients	Concentrated CBD oil from *Cannabis* extract	Synthetic analogue of Δ^9-THC	Synthetic equivalent of Δ^9-THC
Clinical indication	• Seizures associated with Dravet and Lennox-Gastaut syndrome	• Assist with loss of appetite in AIDS patients • Nausea and vomiting associated with chemotherapy agents	
Class	Schedule I	Schedule II	Schedule III
Formulation	Oral solution	Oral capsule	Oral capsule (*Marinol*) Oral liquid (*Syndros*)

FDA Fast Track		
Generic Name	**Ajulemic Acid**	**Nabiximol**
Trade Name	*Anabasum (Formerly Resunab)*	*Sativex*
Active ingredients:	• Synthetic nonpsychoactive cannabinoid	• Ethanol cannabis extract of Δ^9-THC and cannabidiol in 1:1 ratio • Extraction of selected phenotype (clone)
Clinical indication:	As of July 2018: • Phase 1: inflammation • Phase 2: CF, dermatomyositis, SLE • Phase 3: systemic scleroderma	• Phase 3: cancer-related pain • Not approved in the US but approved in Canada for: neuropathic pain associated with MS + adjunctive analgesic to high-dose opioid tx for cancer pain
Formulation:	Oral	Sublingual/spray

METHAMPHETAMINE/STIMULANT USE

Background (*Annual Review of Public Health. 2010;31:385-398; J Psychiatry Neurosci. 2006;31(5):301-313. Curr Drug Abuse Rev. 2010;3(4):239-254; J Neurosci. 2001;21(23):9414-9418*)

- **Alternative names:** vary by region, generally distinguished by appearance/purity. Methamphetamines: *chalk, crank, crystal, ice, meth, speed.* Stimulants: *uppers*
- **Common forms:** Methamphetamine: usually white, bitter-tasting powder or pill. Stimulants: include prescription stimulant, MDMA, ephedrine, synthetic cathinones (bath salts), cocaine
- **Method of use:** both can be sniffed, smoked, injected, and/or taken orally
- **Mechanism of action:** variably ↑ release of DA, blocks reuptake/degradation, + ↑ DA synthesis → potential significant loss of DA transporters, ↑ BBB permeability, ↑ glutamate release
- Protracted abstinence (years) → near full return of DAT levels

Assessment (*Neuropsychopharmacology. 2012;37(3):586-608; J Anal Toxicol. 2016;40(1):37-42*)

- **Acute intoxication:** ↓ sleep, excitability, distractibility, euphoria, ↑ sexuality, anxiety, agitation, akathisia, hypervigilance, violent behavior. SI/HI. Delirium, psychosis
  - *Physical exam:* mydriasis, HTN, tachycardia, hyperthermia, diaphoresis, seizures, tremors, and myoclonus
- **Testing:** Utox (falsely + w/ bupropion, prozac, labetalol, trazodone, Vicks inhaler, ranitidine, high-dose pseudoephedrine) ECG: MI, cardiomyopathy, arrhythmias, BMP: dehydration
- **Long-term/extended daily use:** psychosis (delusions, paranoia hallucinations) may persist even in abstinence, depression/anxiety, persistent fatigue, cognitive impairment: some studies potential memory loss, deficits in executive + motor skills
  - *Physical exam:* "meth teeth"—rotting teeth d/2 chronic dry mouth, poor dental hygiene, bruxism, ↓ saliva; skin changes → acne + excoriations d/2 picking

Signs of Withdrawal (*J Neuropsychiatry Clin Neurosci. 2003;15(3):317-325*)

- No specific physical or life-threatening sx
- **Abstinence syndrome:** anhedonia, sleep issues, psychomotor retardation/agitation, concentration issues, irritability, hyperphagia, typically resolves in 1–4 wk → resolution likely d/2 recovery of stored dopamine, for chronic heavy users may persist for mos

Treatment (*Br J Clin Pharmacol. 2010;69(6):578-592. Neuropsychopharmacology. 2016;41(4):1179. Arch Gen Psychiatry. 2011;68(11):1168-1175. Drug Alcohol Depend. 2008;96(3):222-232. J Psychoactive Drugs. 2000;32(2):157-164*)

- **Acute:** supportive—acute agitation, anxiety, HTN, tachycardia → IV BZD, phentolamine, avoid β-blockers (c/f unopposed α agonism)
- **Long term:** Matrix Model 16 wk program, showed benefit, manualized CBT, individual therapy, social support groups, relapse prevention groups, drug testing + family education. No meds w/ consistent efficacy, some evidence for bupropion + mirtazapine

OPIOID USE DISORDER

Background (Drug Alcohol Depend. 2015;156:104)

- Prolonged use of opioids (prescribed or not) will produce tolerance and physiologic dependence → creates risk for OUD
- OUD is diagnosed by a problematic pattern of use despite consequences, cravings for opioids, and inability to control use
- Pts with OUD are at ↑ risk of morbidity and death d/2 risk of OD, medical complications, injury, suicide

    Method of use: opioids may be taken by mouth, smoked, insufflated, or injected

    Method of action: natural and synthetic agonist to endogenous mu, delta, + kappa opioid receptors in the CNS and PNS

Assessment (APA SUD Practice Guideline; 2006; J Med Toxicol. 2011;7:240)

- **History:** duration, amount, frequency, most recent use, forms + route, last use, longest period abstinent + how, treatment hx, social hx w/ triggers, dependents at risk; check prescription monitoring database if available
  - Medical risk: IN/IV use, sharing paraphernalia, needle licking, exchanging sex for drugs, body packing/stuffing, impaired driving
  - Co-occurring psychiatric + neurologic disorders (incl. hx TBI/anoxic brain injury), **SI/suicide attempt**
  - Readiness for change (precontemplation, contemplation, planning, action, maintenance)
- **Acute intoxication:** ↓ mental status, ↓ respiratory rate and tidal volume, ↓ bowel sounds, constricted pupils (confounded by co-ingestants); **signs of use:** track marks, abscesses, heart murmur, presence of fentanyl patches, injuries
- **Evaluate for medical complications of use:** cellulitis, abscess, osteomyelitis, endocarditis, sepsis, opioid-induced bowel syndrome, hyperalgesia syndrome, toxic leukoencephalopathy w/ inhaled vapor, rhabdo/compartment syndrome
- **Testing:** Utox + extended toxicology (eg, buprenorphine, fentanyl, co-ingestants; consider ECG (esp if methadone), HIV, HCV, renal fxn (risk of rhabdo), TB, STIs

Signs of Withdrawal

Piloerection, diaphoresis, rhinorrhea, lacrimation, tremor, pupil dilation, irritability, N/V/D, insomnia, aches, restlessness (Addiction. 1994;89:1471)

Treatment

Acute Intoxication/OD (N Engl J Med. 2012;367:146; J Toxicol Clin Toxicol. 1996;34:409; World J Emerg Med. 2010;1:75)

- **Naloxone IV** (INIM//SubQ if no IV access): supportive care in resp depression → Bag-mask ventilation before/during administration of naloxone; initial adult dose 0.04 mg IV in pts spontaneously breathing, ↑ doses q2-3 min if no response, titrating to RR > 12; > initial doses for apnea/arrest, *risks precipitated withdrawal, agitation, vomiting, cardiac arrhythmia, pulmonary edema*

- Lasts only 20–90 min, may require repeat dose/continuous infusion → if short-acting opioid → pt awake/alert w/ nl versus ≥ 4–6 h after last naloxone dose + before d/c; if long-acting/modified-release opioid → ↑ risk delayed respiratory depression → consider medical/ICU admission for observation
  - Children/elderly → atypical pharmacokinetics and may need extended monitoring
- Provide education + rescue naloxone; involve friends, family, and treaters
- Consider restriction of visitors or search of body/belongings if risk of in-hospital OD

Withdrawal (J Addict Behav Ther Rehabil. 2015;4:1000138; Am J Emerg Med. 2018 in press; Cochrane Database Syst Rev. 2009;8:CD002025; J Urban Health. 2003;80:189)
- Treat proactively to prevent AMA
- Offer MAT in house if appropriate f/u infrastructure exists, + refer to aftercare
- Can use opioid agonists (methadone, buprenorphine) or α-2 agonists (clonidine, lofexidine); opioid agonist > clonidine to ↓ sx + retain in tx
- Warn pt that **release from hospital/detox is risk factor for OD death** d/2 loss of tolerance ± long half-life of methadone
- Institutional protocols vary, often using Clinical Opioid Withdrawal Scale (COWS)

Clinical Opiate Withdrawal Scale (COWS)

Flow-sheet for measuring symptoms over a period of time during buprenorphine induction.

For each item, write in the number that best describes the patient's signs or symptoms. Rate on just the apparent relationship to opiate withdrawal. For example, if heart rate is increased because the patient was jogging just prior to assessment, the increase in pulse rate would not add to the score.

Enter scores at time zero, 30 min after 1st dose, 2 h after 1st dose, etc.

Resting Pulse Rate: (record beats per minute) *measured after patient is sitting or lying for 1 min*
0—pulse rate 80 or below
1—pulse rate 81–100
2—pulse rate 101–120
4—pulse rate greater than 120

Sweating: *over past ½ h not accounted for by room temperature or patient activity*
0—no report of chills or flushing
1—subjective report of chills or flushing
2—flushed or observable moistness on face
3—beads of sweat on brow or face
4—sweat streaming off face

Restlessness: *observation during assessment*
0—able to sit still
1—reports difficulty sitting still, but is able to do so
3—frequent shifting or extraneous movements of legs/arms
5—unable to sit still for more than a few seconds

Pupil Size:
0—pupils pinned or normal size for room light
1—pupils possibly larger than normal for room light
2—pupils moderately dilated
5—pupils so dilated that only the rim of the iris is visible

Bone or Joint Aches: *if patient was having pain previously, only the additional component attributed to opiates withdrawal is scored*
0—not present
1—mild diffuse discomfort
2—patient reports severe diffuse aching of joints/muscles
4—patient is rubbing joints or muscles and is unable to sit still because of discomfort

Runny Nose or Tearing: *not accounted for by cold symptoms or allergies*
0—not present
1—nasal stuffiness or unusually moist eyes
2—nose running or tearing
4—nose constantly running or tears streaming down cheeks

GI Upset: *over last ½ h*
0—no GI symptoms
1—stomach cramps
2—nausea or loose stool
3—vomiting or diarrhea
5—multiple episodes of diarrhea or vomiting

Tremor: *observation of outstretched hands*
0—no tremor
1—tremor can be felt, but not observed
2—slight tremor observable
4—gross tremor or muscle twitching

Yawning: *observation during assessment*
0—no yawning
1—yawning once or twice during assessment
2—yawning 3 or more times during assessment
4—yawning several times/minute

Anxiety or Irritability:
0—none
1—patient reports increasing irritability or anxiousness
2—patient obviously irritable anxious
4—patient so irritable or anxious that participation in the assessment is difficult

Gooseflesh Skin:
0—skin is smooth
3—piloerection of skin can be felt or hairs standing up on arms
5—prominent piloerection

Score:
5–12 = mild
13–24 = moderate
25–36 = moderately severe
more than 36 = severe withdrawal

Potential Detox Protocol Medication Management	
Sample inpt methadone protocol	**Day 1:** 10–20 mg 1st dose (PO) + 10 mg Q4H prn (PO); max 40 mg (if on BZDs: reduce day 1–10 mg PO Q6H) **Taper:** Take total received in 1st 24 h → ↓ by 20%/d or 5–10 mg/d. May split BID Notes: • QTc: Check ECG before + during 1st 24 h tx • Methadone TID = pain; QD = maintenance • For pts being dc'd to methadone clinic: D/C requires "Last Dose Letter" w/ date + dose received, sealed in enveloped signed across seal
Sample inpt buprenorphine protocol	**Day 1:** wait for COWS 8–10 (risk of precipitating withdrawal) → 4 mg 1st dose → 2 h after 1st dose, 2–4 mg Q6H prn, (if on BZDs: reduce day 1 to 2–4 mg Q8H PRN) max 16 mg/24 h **Taper:** Take total received in 1st 24 h → ↓ by 25%QD. Split to standing BID
Adjunctive "comfort meds"	**Autonomic sx:** clonidine 0.1–0.2 mg TID prn; watch BP (do not give with buprenorphine/methadone during 1st day dosing, will reduce COWS) **GI effects:** cramps—Bentyl 10–20 mg Q6h prn; dyspepsia—Maalox 30 cc Q4H prn (max 80 cc/24 h)/Zantac 150 mg BID; diarrhea—Imodium 4 mg × 1 + 2 mg Q2H prn **Anxiety/insomnia:** hydroxyzine, trazodone

Addiction/OUD Longitudinal Care (JAMA. 2016;315:1624)
- Goals of treatment will vary from complete abstinence to harm reduction, psychosocial treatments ± MAT → agonist MAT (buprenorphine/methadone) versus antagonist MAT (naltrexone)
- Psychosocial interventions with evidence for SUDs: CBT, motivation enhancement therapy (MET), 12-step facilitation (AA, NA), integrated tx for co-occurring d/p, group drug counseling, contingency management
- Random drug screening → assess use + tx adherence: relapse suggests need for ↑ level of care → d/c from tx w/ ↑ risk of OD death
- Education to pt + family about dx, risks (eg, inf → clean needle practices, prevention of OD) (see SAMHSA Opioid Overdose Toolkit: store.samhsa.gov)
- For harm reduction → rx for **rescue naloxone** and teaching on how to use it, incl. family and close contacts
- Pts discharged w/ opioid medication → give short scripts; advise use of lock box

Special Populations (Obstet Gynecol. 2012;119:1070; ACOG. 2017: Committee Opinion #711; Pediatrics. 2016;138:e20161893; Drug Alcohol Depend. 2017;174:9; NIDA. 2014 "Principles of Adolescent substance Use disorder treatment")

- **Pregnant patients:** Agonist MAT → withdrawal a/w poorer maternal and fetal outcomes
- **Children/adolescents:** buprenorphine FDA approved 16+ y/o, most evidence for Adolescent Community Reinforcement Approach (ACRA) and Assertive Continuing Care (ACC)

ACUTE PAIN MANAGEMENT IN OPIOID-DEPENDENT PTS
(Ann Intern Med. 2006;144:127)

- Maintenance MAT will **not** provide adequate control of acute pain
- Maximize nonopioid agents: NSAIDs, acetaminophen, topicals, TCAs
- On methadone maintenance:
  - Basal management → confirm dose w/ methadone program—continue maintenance dose divided to TID (If IM/subQ, give ½ maintenance dose)
  - Add scheduled short-acting opioids (not PRN). Will need > typical doses
  - For breakthrough pain—PRNs given for objective signs of pain (elevated SBP, elevated HR, appearing uncomfortable when not aware of being observed) → adjust standing opiate dose based on PRN use
- On buprenorphine maintenance, choose **one** of the following:
  - Divide daily dose into Q6-8H, ↑ dose until pain controlled (max 32 mg/d)
  - Continue buprenorphine home dose + add scheduled opioid for pain
  - D/C buprenorphine + utilize scheduled opioid → may require > doses as wears off D/2 partial agonism; monitor for sedation as final dose metabolized; reinduce once episode resolved (see buprenorphine, p. 6-42 to 6-46)

TOBACCO USE

General Facts (U.S. Dep of HHS. 2014; MMWR. 2018;67:53; Am J Prev Med. 2014;48:326)

- Leading cause of preventable death, > 480,000 deaths/y in the US
- Tobacco use disorder = use for >1 y + use of ↑ quantities over longer period than intended w/ tolerance + withdrawal upon cessation
- **Any tobacco use poses health risks + any decrease in use confers health benefits**. Encourage pts to cut back/quit whether they meet use disorder criteria or not
- $170 bil/y spent on medical care for smoking-related illnesses + $156 bil/y in lost productivity 2/2 premature death/disability
- ↓ Prevalence in the US; 20.9% in 2005 → 15.5% in 2016
- ~2100 youths/young adults per day convert from occasional to daily smokers
- **See Smoking Cessation chapter for treatment options**

Method of Use (Tob Regul Sci. 2017;3:101; Am J Health Behav. 2011;34:275; U.S. Dep of HHS. 2016; UCSF Ctr for Tob Ctrl Rsrch & Edu. 2018)

- **Smoking tobacco**
  Cigarettes: roll of tobacco wrapped in paper; most commonly used in the US; highly regulated, only flavor addition is menthol
  Cigars: roll of tobacco wrapped in tobacco leaves; regulated by FDA since 2016; variations in flavor/packaging; 3 varieties:
  - Large cigars: hand-rolled (premium) or machine-made (regular), often no filters or tips
  - Cigarillos (medium-sized): mostly machine-made, ± filters
  - Little cigars: predominantly filtered, sold in packs of 20
    Pipes: handheld device through which tobacco is smoked
    Water pipe (hookah, shisha): water-containing chamber through which lit tobacco is vaporized + inhaled; pose many of the same health risks as cigarettes
- **Smokeless tobacco**
  Chewing tobacco (chew, spit tobacco): shredded tobacco leaves held between gum + cheek, discarded by spitting
  Dry snuff (pinch, dip): finely ground tobacco that is snuffed
  Snus: moist snuff in packets held in mouth for absorption; designed so that spitting not required
- **Electronic nicotine delivery systems**
  E-cigarettes (vapes, JUULs): battery-powered devices that use cartridges w/ doses of nicotine for inhaling; do not contain tobacco; long-term health effects not known—↓ levels of carcinogens than cigarettes, ↑ levels of ultrafine particles + toxins linked to CVD + respiratory disease; likely cause increased use of tobacco + other substances in adolescents

Method of Action (Trends Pharmacol Sci. 2006;27:482; NIDA; Ann Rev Phamacol Toxicol. 2009;49:57)

- Nicotine binds nicotinic acetylcholine receptors; mediate cognition, reward, motor activity, analgesia
- ↑ dopamine levels + nucleus accumbens activity

Comorbid Conditions/Risk of Use (MMWR. 2018;67:53; MMWR. 2013;62:81; NASMHPD. 2006; Bipolar Disord. 2011;13:439; J Subst Abuse Treat. 2014;46:194; Clin Psychol Rev. 2010;30:12)

- Psychiatric risk factors:
  Schizophrenia: 70–85% smoking prevalence, 25-y life expectancy gap due mostly to CVD
  Bipolar affective disorder: 50–70% smoking prevalence
  Substance use disorders: 75–97% smoking prevalence among those enrolled in substance abuse treatment; evidence suggests that smoking cessation aids in recovery from other substances
- Demographic risk factors: ♂, age < 65, GED level of education, income < poverty line, American Indian/Alaska Native ethnicity

Signs of Use

- HTN, ↑ HR, ↑ respiratory rate, ↑ appetite, chronic cough, cigarette odor (hair, clothes, breath), yellow discoloration of teeth + nails, dry skin, hair loss/thinning

Signs of Withdrawal

- Anxiety, depression, irritability, restlessness, difficulty concentrating, headache, insomnia, ↑ appetite, weight gain, ↓ HR, + ↓ BP
- Peaks in first 3 d after quitting, subsides over 3–4 wk

Health-Related Complications

- On average, smokers die 10 y earlier than nonsmokers. For every person who dies 2/2 smoking, ≥30 are living w/ serious smoking-related illness
- Respiratory disease: **lung cancer**—smoking a/w ~90% deaths, **COPD**—smoking a/w ~80% deaths
- Vascular disease: **coronary heart disease**—2–4× risk in smokers, **stroke**—2–4× risk in smokers
- Linked to kidney, ureter, bladder, colon, rectal, esophageal, laryngeal, oropharyngeal, tracheal, bronchial, liver, pancreas, stomach, and cervical CA + AML
- Pregnancy: harder to become pregnant, linked to preterm delivery, stillbirth, low birth weight, SIDS, ectopic pregnancy, and orofacial clefts

Drug Interactions (Spec Pharm Serv. 2017; Am J Health Syst Pharm. 2007;64:1917; The Maudsley Prescribing Guidelines in Psychiatry. 12th ed; 2015)

- Tobacco smoke is a potent inducer of cytochrome P450, particularly CYP1A1 and CYP1A2 → medications metabolized in this path may require ↑ doses to achieve therapeutic effects versus if pt quits smoking may require ↓ dose to prevent toxicity

  Clozapine: smoking ↓ plasma levels by up to 50%; for patients who plan to start or stop smoking, obtain a baseline drug level + modify dose to target that level

  Olanzapine: smoking ↓ plasma levels; for patients who quit, consider ↓ dose by 25%

  Chlorpromazine: smoking ↓ plasma levels; for patients who quit monitor closely for side effects, consider ↓ dose if sedation, dizziness, or nausea

  Methadone: smoking may ↓ levels; for patients who quit monitor for side effects, consider ↓ dose if sedation

OTHER SUBSTANCES

BATH SALTS (DESIGNER CATHINONES OR SYNTHETIC STIMULANTS)

Overview (National Institute on Drug Abuse. 2015; online; DEA Drugs of Abuse. 2017; online. Life Sciences. 2014:27-30; Clinical Pharmacology and Therapeutics. 1994:556-562)

- CNS stimulants designed to mimic MDMA and cocaine, contain chemicals related to khat plant (cathinone)
- Marketed on web/in stores as household items (eg, plant food, glass cleaner) not for human consumption to evade DEA
- Packaging suggests ↑ doses → high risk of OD

- **Alternative names:** Bliss, Blue Silk, Cloud Nine, Drone, Energy-1, Ivory Wave, Lunar Wave, Meow Meow Pure Ivory
- **Common forms:** crystalline powder, tablet, capsule or liquid
- **Method of use:** most common = sniffing/snorting, also oral, smoked or injected
- **Method of action:** variable—different for each cathinone; cathinone (nonsynthetic) stimulates ↑ DA and ↓ reuptake of epinephrine, NE, and 5-HT w/ half-life 1.5–2 h; methylene = nonspecific MAO transporter and ↑ release of MAO similar to amphetamine/MDMA, MDPV ↓ uptake of DA, 5-HT + NE

Assessment (National Institute on Drug Abuse. 2015; online; DEA Drugs of Abuse. 2017; online, Pharmacy and Therapeutics. 2012;571-572, 595)
- **Signs of intoxication:**
  - Desired effects: euphoria, alertness, sociability, ↑ sex drive
  - Other psychoactive effects: confusion, panic, psychosis (paranoia/hallucinations/delusions), agitation, violence, headaches, palpations, aggressive behavior, self-destructive behavior
  - Peak effect is 1.5 h s/p ingestion + crash is usually 3–4 h after
- **Physical exam:** tachycardia, HTN, hyperthermia, diaphoresis, seizures
- **Testing:** not detected on routine toxicology screens
- **Long-term/extended daily use:** skeletal muscle breakdown leading to elevated CK, myocarditis; risk of kidney failure, death

Signs of Withdrawal
Depressive and anxious symptoms, difficulty sleeping, tremors, paranoia

Treatment (National Institute on Drug Abuse. 2015; online; DEA Drugs of Abuse. 2017; online, Pharmacy and Therapeutics. 2012;571-572, 595)
- **Acute intoxication:** Benzos—treat agitation and seizures. Avoid antipsychotics due to increased risk of seizure activity. Order ECG, CK, routine labs, and EEG if suspect seizure
- **Withdrawal:** No treatment known
- **Addiction:** No treatment known

DEXTROMETHORPHAN

Overview (J Pediatric Health Care. 2013:135-144; Clini Toxicol. 2007:662-677)
- OTC cough suppressant; D-isomer of codeine (does not bind opioid receptors)
- Causes dissociative + hallucinogenic properties at > therapeutic dose, similar to PCP/ketamine
- Commercial names: Robitussin, Coricidin. Used as adjunct labeled DM. **Alternative names:** Robotripping, Triple C, poor man's PCP, skittles, Purple Drank (w/ codeine)
- *High-risk co-ingestion* (formulated w/ other medications): + acetaminophen: acute liver failure, + chlorpheniramine: anticholinergic toxicity, + guaifenesin (Robitussin DM): N/V/D
- **Common forms:** Syrup, capsule
- **Method of use:** Oral
- **Method of action:** At recommended doses acts on cough center in medulla to elevate threshold for coughing. At high doses NMDA receptor antagonist and 5-HT reuptake inhibitor

Assessment (*J Pediatric Health Care.* 2013:135-144)
- **Signs of intoxication:**
  Dose dependent:
  - Recommended dose (15–30 mg up to 4× daily): drowsiness, dizziness, GI upset
  - 100–200 mg: mild stimulation
  - 200–400 mg: euphoria, hallucinations
  - 300–600 mg: distorted visual perceptions, loss of motor coordination
  - 500–1500 mg: dissociative sedation with similar effect to PCP, LSD, ketamine
- **Physical exam:** nystagmus, dilated pupils, rash, diaphoresis, ataxia, fever, hypertension, shallow respiration, urinary retention, opisthotonos (spasm w/ head and heels bent back and the torso bent forward), tachycardia, hyperthermia
- **Testing:** May cause false + PCP utox
- **Long-term/extended daily use:** risk of addiction and of cognitive dysfunction

Signs of Withdrawal (*National Institute on Drug Abuse.* 2015; online; *DEA Drugs of Abuse.* 2017; online)
Unknown

Treatment (*Clin Toxicol.* 2007:662-677; *National Institute on Drug Abuse.* 2015; online)
- **Acute intoxication:** Activated charcoal can be administered <1 h after ingestion. If sedated or in a coma, give naloxone at high doses
- **Withdrawal:** Treat symptoms, which may include craving, nausea, diaphoresis, tachycardia
- **Addiction:** No approved medication or behavioral treatment

---

GAMMA-HYDROXYBUTYRIC ACID (GHB)

Overview (*National Institute on Drug Abuse.* 2015; online; *DEA Drugs of Abuse.* 2017; online)
- Same as sodium oxybate (Xyrem), prescription med approved for tx of narcolepsy; analogues: gamma butyrolactone (GBL) and 1,4-butanediol (BD) = industrial solvents
- Also sold as supplements marketed for various indications and as "ink stain remover" or "nail enamel remover" for $100 per bottle
- Used in sexual assault d/2 ability to ↑ libido, suggestibility, passivity + amnesia
- Use also for belief GHB + analogues build muscle + cause weight loss
- **Alternative names:** Easy Lay, G, Georgia Home Boy, Grievous Bodily Harm, Liquid Ecstasy, Liquid X, Scoop, Goop
- **Common forms:** Colorless liquid or white powder to be dissolved
- **Method of use:** Swallowed
- **Method of action:** It is a CNS depressant, GHB receptor agonist + weak $GABA_B$ agonist; takes effect in 15–30 min + lasts 3–6 h

Assessment (*National Institute on Drug Abuse.* 2015; online; *DEA Drugs of Abuse.* 2017; online)
- **Signs of intoxication:**
  - Desired effects—euphoria and decreased anxiety
  - Other psychoactive effects—drowsiness, confusion, visual hallucinations, paradoxical excited and aggressive behavior

- In high doses—unconsciousness, seizures (esp. w/ meth co-use), vomiting, nausea, coma, death
- **Physical exam:** respiratory depression, bradycardia, hypothermia
- **Testing:** not detected on routine toxicology screens
- **Long-term/extended daily use:** Regular use can lead to addiction

Signs of Withdrawal
Insomnia, anxiety, tremor, tachycardia, HTN, psychosis

Treatment (National Institute on Drug Abuse. 2015; online; DEA Drugs of Abuse. 2017; online)

- **Acute intoxication:** Intubation is needed to protect airway. Benzodiazepine for seizures. CXR if concern for aspiration
- **Withdrawal:** No treatment known
- **Addiction:** No treatment known

INHALANTS

Overview (Pediatrics. 2007;119:1010; Subst Use Misuse. 2010;45:1335; Addict Sci Clin Pract. 2011;6:19)

Formulations			
	Common Forms	**Alternative Names**	**Methods of Use**
Volatiles	• Solvents (toluene, alkanes, halocarbons): paint thinner, rubber cement, industrial glue, correction fluids, wood finishes, marker tips, spray paint • Fuels: gasoline, propane, kerosene, butane • Aerosol propellants (butane, propane, ethers, halocarbons): air duster, hair spray, cooking sprays, deodorant, spray paint, medical inhalers • Anesthetics: halocarbons such as sevoflurane	Glue, whiteout, spray, air blast, bang, hardware	• Sniffing/snorting • Bagging: placement of inhalant into bag to concentrate large gas volume, associated with morbidity/mortality • Dusting: spraying aerosol directly into nose or mouth • Huffing: placement of inhalant-soaked rag over mouth/nose, also associated with morbidity/mortality • "Snot balls": inhaling fumes off heated rubber cement
Nitrous oxide	Whipped cream, cooking spray, propellant, diverted medical anesthetic	Laughing gas, whippets, buzz bomb	• Inhaled via spacers such as bags, balloons, or refillable dispensers because of cold gas temperature

Formulations *(continued)*			
	Common Forms	**Alternative Names**	**Methods of Use**
Nitrites	Former angina drug, now manufactured for recreational use, billed as cleaning agents or room odorizers	Poppers, snappers, also referred to by brand names (ex, rush, bolt)	• Sniffing from open container or "snapped" glass vials • Huffing

Method of Action *(Clin Toxicol. 2014;52:480; Pharmacotherapy. 2004;24:74-75)*
• Volatiles/N_2O: CNS depressant via positive modulation of GABA-A receptor, NMDA inhibition, affects dopamine + opioid systems. CNS half-life of inhaled toluene is ~20 min, but persists in peripheral fat
• Nitrites: Source of NO, produces smooth + skeletal muscle relaxation w/ vasodilation + feeling of warmth; inhaled half-life < 2 min

Comorbid Conditions/Risk of Use/Epidemiology *(J Stud Alcohol Drugs. 2010;71:205; Addict Behav. 2008;33:970; JAMA Psychiatry. 2016;73: suppl; Drug Alcohol Depend. 2007;88:149; Addict Sci Clin Pract. 2011;6:22)*
• In the US, ~ 10% lifetime use, median onset between 6th and 9th grade; use ↓ after 8th grade, increasing proportion of nitrite and nitrous oxide use in adulthood. 0.2–0.6% community adolescents met criteria for abuse/dependence over past year, ↓ to 0.04% by adulthood
• ↑ rates of solvent/disorder in justice-involved juveniles, American Indian/Alaska Native youth; associated with low SES, especially rural poverty; nitrite use prevalent among men who have sex with men (MSM)
• Comorbidities include MDD, anxiety, conduct/antisocial personality disorders, disordered eating, other SUD, particularly alcohol, marijuana, and stimulants/cocaine; associated with childhood trauma, parental substance use and criminality, personal history of suicidality and interpersonal violence

Signs of Intoxication *(Br J Pharmacol. 2008;154:320; Pediatrics. 2007;119:1011-1014; Clin Toxicol. 2007;45:557-558)*
• **Short-term use/immediate intoxication**
  • CNS depression: initial euphoria, disinhibition progressing to drowsiness as dose increases, with slurred speech, ataxia, tremor, nystagmus (dizziness, blurred vision), visual hallucinations, can progress to seizures, obtundation
  • Mucosal irritation: red, glassy eyes; rhinorrhea/epistaxis, dyspnea, wheezing, nausea/vomiting, perioral or perinasal erythema
  • Inhalant residue: chemical odor on breath, stains on skin or clothing
  • Nitrites: sensations of warmth, headache, flushing, dizziness due to vasodilation and hypotension, may be associated with tachycardia, syncope

- **Testing:** No routine drug screen for inhalants; specialized urine screens detect benzene + toluene. Other lab evaluation includes CMP, calcium, phosphate, CBC, troponin, CK, ABG, urine and serum toxicology to assess other substance use, EKG, CXR (aspiration risk), consider MRI brain if chronic use
- **Longer-term/extended daily use**
  - Common: frequent headache, constitutional symptoms (fatigue, weakness, erratic sleep, anorexia/weight loss), persistent epistaxis/rhinorrhea and sinusitis, "huffer's rash"—perioral/nasal dermatitis with pyoderma, apathy, cognitive slowing, global decline in function
  - Specific neurologic signs: cerebellar or cranial nerve deficits (hearing loss, optic neuropathy), peripheral neuropathy, cognitive deficits (inattention, dysexecutive features, impaired memory, decreased processing speed)
  - Collateral information: stockpiling and storage of inhalants, discarded containers, longitudinal changes in behavior and functioning

Signs of Withdrawal (Subst Abuse Rehabil. 2011;2:71)

- No withdrawal syndrome defined in DSM, most commonly reported symptoms are nonspecific including fatigue, nausea, hypersomnia, anxiety; however, sweating, palpitations, tremor, hallucinations also significantly associated with DSM-IV dependence, may resemble GABA-ergic withdrawal

Treatment (Addiction. 2012;107:280-285; AFP. 2003;68:873; Int J Drug Policy. 2016;31:20; CNS Drugs. 2012;28:931-932)

- **Acute intoxication**
  - No antidote, supportive care, decontamination if extensive skin coverage, prevent self-injury i/s/o AMS
  - Monitor cardiorespiratory status: most common cause of death is arrhythmia; prevention w/ beta-blocker, electrolyte correction, avoid unnecessary stimulation/restraint (startle thought to provoke arrhythmia via catecholamine surge), prevent aspiration
  - Methylene blue if nitrite methemoglobinemia, NAC for large-volume hepatotoxin exposure (ie, chloroform, carbon tetrachloride)
- **Withdrawal:** Case studies have reported successful management w/ BZDs/baclofen
- **Inhalant use disorder:** Education of acute + long-term dangers of use; small studies suggest efficacy for CBT, MI, family therapy, 12-step facilitation, and structured group activity programs (employment, skills training) in adolescent inhalant abuse. Case reports explore lamotrigine, aripiprazole, and buspirone tx

Health-Related Consequences (Clin Toxicol. 2014;52:481-484; BMC Emer Med. 2015;19:3; Pharmacotherapy. 2004;24:73-76; Br J Pharmacol. 2008;154:321; Addict Sci Clin Pract. 2011;6:25)

- **Cardiovascular:** Ventricular arrhythmias, leading cause of death; sensitization of myocardium to catecholamines by volatile hydrocarbons, can occur with 1st use; cardiomyopathy w/ chronic use. Nitrites may interact w/ PDE5 inhibitors (ie, sildenafil) to produce life-threatening hypotension

- **Neuropsychiatric:** *Dementia*; marked deficits in processing speed, attention, and executive function, associated with subcortical white matter injury; may be associated with cerebellar deficits, *cranial and peripheral neuropathies*. Inhalant abuse can cause and elevate future risk of chronic mood and psychotic disorders. Chronic nitrous oxide use is associated with B12 deficiency
- **Respiratory:** Mortality from aspiration, laryngeal edema, and laryngospasm due to local irritant effect; chronic emphysematous changes have been reported
- **Renal:** Toluene → metabolic acidosis, hypokalemia 2/2 renal tubular dysfunction, may potentiate cardiotoxicity + precipitate rhabdomyolysis; acute renal failure is common, decline in function may become chronic
- **Hematologic:** Benzene associated with aplastic anemia, leukemia; inhaled nitrites may trigger hemolysis in G6PD-deficient populations, can cause methemoglobinemia; controversial association with viral cancers and immunosuppression
- **Hepatic:** Mild biliary tract injury acutely, hepatic failure, hepatic and biliary tract carcinomas associated with chronic hydrocarbon exposure
- **Use in pregnancy:** Increased rates of preterm birth and spontaneous abortion; facial deformities, stunted growth, and cognitive/behavioral deficits similar to fetal alcohol syndrome

KETAMINE

Overview (DEA. 2013; "Ketamine" in Drug & Chemical Evaluation Section, Drug Alcohol Dep. 2008;95(3):219-229; Hum Psychopharmcol. 2012;27(2):145-149)
- **Alternative names:** K, Special K, Vitamin K, Kit Kat, Cat Valium, Kiddy Smack, Purple, Jet; when dissociated: K-hole, K-land, baby food
- **Common forms:** Liquid, white powder
- **Method of use:** Snorted, smoked (powder added to tobacco or MJ cigarettes), injected, orally ingested
- **Method of action:** NMDA receptor antagonist, weak agonist of μ-opioid, κ-opioid, and D2 receptors
- **Comorbid conditions/risk of use:** ↑ risk of adverse effects when combined w/ EtOH; can be used as a date rape drug
- Recreational use emerged in the 1970s, occurs in the dance and rave scene; emergence of methoxetamine with similar profile, ↑ duration and intensity
- Used as anesthetic and in treatment-resistant depression (see ketamine under medications, p. 6-11)

Assessment (J Anal Toxicol. 2005;29(5):376-382; Int J Addict. 1990;25:133-139)
- **Short-term use/immediate intoxication:** dream-like dissociated state; hallucinations; ego diffusion; impaired attention, learning, and memory; confusion, sedation, numbing, dizziness; ataxia/immobility, dysarthria, arrhythmia/palpitations, HTN, tremor, abdominal discomfort, nausea/vomiting, in extreme cases sedation leading to respiratory suppression
- **Testing:** Utox up to 2 d after use (14 d for norketamine); quetiapine → false +

- **Longer-term/extended daily use:** limited evidence; ↓ working + episodic memory, ↓ executive function, and psychological well-being (depression, ↑ delusional + dissociative sx); may be reversible upon cessation

Signs of Withdrawal (Addiction. 2006;101(8):1212-1213; NIDA. 2018; in Club Drugs Section)

- Physical withdrawal symptoms are rare in ketamine use and not well studied
- Some case reports suggest withdrawal symptoms of fatigue, poor appetite, drowsiness, craving, anxiety, dysphoria, restlessness, palpitations, tremor, sweating

Treatment (Addict Behav. 2014;39(8):1215-1216; DEA. 2013; "Ketamine" in Drug & Chemical Evaluation Section)

- **Acute intoxication:** Containment and supportive care; close monitoring of cardiopulmonary status, duration of dissociative effects usually 30–60 min
- **Addiction:** No FDA-approved medications. Some studies suggest use of naltrexone given NMDA + opioid receptor mechanism

Health-Related Complications (BJU Int. 2012;110(11):1762-1766; Addiction. 2012;107(1):27-38; NIDA. 2018; in Club Drugs Section, Addiction. 2009;104(1):77-87)

- Urinary frequency, urgency, incontinence, bladder pain and ulcers, hematuria, hydronephrosis and renal impairment, renal papillary necrosis, abdominal pain
- Risk of HIV, hepatitis, and other infections from shared needles

---

MDMA

Overview (National Institute on Drug Abuse. 2015; online; DEA Drugs of Abuse. 2017; online)

- 3,4-Methylenedioxy-methamphetamine
- Synthetic chemical w/ stimulant + hallucinogenic properties
- Metabolized by the liver (CYP 2D6), poor metabolism may cause fatality. 12–36 h half-life
- Can inhibit own metabolism if reconsumed soon after initial ingestion → OD
- **Alternative names:** Molly, Ecstasy, Clarity, Disco Biscuit, E, Eve, Go, Hug Drug, Lover's Speed, XTC, X, STP, Peace, Adam, Beans
- **Common forms:** Most commonly colorful tablets w/ imprinted symbol indicating type. Sold for $20–25 per tablet. Tablets often contain added substances (methamphetamine, ketamine, cocaine, dextromethorphan, ephedrine, caffeine, PCP, heroin). Other forms include capsules, powder, liquid
- **Method of use:** swallowed, snorted, and occasionally smoked. Often taken with other substances ("stacked")
- **Method of action:** Enhances norepinephrine, dopamine, and serotonin release and/or blocks reuptake of these neurotransmitters. Greater serotonin release than stimulants, which is seen in effect of euphoria

Assessment (*National Institute on Drug Abuse. 2015; online; DEA Drugs of Abuse. 2017; online*)

- **Signs of intoxication:** Occurs within 30–45 min of ingestion, lasts approximately 4–6 h, side effects can persist for days. Euphoria/sense of well-being, feelings of closeness, empathy, ↑ sensory perception, distorted time perception, ↑ sexuality. Unwanted effects can include confusion, anxiety, panic, depressed mood, paranoia, insomnia
- Physical exam: tachycardia, hypertension, seizures, hyperactivity, muscle cramping, jaw clenching, tremor, nausea, chills, sweating, blurred vision, **hyperthermia** (2/2 inability to thermoregulate @ high doses) → multiorgan failure/death, **dehydration** 2/2 hyperthermia + crowded, hot conditions where used
- **Testing:** urine, serum + saliva, cross reacts w/ amphetamines, not routinely tested, CMP (dehydration risk, excess water intake, AKI), LFT, CK, ECG
- **Long-term/extended daily use:** use over multiple days = depressed mood, irritability, impaired attention and memory, anxiety. Chronic use 2+ years ↑ risk of permanent cognitive change, primarily memory + learning

Signs of Withdrawal (*National Institute on Drug Abuse. 2015; online; DEA Drugs of Abuse. 2017; online*)

- Reports of cravings. Depression, anxiety, irritability

Treatment (*National Institute on Drug Abuse. 2015; online; DEA Drugs of Abuse. 2017; online*)

- **Acute intoxication:** Address hyperthermia, BZD for seizures, agitation, supportive measures
- **Withdrawal:** No treatment known to mitigate sx
- **Addiction:** More research needed. CBT and behavioral techniques. No approved medication

---

SYNTHETIC CANNABINOIDS

Overview (*National Institute on Drug Abuse. 2015; online; DEA Drugs of Abuse. 2017; online; Curr Psychiatr. 2011;49-57*)

- Designer drugs (nonorganic drugs created in a laboratory) that mimic THC
- Available in gas stations, convenience stores, and online; often branded as a "legal," "safe" alternative to MJ or "herbal incense" or "potpourri" and labeled as not for human consumption to evade law enforcement
- Manufacturers seek to evade legislation banning certain synthetic cannabinoid homologues by creating new synthetic cannabinoids not yet banned, though can be charged via Controlled Substance Analogue Act
- **Alternative names:** Spice, K2, Synthetic MJ, Black Magic/Mamba, Aroma, Scooby Snax, Blaze, Crazy Clown, Fire, Paradise, Demon, Spike, Mr. Nice Guy, RedX Dawn, Ninja, Dream, Genie, Sense, Smoke, Skunk, Cherry Bomb, Chrome, Dr Feel Good, Cowboy Kush, Crystal Skull
- **Common forms:** Chemical is created in powder form, dissolved in solvent, and applied to plant material (to appear as MJ) or concentrated liquid

- **Method of use:** Smoked or vaporized
- **Method of action:** Full agonist of THC CB1 receptor, affinity + potency is usually higher than for THC

Assessment (*National Institute on Drug Abuse. 2015; online; DEA Drugs of Abuse. 2017; online; Curr Psychiatr. 2011;49-57*)

- **Signs of intoxication:** Onset within 10 min, lasts up to 6 h, elevated mood, relaxation, increased appetite
- Adverse/unwanted psychoactive effects include paranoia, hallucinations, anxiety, agitation, SI, SIB
- Physical exam: tachycardia, HTN, tremors, vomiting, AMS
- **Testing:** Not found in standard drug screens 2/2 structural difference from THC/metabolites, rapid metabolism ↓ detection, ECG ± cardiac enzymes, renal function (reports of AKI requiring HD)
- **Long-term/extended daily use:** Case reports of psychosis persisting weeks/months after use, exacerbation of existing psychotic disorder

Signs of Withdrawal (*National Institute on Drug Abuse. 2015; online; DEA Drugs of Abuse. 2017; online; Curr Psychiatr. 2011;49-57*)

- Headaches, anxiety, depression, irritability
- Thought to cause more cravings than MJ

Treatment (*National Institute on Drug Abuse. 2015; online; DEA Drugs of Abuse. 2017; online; Curr Psychiatr. 2011;49-57*)

- **Acute intoxication:** BZD for agitation/seizures, supportive measures
- **Withdrawal:** No treatment known to mitigate symptoms, headache management
- **Addiction:** More research needed

Health-Related Complications (*National Institute on Drug Abuse. 2015; online; DEA drugs of abuse. 2017; online; Curr Psychiatr. 2011;49-57*)

- Complications/death related to contaminants including psychoactive plants, alkaloids, synthetic opioids, MI, Seizure

DEEP BRAIN STIMULATION (DBS)

Indications
- **Severe, drug- and therapy-resistant OCD** (FDA-approved 2009)
  - Many other potential psychiatric applications are being investigated
- Also approved for Parkinson disease (PD), essential tremor, and dystonia

Basics (F1000Res. 2018;7:699; World Neurosurg. 2018;110:133-144)
- **Definition:** invasive neuromodulation using a battery-powered pulse generator implanted in the chest, with leads stereotactically implanted in the brain, generally bilaterally
- Focal, reversible, titratable neuromodulation; an alternative to ablative psychosurgical tx
- **Mechanism:** Likely disrupts/inhibits/overrides pathological activity in cortico-striato-pallido-thalamo-cortical (frontolimbic) circuits (cortical regions thought to be involved include orbitofrontal, medial prefrontal, and cingulate)
- **Targets in OCD** have included ventral capsule/striatum, anterior limb of internal capsule, nucleus accumbens, subthalamic nucleus

Implementation (MGH Psychiatry Update & Board Prep. 4th ed.; 2018:Ch51; Arch Gen Psychiatry. 1999;56:121)
- **Candidacy:** Multidisciplinary evaluation by psychiatry, neurology, and neurosurgery
  - Certain dx? Adeq med and therapy trials? Illness duration? (OCD tends to ↓ with age)
  - Capacity to ↓ accept risks/benefits?
  - Contraindication? (pregnant, has pacer/defib, antisoc PD, SUD <6 mo sober, acute psychosis)
  - General medical clearance for surgery?
- **Stereotactic implantation** of leads and pulse generator by neurosurgery
- **Calibration and control:** Portable, wireless appliance held near pulse-generator in chest. Psychiatrist or neurologist titrates stim (freq, voltage, pulsewidth) q2wk to effect (~3–12 mo). Pt may be allowed to control device w/i clinician-set params. Battery life prior to need for pulse generator replacement is ~3–5 yr; rechargeable models up to 9 yr

Efficacy (PLoS One. 2015;10:e0133591; World Neurosurg. 2013;80:S27.e17-e24; F1000Res. 2018;7:699; Parkinsons Dis. 2017:3256542)
- **OCD:** response (ie, Y-BOCS ↓ by >35%) in >60% of pts, *regardless of brain target*
- **MDD:** unapproved; ↑ mood in OCD and PD pts noted in early trials; small MDD studies have shown clinical response in >50% of pts; however, RCTs have been contradictory
- **Tourette syndrome:** unapproved; 52% ↓ tic severity in meta-analysis including open-label trials; however, RCTs have been contradictory
- **Parkinson disease:** (+ effective for mvmt sx, disability, QOL) Unclear effect on PD psychosis. Psychosis may be a potential adverse effect of DBS, but there are ongoing studies of DBS for SCZ

Complications (MGH Psychiatry Update & Board Prep. 4th ed.; 2018:Ch51; *Neurology.* 2006;66:983; *World Neurosurg.* 2017;97:603-634; *Neurosurg Focus.* 2015;38:E5; *Lancet Neurol.* 2006;5:578; *Front Pharmacol.* 2014;5:139; *Front Neuroeng.* 2014;7:9)

- **Periop (5–10%):** bleed, infection, injury to other structures (eg, sensory nrvs), HA, seizure
- **Device (~10%):** discomfort of pulse generator or leads in head/neck/chest, lead misplacement or migration, other hardware malfunction
- **Stimulus:** hypomania; anxiety, depression, SI (upon cessation); disinhibition (eg, sex, gambling); ?psychosis; palilalia; GI sx (N/V/D); flushing.
- **Glial scar** around leads may chronically blunt efficacy and cause/worsen neuroinflamm inj

Future Directions (*F1000Res.* 2018;7:699; *Brain Stimul.* 2017;10:664-671; *Neurosurg Focus.* 2008;25:E3; *World Neurosurg.* 2018;110:133-144; *Exp Neurol.* 2017;287:461-472)

- **?Tx of** MDD, BPAD, SCZ, anorexia, SUD, PTSD, Tourette syndrome, dementia, epilepsy

Possible targets for these potential applications include:
- *MDD:* subgenual cingulate cortex, ventral capsule/striatum, nucleus accumbens, superolateral medial-forebrain-bundle, inferior thalamic peduncle, lateral habenula
- *Tourette syndrome:* centromedian-parafascicular complex, dorsomedial, ventroanterior, and ventrolateral thalamus; posteroventral and anteromedial globus pallidus internus
- *PTSD:* basolateral amygdala
- *Dementia:* mammillothalamic and mammillotegmental tracts
- "Closed-loop" **stimulator** that dynamically reads and responds to real-time brain activity

ELECTROCONVULSIVE THERAPY (ECT)

Introduction (*Am J Psychiatry.* 2000;157:44)
- Highest rates of response and remission of antidepressant therapies (70–90%)
- Remission rate may be somewhat lower outside of clinical trials, where other factors are less controlled (*Biol Psychiatry.* 2004;55:301-312)
- Considered to be safe during pregnancy (*Obstet Gynecol.* 2009;114(3):703)

Pre-ECT Evaluation (*American Psychiatric Assoc: The Practice of ECT;* 2001)
- Hx/Px by ECT team to verify treatment is indicated, medical evaluation to assess ECT risk
- Indication for ECT related to level of clinical urgency, medication treatment failure, and likelihood of clinical response

Indications for ECT	
First-line therapy *(high acuity)*	Affective d/o w/ psychosis (esp. postpartum)
	Malignant catatonia (including NMS)
	Life-threatening/intolerable SE to meds in moderate-severe illness
	Severe affective episodes req. acute care
	Consider if pt had previous response to ECT
Second-line therapy *(medication failure)*	Medication treatment failure in: • Affective d/o w/o psychosis • Schizophrenia • Some cases of depression/psychosis from med. Illness • Nonmalignant catatonia • Parkinson disease
Last resort *(treatment resistance)*	Treatment resistant: • Dyskinesias • Tourette syndrome • Epilepsy • OCD

See also: *American Psychiatric Association: The Practice of Electroconvulsive Therapy: Recommendations for Treatment, Training, and Privileging*; 2001.

- **Workup:** CBC, CMP, TSH, hCG, ECG; poss. anesthesia c/s
- Delay ECT and seek cardiology c/s if pt has unstable angina, decompensated HF, severe valvular dz

Contraindications to ECT		
N.B. There are no absolute contraindications to ECT		
Strong relative	*Contraindication*	*Timeframe*
	High ICP	Active
	Intracerebral tumor	Active
	Pheochromocytoma	Active
	Cerebral aneurysm	Active
	AVM	Active
	CVA	w/in 3 mo
	MI	w/in 3 mo

(continued)

Contraindications to ECT (continued)		
Other relative	Category	Conditions
	Cardiac d/o	Arrhythmia, unstable angina, myocardial insufficiency, valve abnl, aortic aneurysm
	Neurologic d/o	Intracranial masses, bleeding, ischemia, inflammation, hydrocephalus (incl. NPH), head trauma, craniotomy
	Medical d/o	Clotting abnormality, severe liver or pulm dz (anesthesia risk), esophageal hernia (anesthesia risk, req. intubation)

Preparation for ECT (Am J Psychiatry. 2000;157:44-46)
- **General:** NPO after MN except essential meds (esp. BP meds), VS PM and AM before tx, acetaminophen 1000 mg PO ×1, remove metal objects before tx, void ×1
- **Specific medications:**
  - *Anticonvulsants:* ↓ dose by 50%, then downtaper during admission
  - *Lithium:* d/c night before treatment, then hold acutely
  - *BZDs and weak AEDs:* d/c day prior to treatment, caution with benzodiazepines (monitor for withdrawal, may require taper)
  - *Oral hypoglycemics, SA insulin:* hold AM of treatment (J ECT. 2002;18(1):16)
  - *Warfarin:* d/c if INR >3.5 + CHA_2DS_2-VASc ≤1 (Mayo Clin Proc. 2004;79(11):1936)
  - *β-blocker:* consider atropine w/ induction (Arq Bras Cardiol. 2002;79:149)

Management of Medical Comorbidities in ECT	
Asthma/COPD	Discontinue/downtaper theophylline Continue outpatient bronchodilators/glucocorticoids Provide bronchodilators for asthma exacerbation
Takotsubo cardiomyopathy	Catecholamine surge increases risk during procedure Appropriate cardiac mgmt., involving cardiology May consider β-blockers for cardioprotection
Hypertension	Use medications to manage BP β-blockers sometimes used
ICD	Turn off during ECT (to maintain device's lifetime)
Pacemaker	Keep magnet at bedside
Anticoagulation	Maintain INR ≤3.5
Pregnancy	Consultation with obstetrician and anesthesiologist Noninvasive fetal monitoring if >14–16 wk Nonstress testing if >24 wks

From Mayo Clin Proc. 2007;82:1360; J Clin Psychopharmacol. 1988;8:153; Pacing Clin Electrophysiol. 2004;27:1257; Mayo Clin Proc. 2004;79:1396

Safety and Treatment Course of ECT (Am J Psychiatry. 2000;157:45)
- Very safe (2–4 deaths per 100k treatments) (Convuls Ther. 1997;13(3):125)
- **Administration:** electrodes are placed right unilaterally, bifrontally, or bitemporally/bilaterally (right unilateral and bifrontal may be a/w ↓ cognitive side effects) and an electrical current is used to induce a seizure (typically lasting <60 s) (Br J Psychiatry. 2010;196(3):226-234; Am J Psychiatry. 2012;169:1238-1244)
- **Adverse medical effects:** aspiration PNA, headache (common), nausea, cardiovascular (transient ↑ HR and BP, takotsubo cardiomyopathy), fracture (bone and teeth; low risk) (APA Practice of ECT; 2001)
- **Adverse cognitive effects:** postictal confusion (<60 m), ECT-related delirium (var.), and post-ECT confusion due to prolonged partial seizure (var.); anterograde amnesia (<2 wk), retrograde amnesia (can be wks-mos prior to ECT); 50–80% will report some memory loss; reversible in large majority (99%) of cases (BMJ. 2003;326(7403):1363)
- **Treatment course:** typical acute course of ECT is 2–3×/wk until symptoms improve (~6–12 treatments); 2×/wk vs. 3×/wk have comparable efficacy; continue treatments until remission/plateau or limiting adverse effects; risk of relapse lower with maintenance ECT + pharmacotherapy after acute course; cognitive effects minimal during maintenance ECT (J ECT. 2013;29(2):86)
- **Outcomes:** overall, ECT is a highly efficacious treatment with remission rates of more than 80% (N Engl J Med. 2007;357(19):1939-1945); specific predictors correlated with treatment response include:
  - Higher response rates: shorter depressive episodes, depression with psychotic features, and older age
  - Lower response rates: medication failure during current mood episode (J Clin Psychiatry. 2015;76(10):1374-1384)
- **Special populations—children and adolescents:** to be a candidate for ECT, AACAP guidelines recommend children/adolescents (1) meet criteria for a severe mood disorder, a psychotic spectrum disorder, catatonia, or NMS; (2) have symptoms that are severe/persistent and impairing, or life-threatening; and (3) have failed at least 2 adequate medication trials. Laws vary by state/country regarding ECT consent practices; process may require independent evaluations by multiple physicians (J Am Acad Child Adolesc Psychiatry. 2004;43(12):1521-1539)

TRANSCRANIAL MAGNETIC STIMULATION

Introduction (Lancet. 1985;1(8437):1106-1107)
- A noninvasive and anatomically selective form of brain stimulation
- Application of powerful, rapidly changing magnetic field over the skull alters excitability of neurons in underlying cortical surface without inducing seizure
- Direct effects on superficial cortical neurons lead to changes in functionally connected brain regions (indirect effects)
- FDA approved for treatment-resistant depression (TRD) without psychosis

Treatment Parameters (*Brain Stim.* 2013;6(1):1-13; *Clin Neurophysiol.* 2009;120(12):2008-2039)

- **Brain region targeted (ie, R dlPFC):** Location, depth from skull, and size of target region determine TMS coil type, positioning, and pulse intensity
- **Desired effects on neuronal population:** Low frequency (lf, 1 Hz) stimulation inhibits neurons in ROI, whereas high frequency (hf, 5–20 Hz) stimulates ROI
- **Pulse intensity:** Appropriate intensity determined by baseline cortical excitability (defined as % of motor threshold). Goal is to select intensity that induces desired physiologic changes while minimizing discomfort and seizure risk

Clinical Uses
FDA Approved

- *Depression:* ECT superior to high-frequency rTMS in terms of response and remission, with similar discontinuation rate. In subgroup analysis, ECT outperforms rTMS for psychotic depression, but rTMS noninferior to ECT for nonpsychotic depression (*Prog Neuro-Psych Bio Psych*;51:181-189). Cost-effectiveness modeling suggests rTMS should be tried after one failed med trial (*PLoS One.* 2017;12:10)

Non–FDA Approved, Larger Studies Needed

- *OCD:* Outperforms sham when applied to dlPFC or OFC using heterogeneous protocols with respect to laterality and stimulation frequency (*J ECT.* 2016;32(4):262-266)
- *Schizophrenia:* Evidence that lf-rTMS targeting Wernicke's area decreases auditory hallucinations, and hf-rTMS to dlPFC may decrease negative symptoms (*Innov Clin Neurosci.* 2015;12(7-8):12-19)
- *PTSD:* dlPFC and mPFC are promising targets (*Brain Stim.* 2014;7(2):151-157).
- *Parkinson disease:* Reduction in motor symptoms when hf-rTMS applied to MI, or lf-rTMS applied over other frontal regions (*JAMA Neurol.* 2015;72(4):432-440)
- *Chronic pain syndromes:* Several studies have reported significant pain relief (>30% compared with sham), most successful is hf-rTMS over MI (*Arch Phys Med Rehabil.* 2015;96(4):s156-s172)

Side Effects, Contraindications (*Clin Neurophysiol.* 2009;120(12):2008-2039)
Absolutely contraindicated if metallic implants in head and neck; some consider pacemakers to be a contraindication as well. Reports of seizures, lower risk than with common antidepressants. Headache is common; can see facial muscle contraction or twitching; rarely hypomania in bipolar spectrum patients.

Alternative Stimulation Techniques

- **Transcranial Direct Current Stimulation (TDCS):** Constant direct current applied to electrodes on the head. No FDA approval in the US, but approved to treat major depression in Europe. Meta-analysis of 6 sham-controlled RCTs showed effect sizes similar to that of TMS and antidepressant drugs in primary care setting (*Br J Psychiatry.* 2016;208:522-531)
  - Side effects: Nausea, headache, dizziness, itching. Avoid in patients with seizure disorder

- **Vagal nerve stimulation:** Electrode surgically implanted into left vagus nerve, connected to pulse generator, which sends currents through tractus solitarius to cortical and limbic areas. Not continuous pulses (typically 30 s every 5 min)
  - Side effects include infection at device site, hoarseness, cough, SOB, difficulty swallowing
  - Approved for medication resistant epilepsy and TRD as adjunct only (*Biol Psychiatry.* 2005;58(5):364-373)

BRIEF DYNAMIC/INSIGHT-ORIENTED THERAPIES

Background and Philosophy

- A multitude of brief psychotherapeutic approaches have been developed since the 1970s to target specific conditions, personality structures, or life stages (see chart). Models vary in terms of therapist approach to the patient, number of visits, and formulation of the presenting complaint (ie, as a symptom vs an unconscious conflict)
- All are based on standard psychodynamic principles, with the addition of time-limited nature of treatment and clinician-directed focus on a specific target symptom or conflict rather than encouraging patient free-association
- Goal is to provide the patient with a greater capacity to understand the unconscious or relational patterns that contribute to the current factors causing distress
- The patient's development of insight into conscious and unconscious patterns allows ongoing improvement over time without requiring an indefinite length of therapy
- Models of brief psychodynamic therapy continue to evolve, especially to target specific diagnostic categories or particular life situations

Principles and Techniques

Selected Brief Dynamic Psychotherapies	
(Adapted from Gabbard GO. Textbook of Psychotherapeutic Treatments; 2009)	
Type	**Key Concepts and Techniques**
Time-limited	Centered around lifelong losses as a source of pain; interpretations focus on enabling the patient to master the pain and formulate a new self-image; problem-solving approach
Short-term anxiety-provoking	Identification of an unresolved conflict that emerges through active confrontation by the therapist
Intensive short-term dynamic	Active reenactment of past conflictual relationships, with therapist fostering intense emotional responses; identification of these conflicts and patient's reactions to them in the session helps confront patient's defenses
Supportive-expressive	Focus is on a core conflictual relationship that is brought into conscious awareness; sympathetic listening utilized to identify symptoms and reframe them as coping attempts
Brief adaptive	Focus is on maladaptive personality traits, especially those related to interpersonal function; a highly active therapist makes frequent transference interpretations and works through patient's resistance

(continued)

Selected Brief Dynamic Psychotherapies *(continued)*	
Type	**Key Concepts and Techniques**
Self-psychology	Focus is on intrapsychic representations of others as "self-objects" and developing capacity to see others in more nuanced terms; symptoms resolved by restoring cohesion among fragments of self and self-objects
Dynamic supportive	Maladaptive defenses are challenged, but adaptive defenses are reinforced to reduce anxiety and build self-esteem; the therapist provides active praise and reassurance

Evidence for Effectiveness
- Studied collectively, these therapies have shown clear benefit for depression, PTSD, eating disorders, substance use, personality disorders, and somatic symptom disorders *(Arch Gen Psychiatry. 2004;61:1208; World Psychiatry. 2015;14:137)*
- Incorporating brief psychotherapy on inpatient psychiatric units has been shown to decrease depressive symptoms and improve duration of remission when compared with treatment as usual *(J Affect Disord. 2017;209:105)*
- Brief psychotherapy is a cost-effective treatment of high utilizers of psychiatric services, resulting in both symptom improvement and decreased future treatment utilization *(Arch Gen Psychiatry. 1999;56:519)*

COGNITIVE BEHAVIORAL THERAPY (CBT)

Background and Philosophy
- With the increasing differentiation of psychiatric d/o's following the advent of DSM-III and the rising pressures for empirically testable treatments for them, CBT evolved in the 1980s from the merging of cognitive therapy (which focused on changing inaccurate or unhelpful cognitions) w/ behavior therapy (which aimed to change behavior through interactions w/ the environment), contrasting w/ psychodynamic psychotherapies that had dominated psychiatric practice for decades *(Behav Res Ther. 2015;64:1)*
- CBT refers to a group of evidence-based, manualized psychotherapies in the above tradition involving specific, protocolized strategies targeted to treat clearly defined (typically, disorder-specific) psychopathologies within a limited timeframe *(Front Psychiatry. 2018;9:4)*
- **"Third wave" therapies:** CBT has increasingly expanded to integrate strategies of mindfulness and acceptance into its theory and practice and led to the development of independent therapies

stemming from this tradition, including DBT and ACT *(Psychodyn Psychiatry. 2015;43(3):423)*

- **Transdiagnostic CBT:** More recently, protocols have emerged w/ a broader, more holistic focus in targeting "core" pathologies (eg, neuroticism and emotion dysregulation) common to multiple (and often comorbid) d/o's *(JAMA Psychiatry. 2017;74(9):867)*
- As a whole, CBT is the psychotherapy w/ the greatest amount (and arguably the highest quality) of empirical research to support its use in multiple d/o's, populations, and settings *(Front Psychiatry. 2018;9:4)*

Principles and Techniques *(Braz J Psychiatr. 2008;30(suppl II):S54)*

- **Central hypothesis:** The way you perceive and process reality influences the way you feel and behave; accordingly, change dysfunctional thoughts and behaviors (through empirical, critical, problem-solving approaches) to improve how you feel
- **Cognitive behavioral "triangle":** Environmental stimuli → automatic negative thoughts ↔ negative emotions ↔ response behaviors (in any order)
- **Durable mechanism of action:** Demonstrated at least in depression, CBT has an enduring effect persisting beyond the end of the acute treatment that is similar to initiation plus long-term continuation of antidepressant pharmacotherapy *(BMJ Open. 2013;3:e002542)*
- **Concepts**

  Automatic negative thoughts: Spontaneous thoughts on the edge of awareness representing immediate interpretations of reality whose presence most people are not aware of and whose accuracy is generally taken for granted; CBT teaches monitoring and questioning of these

  Core beliefs (or *schemas*): Acquired early in life through personal experience and identification w/ important others, these internal cognitive structures comprise ideas, memories, and knowledge from our most basic beliefs (assumptions, implicit rules) about the world and help us organize and make sense of new data we encounter, thus filtering and shaping how we perceive and conceptualize new stimuli

  Diathesis-stress model: Certain core beliefs increase vulnerability to emotional disorders that may be precipitated by additional stressors (eg, environmental reinforcement)

  Cognitive distortions: eg, catastrophizing, emotional reasoning, dichotomous thinking, selective abstraction, mind reading, labeling, minimization and maximization, and imperatives

- **Phases of treatment** *(Spine J. 2008;8(1):40)*
  1. Assessment: Diagnosis, degree of impairment, treatment-planning, informed consent
  2. Reconceptualization: Identification and interrogation of maladaptive cognitions
  3. Skills acquisition: Coping w/ difficulties, avoiding cognitive distortions
  4. Skills consolidation and application training: Strengthening acquired skills through practice

5. Generalization and maintenance: Expanding applications of skills and planning to support continued coping after acute treatment's end
  6. Posttreatment assessment and follow-up: Evaluation and monitoring of ongoing skills use
- **Interventions** (*Braz J Psychiatr.* 2008;30(suppl II):S54)

  Cognitive: identification, questioning, and modification of automatic thoughts; reattribution (testing assumptions and thoughts by considering alternative causes of events), cognitive restructuring (identifying, disputing irrational and maladaptive thoughts); cognitive rehearsal, and other imaginal cognitive procedures

  Behavioral: activity scheduling (behavioral activation); mastery and pleasure ratings; graded-task behavioral assignments; reality testing experiments; role-playing; social skills training; and problem-solving skills training

Evidence-Based Applications (*Cognit Ther Res.* 2012;36(5):427; *Clin Psychol Rev.* 2006;26:17)

- Strongest evidence is for anxiety d/o's, somatoform d/o's, BN, anger dyscontrol, and general stress
- **Large effect sizes in:** adult and adolescent unipolar depression, GAD, panic d/o w/ or w/o agoraphobia, social phobia, PTSD, OCD, and childhood depressive and anxiety d/o's
- **Medium to large effect sizes in:** somatoform disorders (hypochondriasis, BDD)
- **Medium effect sizes in:** marital distress, anger, childhood somatic disorders, and chronic pain
- **Small to medium effect sizes in:** short-term tx of bipolar d/o (though well-supported in bipolar depression); unclear if superior to other tx in the long-term tx of bipolar d/o
- Highly effective for cannabis and nicotine use d/o's; less effective for opioid and alcohol use d/o's
- Superior to other therapies for BN; less evidence in other eating d/o's
- For insomnia ("CBTi"), superior efficacy on multiple outcomes versus other interventions
- In psychotic d/o's, efficacy especially for positive sx and other 2° outcomes; inferior to other tx (pharmacotherapy, family intervention) for chronic sx, relapse prevention
- Somewhat superior to antidepressant pharmacotherapy for depression in adults (though combination of psychotherapy and pharmacotherapy often superior to either modality alone) (*JAMA Psychiatry.* 2014;71(6):706)
- Self-guided Internet-based CBT (iCBT) has been shown to be effective for sx of depression and may provide an empirically supported first-step treatment option w/ the potential to expand access and reduce costs (*JAMA Psychiatry.* 2017;74(4):351)

COGNITIVE PROCESSING THERAPY

Background and Philosophy (Resick PA, Monson CM. Cognitive Processing Therapy: Veteran/Military Version; 2006)

- Definition: A form of CBT to treat PTSD that helps patient address avoidance by providing psychoeducation, and guiding pt through the traumatic event, while nonjudgmentally challenging negative thoughts and emotions
- Rooted in 2 theories:
  - Information processing theory: problematic thoughts, behaviors, and emotions that result from past trauma are due to avoidance of distressing thoughts and emotions related to the trauma
  - Social cognitive theory of PTSD: primary emotions result directly from response to the event (fear), whereas secondary emotions are based on interpretations of the event (guilt/shame)
- By challenging automatic thoughts and emotions, pt learns to not overgeneralize
- Originally developed to treat PTSD in sexual assault survivors; later found to be effective in other types of trauma

Principles and Techniques

- Psychoeducation: In the first session, pt learns more about their specific symptoms and about the theories of PTSD (see above)
  - Impact statement: Pt writes down perceived impact of the trauma on his life
  - A-B-C chart: Activating event (something happens) → Belief/stuck point (I tell myself something) → Consequence (I feel or do something)
  - Socratic dialogue (CARD): (1) **C**larify situation and pt's automatic thoughts; (2) understand pt's **A**ssumptions about the event and his role in it; (3) elicit **R**eal evidence for their assumptions; (4) elicit pt's resulting **D**eeper beliefs about himself and meaning of the event
  - Challenge questions: nonjudgmental questions meant to help pt assess accuracy of automatic thoughts

Evidence for Effectiveness

- Retrospective review within the VA showed CPT and prolonged exposure therapy equally effective in decreasing PTSD checklist scores in veterans with PTSD (Psychol Rep. 2018;121(2):282-302)
- When full protocol compared to constituent components, substantial improvement in PTSD, and depressive sx seen in all groups; however, cognitive therapy group showed greater reduction in sx than writing assignment alone (J Consult Clin Psychol. 2008;76(2):243)
- In a 2015 review of 5 RCTs evaluating CPT, CPT outperformed treatment-as-usual control conditions in achieving meaningful symptom reduction. However, mean posttreatment scores for CPT remained at or above clinical criteria for PTSD, and approximately two-thirds of patients receiving CPT retained their PTSD diagnosis after treatment. Benefits only marginally better than nontrauma-focused psychotherapy (JAMA. 2015;314(5):489-500)

DIALECTICAL BEHAVIOR THERAPY (DBT)

Background and Philosophy (*Am J Psychother.* 2015;69(2):97; *Linehan M. DBT Skills Training Manual. 2nd ed.;* 2015)

- DBT emerged in the 1990s out of attempts by psychologist Marsha Linehan to apply behavioral therapeutic principles and techniques to the treatment of complex, multidiagnostic pts with severe suicidal behaviors (*Am J Psychother.* 2015;69(2):97)
- DBT was the first psychotherapy to demonstrate effectiveness for BPD with controlled trials and remains a major evidence-based treatment for BPD (alongside other specialist psychotherapies MBT, TFP, and SFT, as well as generalist models GPM and SCM) (*JAMA Psychiatry.* 2017;74:319; *Curr Opin Psychol.* 2018;21:127)
- **Philosophy:** Uses the concept of the dialectic (synthesizing opposites) to integrate change-oriented behaviorist principles with acceptance-based techniques, including mindfulness (derived from contemplative practices such as Zen)
- **Goal:** To create a "life worth living" by helping pts change problematic cognitive, behavioral, emotional, and interpersonal patterns while helping them tolerate the distress that might otherwise interfere with the pursuit of treatment goals
- **Model of BPD:** Nonpejorative, evidence-based, and treatment-guiding "biosocial theory" of an emotion regulation system d/o stemming from reinforcing transactions between biological vulnerabilities (high affective intensity and reactivity, impulse control deficits) and environmental risk factors (invalidation, reinforcement of affective lability)

Principles and Techniques (*Prof Psychol Res Pr.* 2013;44(2):73; *Am J Psychother.* 2015;69(2):97)

- **Hierarchical stages of treatment**
  Pretreatment: Psychoeducation, informed consent, goal-setting, commitment generation
  Stage 1: Achieve stabilization through behavioral control by mitigating life-threatening and treatment-interfering behaviors while reducing quality-of-life–interfering behaviors (eg, substance abuse) and replacing dysfunctional behaviors w/ skillful ones
  Stage 2: Reduce emotional suffering (related to BPD as well as 2/2 comorbid d/o's) while preserving the goal of experiencing a full range of emotions
  Stage 3: Ameliorate "ordinary" (ie, less pathological) problems in living while improving self-respect and quality of life
  Stage 4: Develop awareness of self, foster a sense of fulfillment, find joy
- **Modularity:** To afford the flexibility required to tackle the complex clinical problems for which it was developed, DBT's intrinsic modularity allows therapists to isolate and apply (or omit) specific interventions according to treatment-guiding principles and hierarchical priorities

- **Components of Therapy**
  - *Individual psychotherapy*: Review of daily Diary Card (tool for monitoring affect ratings, problematic behaviors, and skills practice) identifies highest priority targets of treatment, which are collaboratively scrutinized (via chain and solution analyses) for opportunities to replace maladaptive behavior w/ newly acquired skills; role-playing, imaginal rehearsals, and commitment-generating interventions support adoption of skillful behaviors
  - *Skills training*: Protocol-based weekly group therapy that provides a dedicated setting for the didactic teaching of behavioral skills that require practice to replace maladaptive behaviors
  - *Between-sessions phone coaching*: Addresses reality that suicidal pts often need more therapeutic contact than is afforded by weekly individual sessions and prevents the reinforcing of suicidal behaviors that may take place if phone calls are reserved for when pts are suicidal
  - *Consultation team*: Serves to improve treatment by bolstering therapist adherence to evidence-based practice, managing burnout, providing support for those treating pts imminently at risk for suicide or presenting with other severely dysfunctional behaviors

- **DBT skills**
  - Acceptance skills
    - Mindfulness: "Core" skills (wise mind, describe/observe/participate, etc), to practice intentionally attending to the present experiencing and observing of oneself and one's environment with curiosity and w/o judgment
    - Distress tolerance: Skills for enduring distress w/o impulsively, destructively trying to avoid it
  - Change skills
    - Interpersonal effectiveness: Skills for handling interpersonal conflict constructively, developing healthy relationships and ending destructive ones, and effectively reinforcing others' behaviors
    - Emotional regulation: Psychoeducation and skills for identifying and making sense of emotions, decreasing vulnerability to negative affect, modifying emotional responses, and coping with difficult affects

Evidenced-Based Applications

- **Adaptations of DBT:** Varying levels of evidence support the utility of DBT applied in TRD (adults and geriatrics), eating disorders (BN, BED, BPD w/ comorbid AN), BPD w/ comorbid SUDs, ADHD, adolescents w/ self-injurious and suicidal behaviors, and a range of populations in forensic settings (*Prof Psychol Res Pr.* 2013;44(2):73)
- **Stand-alone DBT skills training:** Preliminary evidence indicates some effectiveness for sx of Axis I d/o's (MDD, ADHD, BED), but data are more mixed for BPD sx (suicidality); nevertheless, stand-alone skills training is being implemented widely and unsystematically for a variety of sx, d/o's, and populations (*J Clin Psychol.* 2015;71:1)

- **Source of DBT's effectiveness?** Overall, evidence supports benefits of full DBT over isolated components thereof, although evidence is increasing for role of skills training in reducing depressive and other sx, and importance of specialized training of clinicians for assessment and management of suicidal behaviors (*JAMA Psychiatry.* 2015;72(5):475)

GOOD PSYCHIATRIC MANAGEMENT (GPM)

Background and Philosophy (*J Pers Disord.* 2008;22(1):22-41)
- **History:** Developed by John Gunderson in 1990s as a simple tx for borderline personality disorder (BPD) provided by nonspecialists in response to mounting public health need
- **Theory**
  The core sxs of BPD stem from hypersensitivity to interpersonal situations leading to a repeating cycle of idealization/isolation:
  1. Idealization: pt feels connected and idealizes the other in an important relationship
  2. Threat: pt perceives a threat (real or imagined) to the relationship and responds with maladaptive behavior (eg, rage, devaluation, self-injury)
  3. The other withdraws (eg, breaks up, stops answering texts) or responds with anger
  4. Isolation: pt feels alone, leading to dissociation and/or suicidal ideation
- **Guiding philosophy**
  Assumes that symptoms of BPD will improve with a shift to a more supportive interpersonal context
  The GPM therapist provides that context by acting as (1) a supportive, reliable figure in the pt's life and (2) a case manager to problem-solve real-life issues and assist pt efforts to find a more supportive environment in the real world (eg, employment)

Principles and Techniques
6 Key Principles of GPM (*Curr Opin Psychol.* 2018;21:127-131)
1. Be active, not reactive: the therapist should challenge silence, passivity, avoidance and not overreact in the face of provocation
2. Support via listening and selective validation: the therapist should see the patient's description as valid and understandable
3. Focus on "getting a life": enable pt efforts to obtain gainful employment (through case management) if the pt is unemployed. Stable work is an urgent priority in tx and trumps focus on relationships
4. The therapy relationship is real and professional: the therapist should be a real person with real feelings and disclose when helpful (eg, "you scared me"; "I would be angry")

5. Change is expected: continuation of therapy should be contingent on pt improvement; failure to improve should prompt the question of termination
6. Accountability: if pt fails to meet an agreed-upon goal or homework assignment, this should be pointed out and discussed

Other Techniques
- Psychoeducation: early in tx, the therapist should deliver the diagnosis of BPD and explain the prognosis
- Develop interpersonal insight: therapist consistently points out relationship between sxs and interpersonal stressors
- Minimize iatrogenesis: taper unnecessary medications; if meds are necessary, prescribe medications with safe SE profile (eg, SSRIs)

Evidence-Based Application
- Single blind RCT of 180 pts randomized to receive either 1 y of DBT or 1 y of GPM showed GPM is equally efficacious to DBT in terms of major tx outcomes including suicidal ideation, ER visits, and health care utilization (*Am J Psychiatry.* 2009;166:12)
- Benefits are observable within 10 weekly sessions (*Psychother Psychosom.* 2014;83:176-186)
- Durable improvements (in suicidality, self-harm) are seen at 2 y follow-up after GPM tx had stopped, although functional impairment (ie, unemployment) persisted (*Am J Psychiatry.* 2012;169:650-661)
- **Indications for GPM**: some have argued that GPM is particularly well-suited as a first-line tx for straightforward cases of BPD, given relatively minimal training investment for clinicians (one-day workshop), and that refractory pts can be referred to more intensive specialized tx (*Harv Rev Psychiatry.* 2016;24:342-356)

INTERPERSONAL PSYCHOTHERAPY (IPT)

Background and Philosophy (*Arch Gen Psychiatry.* 1994;51:599; *World Psychiatry.* 2004;3:136)
- Developed in the 1970s by Myrna Weissman and Gerald Klerman as a treatment for depression that also improved patients' abilities to manage interpersonal situations, to improve relationships, and to mobilize social supports
- Biopsychosocial factors interact to contribute to mental illness, medical illness, personality structures, and culture at large, in complex ways that can be difficult to access
- Mental illness causes interpersonal and social difficulties; addressing these difficulties affects the wider range of factors causing illness, leading to resolution of symptoms
- Symptoms are explicitly medicalized; patients are told they are suffering from an illness that can and will respond to treatment

- Focus is on specific interpersonal events that occur in a patient's life, rather than on unconscious or intrapsychic factors
- Treatment progresses through time-limited stages focusing on 1 of 4 interpersonal foci: grief, interpersonal disputes, role transitions, and interpersonal deficits

Principles and Techniques (*Comprehensive Guide to Interpersonal Psychotherapy. New York: Basic Books; 2000*)

- IPT is explicitly framed to the patient as a structured, time-limited intervention (12–16 wk) that will result in symptom relief by the end of the treatment
- At the first session, the patient and clinician jointly complete an inventory of patient's important relationships and recent life changes along with a standardized symptom checklist (eg, PHQ-9, QIDS) to determine a choice of focus (see chart)
- In addition to standard techniques common to all psychotherapies (eg, nondirective exploration, identifying and labeling affect, clarification, and restatement), the therapist actively engages patients around 3 domains to shape interpersonal functioning: communication analysis, decision analysis, and role-playing
- Tasks specific to each treatment focus are accomplished over the course of therapy, either in sessions or as worksheets for the patient to complete between sessions
- Explicit focus on identifying progress and anticipating upcoming termination of treatment

Selecting an IPT Treatment Focus	
Grief	Death or other loss of a person close to the patient
Interpersonal disputes	Difficult personal relationships (eg, spouse, sibling, coworkers) that are characterized by unequal role expectations between individuals
Role transitions	Change in a defined role (eg, job loss, retirement, new baby, graduation, marriage)
Interpersonal deficits	Long history of challenging relationships owing to patient's poor communication or lack of coping skills; in contrast to the other foci, there is often no acute trigger for symptom onset

Evidence for Effectiveness

- Extensively studied as treatment of major depressive disorder, with multiple randomized controlled trials demonstrating efficacy either as an independent treatment or in conjunction with medication (*Am J Psychiatry.* 2011;168:581)
- More recent investigations have shown IPT to be equivalent to CBT in the treatment of anxiety disorders and eating disorders (*Am J Psychiatry.* 2016;173:680)

MENTALIZATION-BASED TREATMENT (MBT)

Background and Philosophy
- Developed by Anthony Bateman and Peter Fonagy in the early 2000s for treatment of borderline PD, also being studied for narcissistic PD, depression, PTSD, and eating disorders
- Mentalizing is the process of trying to "read" internal states (thoughts, feelings, desires, attitudes, goals, needs, etc) of oneself and of others (World Psychiatry. 2010;9:11-15)
- Mentalization is also defined as making sense of what is going on within oneself and others in terms of mental states

Principles and Techniques (World Psychiatry. 2010;9:11-15)
- Core principles
  - Poor mentalizing results in self-destructive behaviors
  - One of the core features of BPD is a fragile mentalizing capacity
  - Aim is to learn to question assumptions one makes about one's own and others' internal states, "take the inquisitive stance," as incorrect mentalizing often leads to distress, mistrust, and emotional destabilization
- Goals of treatment
  - To enable patients to see oneself from the outside and others from the inside
  - Achieving standard outcomes of BPD-targeted treatments including reduction of suicidality and self-harm, hospitalizations, mood symptoms
  - To gain self-awareness and other-awareness
  - To understand misunderstandings and to feel less misunderstood
- Techniques
  - Often employed as a combination of individual therapy as well as an intensive experiential group (in which the goal is to practice mentalization of self and others through examining points of discrepancy and rigidity arising within and between group members)
  - May be used in inpatient/partial hospital/outpatient settings
  - Initial task is to stabilize emotional expression/affect regulation, as one cannot consider internal representations without this, and uncontrolled affect leads to impulsivity
  - Focus on mentalizing rather than behaviors, cognitions, or insight
  - Work includes developing a written formulation of the patient's mentalizing deficits, sharing this document with the patient early in treatment, and referring to it throughout the work together
  - Address the 3 types of nonmentalizing in patients:
    1. Psychic equivalent: belief that one's interpretation is fact, treating thoughts as facts (eg, "He definitely hates me. I just know it.")
    2. Pretend mode: ideas do not bridge between inner and outer reality, mental world decoupled from external reality (eg, "yes-ing" provider, endless inconsequential talk and meaningless statements)

3. Teleological mode: using outcome to determine cause after the fact (eg, "you did not call me back right away therefore you hate me," jumping to conclusions about the why based on the action)
- Key interventions include empathic validation; clarification, exploration, and challenge of mentalization; affect identification and affect focus; mentalizing the therapeutic relationship

Evidence-Based Applications
- RCT of MBT outpatient versus structured clinical management for BPD × 1.5 y showed decreased hospitalizations, suicide attempts, life-threatening self-harm, medication use, overall symptoms, depressive symptoms, increased GAF scores, and interpersonal/social functioning (Am J Psychiatry. 2009;166:1355-1364)
- Possible greater improvement for BPD pts with more significant other PD comorbidities and more pervasive interpersonal problems (Br J Psychiatry. 2013;203:221-227)
- RCT of MBT partial hospitalization programs versus treatment as usual for BPD showed decreased suicidal/self-harming acts, hospitalizations, depressive symptoms, increased social and interpersonal functioning, no cost difference between groups, decreased mental health service utilization, decreased medication use, increased GAF scores, increased employment, and increased school enrollment (Am J Psychiatry. 1999;156:1563-1569; Am J Psychiatry. 2003;160:169-171; Am J Psychiatry. 2008;165:631-638)

MINDFULNESS-BASED THERAPIES

Background and Philosophy
- **Definition**: "mindfulness means paying attention in a particular way: on purpose, in the present moment, and nonjudgmentally" (Kabat-Zinn J. Wherever You Go, There You Are: Mindfulness Meditation in Everyday Life; 2009)
Mindfulness meditation: exercises to evoke, sustain, and create a habit of mindfulness
- **Origin** in Eastern religions, spirituality—increasingly practiced in secular contexts
- **Common goals** of mindfulness-based therapies:
  Cultivate equanimity in the face of external and internal stressors
  Interrupt maladaptive mental habits through grounding in the present moment
  Learn to approach oneself and others with openness and nonviolence
- **How mindfulness works:**
  Induces the relaxation response (balances the autonomic nervous system and calms the mind) (Benson H. The Relaxation Response; 1992)
  Decreases mind-wandering and rumination, both linked to negative mood; reduces activation in the default mode network (PNAS. 2011;108(50):20254-20259)

Develops the ability to engage with thoughts and feelings more objectively, as if from a third-person perspective (ie, *cognitive defusion* or *decentering*, mediated through frontal lobe inhibition of amygdalar activity) (*Psychol Addict Behav.* 2013;27(2):351-365)

Promotes tolerating and accepting unpleasant states of mind rather than trying to avoid them, which is typically counterproductive

Promotes insight into one's habits and patterns of mind through sustained, direct observation

Replaces automatic reactions with intentional responses; strengthens frontal lobe executive function (*Perspect Psychol Sci.* 2011;6(6):537-559)

Principles and Techniques
- **Leading mindfulness-based therapies**

  Mindfulness-based stress reduction (MBSR) (*Gen Hosp Psychiatry.* 1982;4(1):33-47)

  Mindfulness meditation, body scanning (noticing the body's various sensations nonjudgmentally), and yoga led by certified instructors

  Structured with 8 weekly group sessions and daily practice homework

  Mindfulness-based cognitive therapy (MBCT) (*Z Segal et al., Mindfulness-Based Cognitive Therapy for Depression: A New Approach for Preventing Relapse;* 2002)

  Integrates approaches from cognitive behavioral therapy (CBT) and MBSR

  Disrupts maladaptive thought patterns that arise in reaction to dysphoria

  Mindfulness-based relapse prevention (MBRP) (*J Cogn Psychol.* 2005;19(3):211-228)

  Teaches mindfulness and other CBT strategies to identify, manage, and reduce vulnerability to triggers for relapse in patients with substance use disorders

  Reduces craving and helps patients handle stressors without substance use

  Acceptance and commitment therapy (ACT) (*S Hayes et al., Acceptance and Commitment Therapy: An Experiential Approach to Behavior Change;* 1999)

  Helps patients accept their negative thoughts and feelings rather than struggling to eliminate, avoid, control, or explain them

  Patients then focus on exploring and acting in accordance with their values

  Dialectical behavior therapy (DBT) (*Bull Menninger Clin.* 1987;51(3):261-276)

  "Dialectic" is about navigating both acceptance and change, and replacing "all or nothing" cognitive distortions with more nuanced thought/behavior patterns

  Mindfulness, distress tolerance, interpersonal effectiveness, and emotion regulation skills are typically taught in a group therapy setting

- **Comparison to other therapies**
  Distinctive for often emphasizing connection between mind and body

  Shares with many therapies a fundamental arc: patients become more aware of habitual patterns, see those patterns in a new light, and are empowered to regulate their behavior in a more flexible, conscious way

Evidence for Effectiveness
- A wide range of therapeutic targets including chronic pain, anxiety, depression, PTSD, psychosis, substance use disorders, and coping with serious illness
- Efficacy is controversial; thousands of research articles but many of questionable quality; research expanding exponentially in recent years (*BMJ. 2015;351; JAMA. 2015; 314(13):1327-1329; Perspect Psychol Sci. 2018;13(1):36-61*)
- MBSR is best validated for physical, psychiatric symptoms in patients with chronic pain (*JAMA. 2016;315(12):1240-1249; Ann Intern Med. 2017;166(7):493-505*)
- MBCT prevents relapse in recurrent major depressive disorder as effectively as antidepressant medication (*Clin Psychol Rev. 2011;31(6):1032-1040*)
- MBRP outperforms usual treatment in reducing substance misuse (*J Subst Abuse Treat. 2017;75:62-96*)
- DBT is the gold standard treatment for borderline personality disorder with strong evidence for reducing suicidality (*Arch Gen Psychiatry. 2006;63(7):757-766*)

MOTIVATIONAL INTERVIEWING (MI)

Background and Philosophy (*Behav Cogn Psychother. 1995;23:325; J Teaching Addict. 2006;5(1):3*)
- **Overview:** MI is an evidence-based form of counseling that elicits change in behavior by actively and nonjudgmentally guiding the pt in clarifying his own motivation for change through collaborative examination and resolution of his ambivalence
- **Basic assumptions:** (*Int J Behav Nutr Phys Act. 2012;9:19*)
  Persisting ambivalence is the main barrier to precipitating behavior change

  The pt is more likely to act on ideas he has expressed himself
- **Ambivalence:** An unresolved conflict between 2 courses of action, each of which has its own perceived costs and benefits; simultaneously feeling 2 ways about something (eg, wanting, on the one hand, to use a substance while, on the other hand, wanting at the same time *not* to use it)
- **Guiding philosophy:** The "spirit of MI"
  Motivation and readiness to change behavior are clarified within the pt; they cannot be imposed by the clinician

Clinician's role is to guide the pt actively yet respectfully in collaborative examination, clarification, and resolution of ambivalence, not to issue authoritative injunctions

Partnership, based on mutual respect of autonomy, joins the pt and clinician; clinician communicates that he sees that the pt already "ha[s] what [he] need[s]" to change

Trying to convince the pt of the benefits of changing behavior is not effective, nor is coercing, confronting, debating, or arguing w/ the pt

Resolution of ambivalence is the pt's job, not the clinician's; pt has the full right to choose his behavior and its consequences

Readiness to change a behavior is not a static trait; it is a shifting state that fluctuates as a function of interpersonal interaction, including between pt and clinician

Listening for, pulling for, and reinforcing motivational speech from the pt himself is what leads to behavior change

- **Stages of behavior change:** Change is a process, and often, it is a cycle (*Am J Health Promot.* 1997;12(11):38)

    Precontemplation: Pts do not intend to take action toward behavior change in the foreseeable future; pts may be under-informed about risks and/or demoralized by prior failed attempts to change; pts often avoid thinking/talking about their risky behaviors

    Contemplation: Pts generally intend to change sometime in the foreseeable future—but not immediately; with heightened ambivalence; pts are more consciously aware of the pros and cons of changing behavior, which can keep them stuck in this stage, sometimes chronically

    Preparation: Pts are determined to make behavior changes in the immediate future and have created (or are in the process of creating) a specific plan of action for change

    Action: Pts have now taken action to realize meaningful, risk-reducing behavior changes

    Maintenance: After execution of behavior change, pts are working actively to prevent relapse

- **Change talk and commitment talk:** (*J Teaching Addict.* 2006;5(1):3; *Int J Behav Nutr Phys Act.* 2012;9:19)

    Change talk: Pt's verbal indications of reasons, need, desire, capacity, or commitment to change

    Commitment talk: Pt's emphatic verbal indications of decision or contract about a plan for change (eg, "I will…" rather than the change talk of "I need to…" or "I'll try to…")

Principles and Techniques

- **Alliance → change talk → planning and commitment talk:** (*Int J Behav Nutr Phys Act.* 2012;9:19)

    1. Exploring: Elicit pt's history and narrative, develop alliance w/o pushing for change

    2. Guiding: Move conversation to possibility of change, evoke change talk, and summarize

3. Choosing: Once any commitment is made, help pt develop goals and plan (anticipate obstacles, monitoring, contingencies)

- **Principles:** (SAMHSA, *Enhancing Motivation for Change in Substance Abuse Treatment*; 1999)

  Express empathy: Communicating understanding of the pt's perspective (including benefits of not changing behavior) w/ interventions such as reflective listening

  Support self-efficacy: Explicitly accepting and affirming the pt's strengths, difficulties, and autonomy

  Develop discrepancy: Eliciting incongruencies between pt's goals, values, and current behaviors; help pt see gaps between where he is and where he wants to be

  Avoid argument: Preventing the provocation of resistance (ie, arguments for maintaining the status quo) by monitoring and staying close to the pt's current stage of change w/o pushing for change prematurely or w/o permission

  Roll with resistance: Defusing any unavoidable resistance by reflecting it back to the pt, emphasizing his choice and control, and joining with the resistance (rather than by opposing—and thereby strengthening—resistance)

- **"OARS" counseling skills:** (*J Teaching Addict.* 2006;5(1):3)

  Open-ended questions: Pose questions that require more than single-word responses

  Affirming: Express recognition of the pt's strengths, motivations, intentions, and progress

  Reflecting: Show you are listening and understanding the pt's message by synthesizing and expressing it back to him

  Summarizing: Highlight meaningful and/or useful content discussed so far to guide dialogue going forward

Evidence for Effectiveness (*J Clin Psychol.* 2009;65(11):1232; *Annu Rev Clin Psychol.* 2005;1:91)

- **Language matters:** MI upregulates change talk and decreases resistance; resistance is inversely related to behavior change; change talk predicts commitment talk; increasing strength of commitment talk predicts behavior change (*J Teaching Addict.* 2006;5(1):3)
- High variability in effect sizes seen between studies, but numerous controlled trials suggest MI is 10–20% more effective than no treatment and is at least as effective as other evidence-based treatments for reducing a diversity of problematic and risky behaviors and bolstering pt engagement in treatment
- Dose–response effect demonstrated: more MI sessions lead to more behavior change
- Behavior changes resulting from MI shown to be durable at least up to 1 y after treatment
- Effectiveness has been shown for various adaptations of MI, although the highest effectiveness may emerge when it is used in conjunction with other treatments, and least effectiveness is seen when MI is delivered in a group format
- Effectiveness of MI has been demonstrated across a diversity of pt populations and across a spectrum of severity of problematic behaviors

PSYCHODYNAMIC PSYCHOTHERAPY (PDP)

Philosophy and Background (Gabbard GO, Psychodynamic Psychiatry in Clinical Practice; 2014)

- **Definition:** psychodynamic psychotherapy focuses on revealing the content of the pt's unconscious, and through these revelations, alleviates psychiatric symptoms
- **The unconscious:** desires, thought processes, memories, and conflicts, which are not available to introspection
- Psychodynamic psychotherapy assumes **psychic determinism:** many behaviors (especially pathological ones) are determined by unconscious processes
- **History:**

  Rooted in *Drive Theory* (Freud, 1890s): postulates that the unconscious has 3 parts: id (sexual and aggressive drives), superego (asserts conscience and personal ideals), and the ego (restrains the id to conform to social rules), and that psychopathology arises from conflict between these parts

  In contrast to drive theory, *Object Relations Theory* (Klein, Fairbairn, Winnicott, et al., 1940s) postulates that psychopathology derives from conflict between "internalized objects" (ie, internalized representations of important relationships)

  Self-psychology (Kohut, 1970s): maintains that empathic failure in early caregivers, leads pts to fail to develop a coherent sense of self, and causes them to seek out external validation from others in adulthood

  Attachment Theory (Bowlby, 1970s): proposes that the attachment style between the infant and mother (which is a mix of environmental and genetic factors) persists through adulthood and can lead to psychopathology

Principles and Techniques

- **7 key principles distinguish PDP from other therapies:** (Am Psychol. 2010;65:98-109)

  Focus on affect: in comparison with other therapies with a more cognitive focus, PDP prioritizes uncovering of emotional insights

  Exploration of attempts to avoid unpleasant thoughts and feelings: PDP therapists actively point out and seek to understand avoidance of distress (classically called *defense* and *resistance*), eg, missing sessions, changing the topic

  Identification of recurring themes: PDP addresses repeating behavioral patterns and seeks to understand their patterns

  Discussion of past experiences: PDP focuses on the exploration of how past experiences connect to present-day problems

  Focus on interpersonal relations: PDP emphasizes how interpersonal patterns lead to ongoing symptoms

  Focus on the therapy relationship: PDP assumes that global interpersonal patterns will emerge within the pt–therapist dyad; the pt will develop feelings about the therapist (*transference*), and the therapist will develop feelings about the pt (*countertransference*), the content of which should be analyzed

Exploration of fantasy life: PDP encourages patients to speak freely without an agenda and without self-censorship (*free-association*) to uncover unconscious wishes and fears

- Technique: therapist interventions exist on a supportive-uncovering continuum; ↑ pt distress → ↑ supportive interventions (*Am J Psychother.* 2009;60:233-259)

Affirmation/praise (most supportive): explicitly support the pt's behavior, eg, "you made the right choice"

Empathic validation: explicitly convey understanding of an emotional reaction eg, "you must have felt awful then"

Confrontation: call attention to the possibility of an unconscious process at work, eg, "I notice you changed the subject when you began talking about your ex-wife. What happened there?"

Clarification: clarify a recurring pattern, eg, "It reminds me of last week, when you were also having difficulty talking about your mother leaving home when you were little"

Interpretation (most uncovering): suggest that a conscious thought, feeling, or behavior is due to an unconscious force, eg, "I wonder if the pain of your separation from your ex-wife reminds you of your mother leaving home"

Evidence for Effectiveness

- Robust evidence from meta-analyses that short- and long-term psychodynamic psychotherapy improves symptoms for a variety of diagnoses with moderate effect including mood disorders, anxiety disorders, personality disorders, and somatization (*Cochrane Database Syst Rev.* 2006;18; *Arch Gen Psychiatry.* 2004;61:1208-1216; *Psychother Psychosom.* 2009;78:265-274; *JAMA.* 2008;300:1551-1565)
- In contrast to other therapies, benefits seem to accrue with longer treatments
- Limited evidence that psychodynamic therapies are less effective, and associated with high dropout rates, for pts w/ psychosis and borderline personality disorder (*J Nerv Ment Dis.* 1989;177:38-42; *Schizophr Bull.* 1984;10:564-598)

DEFENSES

Defenses are unconscious psychological mechanisms which (1) manage some overwhelming feeling (eg, grief, anxiety, anger) and/or (2) maintain self-esteem

- Defenses are classified based on the developmental stage at which they first appear and the extent to which they preserve reality and maintain integrity of relationships (ie, ↑ mature → ↑ integrity and correspondence with reality)
- Pathology is not measured by the *presence* of immature defenses (as it is normal to revert to immature defenses under stress), but by the *absence* of mature defenses

Defense Mechanisms (J Abnl Psych. 1994;103:44)		
Psychotic Defenses	**Definition**	**Example**
Denial	Blocking unpleasant or difficult external stimuli from consciousness	*A lawyer, after being given a diagnosis of lung cancer is recommended follow-up with an oncologist a week later. Instead, he misses the appointment and continues his usual routine, as if nothing has happened.*
Delusion	Believing that something mistaken is true even against evidence to the contrary	*An author becomes convinced that his critics are conspiring to poison him after negative reviews of his most recent book are published.*
Immature Defenses	**Definition**	**Example**
Acting out	Conveying unconscious feelings through action rather than words	*A pt who is unconsciously upset with her therapist shows up 20 min late to her appointment.*
Dissociation	Detaching from physical and emotional sensations, usually in response to painful stimuli	*A pt begins to feel outside his body when discussing details of a prior traumatic experience.*
Projection	Attributing unpleasant thoughts or feelings in oneself on to others	*A husband who harbors an attraction to his secretary accuses his wife of cheating.*
Splitting	Failing to see both positive and negative qualities in a single person, group of people, or institution	*A pt tells his therapist that while he likes working with her, he absolutely detests the support staff for their incompetence.*
Neurotic Defenses	**Definition**	**Example**
Intellectu-alization	Focusing on the cognitive components of a situation while avoiding the emotional components	*A physician who is just diagnosed with leukemia queries prognostic and life expectancy data on PubMed.*
Repression	Blocking unpleasant internal stimuli (eg, memories, desires) from consciousness	*A pt believes that he was abused as a child but can't recall any of the details.*

(continued)

Defense Mechanisms *(continued)*		
Psychotic Defenses	**Definition**	**Example**
Reaction formation	Behaving the complete opposite from internal, uncomfortable desires	*A woman constantly criticizes her coworker to whom she is secretly attracted.*
Displacement	Transferring uncomfortable impulses from one person to another	*A father who is humiliated by his boss at work returns home to yell at his child.*
Somatization	Converting uncomfortable emotions into uncomfortable physical sensations	*A pt, when describing his mother's harsh criticism in session, begins to experience a headache.*
Mature Defenses	**Definition**	**Example**
Suppression	Consciously blocking unpleasant stimuli from consciousness to contend with immediate needs	*A fireman responds to a fire and sees the bodies of several victims. He deals with the fire, then, a day later, seeks counseling.*
Humor	Focusing on the humorous aspects of a painful emotion/ situation	*A man undergoing chemotherapy laughs with his grandchildren about his baldness.*
Sublimation	Redirecting unacceptable emotions into socially acceptable behaviors	*A teenage boy, angered by the death of his mother a year earlier, finds an outlet for his anger by rising through the ranks of his basketball team.*

SUPPORTIVE THERAPY

Background and Philosophy

- First defined in 1939 in the context of social work, definition broadened in the 1950s in the context of psychoanalysis, to support the patient in their current struggles rather than trying to deepen their understanding of unconscious drives (*Nord Psychol.* 2007;59(2):181-188)
- Objectives of supportive therapy are more limited than psychodynamic therapy, with the focus on ameliorating conscious, rather than unconscious, problems, and conflicts
- Help pt cope with symptoms, prevent relapse of illness, or deal w/ transient problem

Principles and Techniques

Core Principles (Winston A, Rosenthal R, Pinsker H. *Introduction to Supportive Psychotherapy.* Washington, DC: American Psychiatric Publishing, Inc; 2004)

- Therapist directly attempts to ameliorate symptoms and maintain, restore, or improve self-esteem, ego function, and adaptive skills
- Therapeutic alliance is key, as therapist is the figure of stability in pt's chaotic or difficult world, and continued positive interactions with therapist combat pt's hopelessness and expand the pt's self-mastery

Techniques

- Support pt's defenses unless maladaptive, rather than analyzing them
- Discuss origins of defense/type of problem only as creation of a narrative, rather than to unearth unconscious material, with the goal of overcoming the problem
- Transference/countertransference not usually addressed in sessions unless interfering with therapeutic alliance/disrupting treatment
- Incorporate teaching (psychoeducation), encouragement, modeling, advice giving (ideally following collaborative discussion), and anticipatory guidance surrounding potential problems and solutions
- Goals include amelioration of symptoms as well as improvement/ enhancement of adaptation, self-esteem, and overall functioning
- Basic strategies include formulating the case, being a "good parent," fostering and protecting the therapeutic alliance, managing the transference, holding/containing the patient, lending psychic structure, maximizing adaptive coping mechanisms, providing role model for identification, decreasing alexithymia (giving pts language to describe mood), making interpersonal connections, raising self-esteem, ameliorating hopelessness, focussing on the here and now, encouraging pt activity, educating pt and family, and manipulating the environment (eg, communicate with social services if needed) (*J Psychother Pract Res.* 9(4):173–189)

How to Start?	
(Winston et al., *Introduction to Supportive Psychotherapy*; 2004)	
Ideal therapeutic candidate	Pt in crisis and/or w/ chronic illness with concomitant impairment of adaptive skills and psychological functions
Relative contraindications	Organic mental disorders, eg, delirium, intoxication, dementia. OCD, Tourette syndrome, panic disorder, bulimia have stronger evidence for alternative modalities
Frequency, number of sessions	Weekly, during crisis or indefinitely if pt with chronic illness
Therapeutic stance	Conversational, active, alliance-strengthening
Boundaries	Judicious use of disclosure allowed if purposeful/in the interest of pt's treatment

Evidence-Based Applications
- Few if any quality studies evaluating the supportive therapy modality alone, often used as comparative therapy type in studies on populations known to benefit from other types of therapy (eg, OCD)
- Extensive research demonstrates effect of any specific psychotherapy is attributable to supportive common factors among the psychotherapies, having a "helping relationship" with the therapist (*Harv Rev Psychiatry*. 20(5):259-267)
- Naturalistic, nonrandomized 30-y study demonstrated supportive interventions were significantly more effective and accounted for more achieved outcomes (including structural changes) than anticipated (*J Consult Clin Psychol*. 57(2):195-205)
- Meta-analysis of supportive therapy in depression demonstrated effective treatment of depression in adults, equivalent to other psychotherapy modalities when controlling for researcher alliance (*Clin Psychol Rev*. 32(4):280-291)
- Multisite trial of dynamic versus supportive therapy in schizophrenia found decreased relapse and rehospitalization and improved social functioning with supportive therapy (*Schizophr Bull*. 10:520-563; *Schizophr Bull*. 10:564-598)

GROUP THERAPY

Background and Philosophy
- **Overview:** Group therapy is the treatment of psychological problems in a group context rather than individual
- **Scope:** Conditions treated by group therapy range from adjustment (coping with chronic medical conditions, bereavement) to personality disorders, mood disorders, and substance use disorders. Relative contraindications include severe paranoid propensities or crisis situations better served by higher levels of care
- **Approach:** A variety of approaches can be utilized, including but not limited to behavioral and cognitive-behavioral, psychoanalytic and interpersonal, and psychoeducational. Groups can range from manualized skills-based education sessions (eg, DBT, CBT, ACT, mentalization) to peer-led self-help meetings (eg, AA, DBSA), to process-oriented interpersonal groups (eg, psychoanalytic, psychodynamic)

Principles and Techniques
- **Core therapeutic principles** (*Yalom I, The Theory and Practice of Group Psychotherapy*; 2005)

  Universality and cohesiveness: Members feel that they are not going through challenges alone and can cultivate a sense of belonging

  Self-understanding and interpersonal learning: Feedback from group members can improve insight and translate into growth

  Development of socializing techniques: The group is structured to promote effective communication and dissuade maladaptive behaviors

Corrective recapitulation of primary family experience: Dynamics present in a member's family system can be unconsciously reenacted by group, and if recognized, can give insight to avoid repeating unhelpful patterns

Imparting information: Leader and group members can provide advice or education

Existential factors: Taking responsibility for consequences of decisions

Altruism: Helping others in the group can boost members own sense of purpose and self-esteem

Instillation of hope and imitative behavior: Seeing success of other members can foster hopefulness for improvement and can set examples of successfully implemented knowledge and skills

Catharsis: Sharing allows for release of intense emotions to promote healing

- **Developmental stages and techniques** (*Int J Group Psychother.* 2008;58(4):455-542)
  1. **Forming or "Preaffiliation":** Tentative sharing and self-disclosure will begin; anxiety is common. Leader identifies similarities between members, clarifies group purpose/roles, and suggests guidelines for participation
  2. **Storming or "Power and Control":** Emotional engagement increases, and conflict is expected; subgroups and pairing may occur as members try to create hierarchy. Leader reiterates ground rules, encourages connection and interpersonal feedback, and invites expressions of negative affect to work toward conflict resolution
  3. **Norming or "Intimacy":** Having weathered the storming phase, trust and commitment increase and allows for vulnerability and enhanced cohesion. Leader is less active, balancing confrontation and support to allow optimal learning
  4. **Performing or "Differentiation":** Acceptance of differences between members, awareness of strengths and weaknesses; themes may include the time-limited nature of the group. Leader allows group to run independently and may help members to magnify differences and express empathy
  5. **Adjourning or "Separation":** Sadness and anxiety regarding the loss of the group, recurrence of presenting problems may occur, with focus on future and maintaining gains. Leader assists with summative evaluation of progress, preparing for postgroup, and facilitates goodbyes

Evidence for Effectiveness (*Focus.* 2016;14(2):229; *Int J Group Psychother.* 1986;36(2):171; *Group Dyn.* 1998;2(2):101; *J Couns Psychol.* 2005;52:310)

- Meta-analyses reviewing group versus individual therapy showed that groups are at least as effective and occasionally more effective than individual care (diagnoses effectively treated include adjustment disorders, MDD, personality disorders, phobias, and anxiety disorders, among others)

- Measures of group cohesion have been correlated with clinical improvement
- Studies found that groups may be more cost efficient, as more patients can be treated for the same amount of time, particularly helpful when mental health resources are scarce

COUPLES THERAPY

Background and Philosophy

- Couples therapy focuses on problematic patterns in a relationship (see also "Family Therapy" section) rather than an individual
- Guiding philosophy:

  Relationship distress and mental health symptoms can be chronic; an individual's symptoms affect (and are affected by) the partner and the relationship (Am J Psychiatry. 1990;147(9):1128-1137)

  Distress between partners → tension and interpersonal hostility → loss of intimacy and emotional connection → depression and dissatisfaction within the partnership

  Couples therapy attempts to decrease relationship distress by exploring, processing, and changing problematic patterns

  There are many different types of couples therapy that draw from different theoretical backgrounds (eg, family systems theory, cognitive behavioral therapy, and attachment theory) (Am J Fam Ther. 2003;31(5):345-353)

- **Common problems:** Poor communication, lack of support between partners, not fulfilling expected marital roles, poor understanding about an individual's mental health condition with interpersonal sequelae (eg, blame and criticism toward a depressed person's negativity)

Principles and Techniques (Ryan CE, Keitner GI, Epstein NB, Evaluating and Treating Families: The McMaster Approach; 2005)

- Explore the nature and quality of the relationship, life changes, each partner's understanding of the situation, awareness of treatment strategies, and expectations of the partner
- Evaluate the couple's functioning (unique to each couple):
  - Problem-solving (ability to resolve problems together)
  - Communication (exchanging information with each other)
  - Roles (repeated behaviors by individuals to fulfill family functions)
  - Affective responsiveness (ability to respond to feelings experienced by the other)
  - Affective involvement (degree of interest and valuing the other's activities)
  - Behavioral control (rules of accepted behavior within partnership)
- Identify potentially dysfunctional patterns, acknowledge unacknowledged feelings, reframe challenges using underlying feelings, elucidate how each contributes to problematic dynamics (eg, acting in ways that irritate or alienate the partner, or selectively seeking negative feedback, leading to rejection and poor self-image, followed by guilt

and resentment), promote acceptance of each other's experiences, facilitate expression of needs and wants, and generate solutions to restore positive interactions and shared activities

- Tolerating elicitation of strong affect within the relationship (eg, anger, fear, disappointment, attraction)
- Problems with sexual functioning are more likely to be successfully addressed in couples therapy if they are secondary to relationship distress. If sexual dissatisfaction is the cause of relationship distress it is more likely to respond to sex therapy *(Kay J, Tasman A, Couples Therapy, in Essentials of Psychiatry. 2006:894-902)*
- Contraindications: primarily risk of violence, otherwise at discretion of therapist if there are secrets/confidentiality that interfere with treatment

Evidence for Effectiveness

- There are many different modalities in couples therapy (eg, cognitive restructuring, behavioral therapy, emotional expressiveness training) that are superior to control, but they are not significantly different from each other *(J Consult Clin Psychol. 1990;58(5):636-645)*
- Consistent evidence for using couples therapy to treat depression in one or both members of the partnership. Risk of depression is up to $25\times$ greater in distressed relationships versus untroubled relationships *(J Soc Clin Psychol. 1994;13(1):33-41)*. Poor response by family members to a depressed patient leads to lower likelihood of recovery and higher risk of relapse *(Am J Psychiatry. 1995;152(7):1002-1008)*
- Meta-analysis of 8 randomized trials ($n = 567$ couples) showed couples therapy efficacious for treating depression and reducing relationship distress with large effect size compared with wait list control; individual therapy was equally effective for treating depression (but not reducing relationship distress) *(Cochrane Database Syst Rev. 2006;CD004188)*

MONOAMINE OXIDASE INHIBITORS (MAOIs)

General Facts (*J Clin Psychiatry.* 2007;68:35-41; *CNS Drugs.* 2013;27:789-790)

- Discovered in 1952 when iproniazid, a medication used to treat tuberculosis, was noted to have antidepressant qualities
- Iproniazid found to inhibit monoamine oxidase (MAO), an enzyme involved in catabolism of serotonin (5HT), dopamine (DA), and norepinephrine (NE)
- Inhibition of MAO in the brain was found to increase synaptic availability of these neurotransmitters → development of MAOIs for depression
- Examples of MAOIs: isocarboxazid, phenelzine, selegiline, and tranylcypromine, rasagiline (used in Parkinson's disease)
- Generally 4th line for the treatment of depression owing to significant side-effect profile
- Dreaded complications of MAOIs include hypertensive crises and serotonin syndrome

Mechanism of Action (*Neuropsychopharmacology.* 1999;20:226-247)

- MAO is found in many parts of the body including the brain, GI tract, liver, and more

MAO Subtype	Location	Neurotransmitters (NTs)	Special Considerations
MAO-A	Intestine, brain	5HT, NE, Epi	Degrades tyramine (Tyr), which can act inappropriately as NT
MAO-B	Platelets, brain	Dopamine, tyramine	N/A

- MAOIs irreversibly inhibit MAO-A, MAO-B, or both and bind to MAO for the life of the enzyme (14–28 d); ~7–14 d for new MAO to be made for activity/function to return

Indications (*J Clin Psychiatry.* 2010;71(suppl E1):e08; *J Psychopharmacol.* 2003;17(2):149-173)

- Owing to significant drug/food interactions, MAOIs are used rarely; usually reserved for treatment-resistant depression (2 or more unsuccessful trials of other antidepressants)
- May be useful for patients with atypical depression (hyperphagia, hypersomnia, leaden paralysis, rejection sensitivity)
- Selegiline and rasagiline also used in Parkinson's disease

Adverse Effects (*J Psychiatr Pract.* 2004;10:239-248; *J Clin Psychiatry.* 1996;57:99-104; *CNS Spectr.* 2008;13:855-870; *Biol Psychiatry.* 2003;54:1099-1104; *Am J Psychiatry.* 1991;148:705-713; *J Clin Psychopharmacol.* 1989;6:397-402)

- Common: Insomnia, sedation, orthostatic hypotension, dizziness, and nausea

Adverse Effects	Pathophysiology	Special Considerations	Drug Interactions
Hypertensive crisis	MAO-A metabolizes dietary tyramine in gut MAOI causes tyramine to build up and enter bloodstream acting as a false NT → release of NE, ↑ BP → hypertensive crisis → stroke → death	Dietary restrictions: aged cheeses, cured meats, soy sauce, tofu, tap beer, etc Transdermal MAOIs (selegiline) can be used to avoid 1st-pass metabolism in the gut → dietary restrictions not required when using the minimum effective dose of the Selegiline transdermal patch	Can be precipitated by sympathomimetics, including decongestants (over the counter), amphetamines (methamphetamine and other stimulants); bupropion; meperidine
Serotonin syndrome	MAOIs block catabolism of 5HT, build up, and when MAOIs used in conjunction with other strong serotonergic effects → serotonin syndrome	Other serotonergic medications should not be taken for 5 ½ lives prior to instituting MAOI treatment. Eg: fluoxetine requires 5-wk wash-out period	Antidepressants Linezolid Synthetic opioids Triptans Other serotonergic agents

Efficacy (*J Psychiatry Pract.* 2009;15:45-49; *Acta Psychiatr Scand.* 2007;115:360-365)
- In the STAR*D trial, MAOIs were introduced as 4th-line treatment for refractory depression with a remission rate of 6.9% in people who had not achieved remission with 3 prior trials of medication

Prescribing (*J Clin Psychiatry.* 2010;71(suppl E1):e08; *CNS Spectr.* 2006;11:363-375)
- Tranylcypromine: Initial 10–30 mg, target dose 20–40 mg, increase by 10 mg q2–3wk, max dose 60 mg daily
- Phenelzine: Initial 15–45 mg, target dose 15–60 mg, increase by 15 mg q2–3wk, max dose 90 mg daily
- Selegiline transdermal: Initial 6 mg daily, goal dose 6 mg, increase by 3 mg q2wk, max dose 6–12 mg daily (when using the Selegiline patch at greater than 6 mg daily, a low-tyramine diet is required, given very little data regarding safety profile)
- Isocarboxazid: Starting dose 10–20 mg/d, max daily dose 30–60 mg

TRICYCLIC ANTIDEPRESSANTS

General Facts

- Tricyclic antidepressants (TCAs) are older medications that are generally considered 2nd or 3rd line for depression as they have many side effects
- **Mechanism of Action:** Block reuptake of 5-HT and NE → increase downstream DA in the frontal cortex; histamine (H1) blockade → insomnia; presynaptic alpha blockade → sedation and anxiolysis
- **Metabolism:** Oxidized in the liver; can phenotype to rule out CYP2D6 variant, which may impart extreme sensitivity to side effects

Indications

Depression: Most TCAs treat depression, **amitriptyline** and its metabolite **nortriptyline** are most used. In 2018 meta-analysis of antidepressants, amitriptyline was one of the most efficacious agents (OR 2.13) without increased rate of dropout (*Lancet. 2018;391:1357-1366*). In contrast, clomipramine not as efficacious, more poorly tolerated. In a 2003 trial, up to 40% of patients who had failed treatment with 2–4 antidepressants responded to 6 wk of **nortriptyline** (*J Clin Psychiatry. 2003;64:35-39*)

Insomnia (sleep maintenance): **Doxepin** is preferentially antihistaminergic at low doses (5–10 mg). A 2010 long-term polysomnographic study showed utility for sleep maintenance and early morning awakening in the elderly (*Sleep. 2010;33:1553-1361*)

PTSD: **Imipramine** has a weak recommendation by the US Dept of Defense/VA as monotherapy (in contrast to other TCAs), although SSRIs remain 1st-line (*VA/DoD Clinical Practice Guideline for the Management of PTSD. 2017:1-34*)

OCD: **Clomipramine** is the only TCA with FDA approval for OCD. A 2016 meta-analysis found that it may be more efficacious than SSRIs in pediatric patients (*JAACAP. 2016;55:851-859*)

Nicotine dependence: In 2008 RCT, **nortriptyline** performed similarly to nicotine replacement, but little evidence to support combo (*BMJ. 2008;336:1223-1227*)

Cataplexy syndrome: Multiple small-scale studies have supported use of **clomipramine** and **protriptyline** in preventing loss of voluntary muscle tone in syndromes such as narcolepsy (*Nat Sci Sleep. 2017;9:39-57*)

Enuresis: **Imipramine** thought to work via anticholinergic effects and an unknown central mechanism. However, 2016 Cochrane review found TCAs to be no more effective and less tolerable than desmopressin, less effective than bed-wetting alarm (*Cochrane Database Syst Rev. 2016;1:CD002117*)

Anxiety disorders: TCAs as a group were found to have a lower effect size (nonsignificant) than SSRIs, SNRIs, and BZDs in a 2015 meta-analysis *(Int J Clin Psychopharmacol. 2015;30:183-192)*

Adverse effects

Overall, more common in TCAs than other antidepressants; best to minimize TCA use in geriatric and pediatric populations

Common: GI upset, sedation, hypotension, anticholinergic effects (constipation, urinary retention, dry mouth, dry eyes), sexual dysfunction, hyponatremia

Uncommon: arrhythmias, seizures (especially when coadministered with tramadol), paralytic ileus, confusion and delirium, liver failure

Note: generally avoided in geriatric and pediatric patients

Monitoring

EKG baseline (in >50 y/o); baseline and periodic weights, consider FLP, HbA1c; BMP + Mg in patients at risk of arrhythmia

Overdose *(Emerg Med J. 2001;18:235-241)*

- TCAs can be lethal in overdose and may require ICU admission
- **Toxic effects** include the following:

  Anticholinergic effects: may result in toxic megacolon, impaired thermal regulation, fever, and delirium

  Alpha-receptor blockade: may result in severe hypotension necessitating IV fluid administration and pressor support

  Sodium-channel blockade: may result in myocardial membrane instability, subsequent arrhythmias, and impaired cardiac contractility

  Norepinephrine reuptake blockade: likely mediator of tachycardia, seizures, and altered mental status

- **Workup of suspected ingestions** includes the following:

  Exam: Altered mental status, tachycardia, hypotension, flushing, dry skin

  Serum TCA level: >1000 µg/L associated with worse outcomes

  EKG + cardiac monitor: Wide complex tachycardia, increased QTc; monitor until normal for 12–24 h

  BMP + ABG/VBG: Metabolic/respiratory acidosis

- **Management of overdose:**

  Reduce absorption via gastric lavage (if <1 h after) and activated charcoal

  Stabilize cardiac membrane, treat acidemia, reduce bioavailable TCA via serum alkalization with sodium bicarbonate

  Reduce risk of arrhythmia via electrolyte repletion (Mg > 2, K > 4); no role for antiarrhythmics

  Treat dangerous hypotension with IV fluids and pressor support as necessary

  Intubate for airway compromise (GCS ≤ 8)

  Treat seizures with benzodiazepines

  Note: most complications of overdose will occur within 6 h of overdose

Prescribing

Tertiary Amines						
Name	Half-Life (h)	Start (mg/d)	Goal (mg/d)	Freq	Titration	Nota Bene (NB)
Amitriptyline	10–28	25	50–150	qPM	+25 mg q3–7d	Often used in chronic pain syndromes (eg, migraines, fibromyalgia)
Clomip-ramine	17–28	25	100–250	qPM	+25 mg q5d	
Doxepin	8–24	25	75–300	qPM	+25 mg q3–7d	Often used in topical formulation for pain (pruritic, neuro-pathic)
Imipramine	20	150	50–300	qPM	+25 mg q3d	

Secondary Amines						
Name	Half-Life (h)	Start (mg/d)	Goal (mg/d)	Freq	Titration	NB
Desipramine	24	25	100–300	qPM	+25 mg q3–7d	Better tolerated than parent drug, imipramine
Nortriptyline	36	10–25	75–300	qPM	+25 mg q3–7d	Better tolerated than parent drug, amitrip-tyline
Amoxapine	8	75	200–400	B/TID	+75 mg q7d	Risk of EPS due to metabolites structurally similar to neuro-leptics

(continued)

Secondary Amines *(continued)*						
Name	Half-Life (h)	Start (mg/d)	Goal (mg/d)	Freq	Titration	NB
Protriptyline	74	15	15–60	TID	+5 mg q3d	Manufacturer reports onset is faster than other TCAs (<1 wk)
Maprotiline	51	25	75–225	qPM	+25 mg q3–7d	

SEROTONIN AND NOREPINEPHRINE REUPTAKE INHIBITORS (SNRIS)

General Facts
- **Summary**: SNRIs are 1st line for a wide variety of the most prevalent psychiatric conditions and highly utilized in chronic pain syndromes

Mechanism of Action
Inhibit presynaptic serotonin (5-HT) (SERT) and norepinephrine (NET) transporter proteins, increasing the availability of 5-HT and NE in the synaptic cleft. Many SNRIs display dose-dependent and sequential reuptake inhibition (ie, 5HT 1st, then NE)

Indications
FDA approved for at least 1 agent: MDD, GAD, panic disorder, social anxiety disorder, fibromyalgia, diabetic peripheral neuropathy, chronic MSK pain
Off-label: PTSD, PMDD, stress urinary incontinence

Adverse Effects
- Common effects: nausea (most common, diminishes over time), dizziness, diaphoresis, constipation, headaches, insomnia, HTN, hyponatremia (SIADH), slightly increased bleeding risk with NSAIDs, bone resorption, moderate sexual side effects (anorgasmia, delayed ejaculation, decreased libido)
- QTc prolongation: not as associated with QTc prolongation, except venlafaxine (*Ann Pharmacother.* 48(12):1620-1628)
- Discontinuation syndrome: more common with SSRIs but can occur with SNRIs (more common w/venlafaxine and desvenlafaxine). Dizziness, headache, tremors, insomnia, GI upset, and paresthesias can occur within 1–3 d of suddenly stopping an SNRI, generally lasts no longer than 1–3 wk. Can be treated by restarting the agent with a gradual taper. Risk is strongly related to half-life (shorter half-life = higher risk)
- Serotonin syndrome (SS): Overdoses and polypharmacy with other serotonergic agents (eg, MAOIs, TCAs, triptans, meperidine, and linezolid) can cause a potentially life-threatening psychomotor syndrome (*NEJM.* 2005;352:1112)

SELECTIVE SEROTONIN REUPTAKE INHIBITORS (SSRIs)

General Facts
- The 6 SSRIs are 1st line for a wide variety of the most prevalent psychiatric conditions. They are cheap, extensively studied, well tolerated, and relatively safe in overdose and pregnancy

Mechanism of Action
- Inhibition of the serotonin (5-hydroxytryptamine, 5-HT) transporter (SERT) increasing the availability of 5-HT in the synaptic cleft

Indications
- *FDA approved for at least 1 agent:* major depressive disorder (MDD), premenstrual dysphoric disorder (PMDD), generalized anxiety disorder (GAD), panic disorder (PD), social anxiety disorder (SAD), obsessive–compulsive disorder (OCD), posttraumatic stress disorder (PTSD), vasomotor symptoms of menopause, bulimia nervosa, bipolar depression (only olanzapine/fluoxetine combination therapy)
- *Off-label:* Premature ejaculation, substance-induced mood disorders, persistent depressive disorder, binge eating disorder, anorexia nervosa, pathological gambling, fibromyalgia

FDA-Approved Indications for SSRIs								
Generic (Brand)	MDD	PMDD	GAD	PD	SAD	OCD	PTSD	Other
Sertraline (Zoloft)	X	X		X	X	X	X	
Escitalopram (Lexapro)	X		X					
Citalopram (Celexa)	X							
Fluoxetine (Prozac)	X	X		X		X		Bulimia nervosa Bipolar depression*
Paroxetine (Paxil)	X	X	X	X	X	X	X	Vasomotor symptoms of menopause (Brisdelle)
Fluvoxamine (Luvox)						X		

*Only in combination with olanzapine.

Adverse Effects
- **Common effects**: GI upset (nausea, vomiting, diarrhea), headaches, tremors, jitteriness, somnolence, insomnia, hyponatremia (SIADH), slightly increased bleeding risk with NSAIDs, sexual side effects (anorgasmia, delayed ejaculation, decreased libido)

- **Weight gain** (*JAMA Psychiatry.* 2014;71:889): No consistent weight gain in short-term RCTs (4–12 wk), but retrospective cohorts indicate that they may cause modest gains of up to 1 kg on average after 1 y
- **QTc prolongation** (*Psychosomatics.* 2013;54:1): Largest concern with citalopram (10–20 ms) and to a lesser extent escitalopram (5–10 ms). Not clearly a class effect with other agents being relatively safe
- **Treatment emergent affective switching** (*Am J Psychiatry.* 2004;161:163): Although controversial, unipolar antidepressants may induce manic episodes in bipolar depression. Screening for prior manic or hypomanic episodes is recommended before treatment (always in conjunction with a mood stabilizer)
- **Discontinuation syndrome** (*Drug Saf.* 2001;24:183): Dizziness, headache, tremors, insomnia, GI upset, and paresthesias ("brain zaps") can occur within 1–3 d of suddenly stopping an SSRI. Generally, lasts no longer than 1–3 wk. Can be treated by restarting the agent with a gradual taper or cross-tapering to fluoxetine (half-life 3–5 d). Risk is strongly related to half-life (shorter = higher risk). SSRIs are not addictive, and this syndrome is not life-threatening
- **Serotonin syndrome (SS)** (*NEJM.* 2005;352:1112): Overdoses and polypharmacy with other serotonergic agents (eg, MAOIs, TCAs, triptans, meperidine, linezolid) can cause a potentially life-threatening psychomotor syndrome
- **Overdose (OD) effects** (*Am J Psychiatry.* 2017;174:438): Generally very safe. Most common effects are drowsiness and GI upset. A review of nearly 1 million single agent antidepressant exposures showed that citalopram was significantly more dangerous than sertraline, escitalopram, or fluoxetine (4.2 deaths per 10,000 ODs vs 0.9, 0.9, and 0.8, respectively). For comparison, amitriptyline caused 37.5 deaths, acetaminophen 25.8, and diphenhydramine 4.8 per 10,000 exposures

Controversies
- **Black box warning** (*NEJM.* 2007;356:2343): The FDA requires all antidepressants to carry a black box warning about increased suicidal thinking and behavior in children and young adults <24 y. A meta-analysis of 372 RCTs (n = 99,839) showed an increase of 14 exacerbations per 1000 patients <24 y, no increase in patients 24–65 y, and a decrease of 6 cases among patients >65 y. No completed suicides among children were noted. Proposed explanations include activating side effects and an early energy response that precedes a delayed effect on mood. The risk is generally considered to occur transiently in the initial weeks of treatment, although data evaluating long-term risk are lacking
- **Teratogenicity** (*Acta Psychiatr Scand.* 2013;127:94): SSRIs are generally considered safe in pregnancy, and continuation is recommended for high-risk women. Paroxetine was previously thought to carry a higher risk because of possible cardiac malformations, but this is no longer widely accepted (inconsistent evidence).

No teratogenic effects are convincingly established, although persistent pulmonary hypertension has been intermittently associated. Late exposure can cause a poor neonatal adjustment syndrome with transient and self-limited discontinuation-like symptoms after delivery

- **Separation from placebo** (Br J Psychiatry. 2012;200:97): Some researchers allege that the SSRIs do not consistently separate from placebo to a clinically meaningful degree when unpublished data are taken into account (PLoS Med. 2008;5:e45). Larger-network meta-analyses indicate a true small-to-moderate effect size that is comparable to the treatments of other chronic diseases such as asthma, hypertension, and multiple sclerosis

- **Comparative efficacy:** Traditionally all unipolar antidepressants were thought to have equivalent efficacy and tolerability on a population level (see the STAR*D trial results). Emerging evidence from network meta-analyses by members of the Cochrane Collaboration suggests that sertraline and escitalopram may have a slight edge for adults and fluoxetine for children (Lancet. 2009;373:746; Lancet. 2016;388:881; Lancet. 2018;391:1357)

SSRIs: Prescriber's Pharmacology				
Medication	Half-Life (h)	Start (mg/d)	Goal (mg/d)	Nota Bene (NB)
Sertraline	26	50	50–200	Generally well tolerated despite significant GI upset Well studied in the presence of cardiac disease Good 1st-line agent for adults
Escitalopram	27–32	10	10–20	Clean metabolism with few drug interactions Good 1st-line agents for adults QTc prolongation but less than citalopram
Citalopram	35	20	20–40	Slightly more dangerous in overdose Used in STAR*D as the 1st-line agent Dose reduced from 60 mg by the FDA for QTc prolongation (highest risk among SSRIs) 20 mg max in geriatrics recommended by FDA

SSRI 6-9

(continued)

SSRIs: Prescriber's Pharmacology *(continued)*				
Medication	**Half-Life (h)**	**Start (mg/d)**	**Goal (mg/d)**	**Nota Bene (NB)**
Fluoxetine	72–216*	20	20–60	Very long half-life, low risk of dc syndrome Strong CYP2D6 inhibitor Good 1st-line agent for children
Paroxetine	21	20	20–60	Short half-life, high risk of dc syndrome Strong CYP2D6 inhibitor Anticholinergic, possibly more weight gain/sedation IR, CR (immediate, continuous) formulations
Fluvoxamine	14–16	50	100–300	Short half-life, high risk of dc syndrome Only SSRI not approved for MDD (just OCD) Most expensive SSRI Extensive drug interactions Can augment clozapine via CYP1A2 inhibition IR, CR (immediate, continuous) formulations

All SSRIs are dosed QD except fluvoxamine IR, which is BID (CR is QD). Titrate in increments of their starting dose as fast as every 3 d inpatient and every 7 d outpatient. Starting doses should be halved in the presence of panic disorder or severe anxiety to prevent discontinuation. Effective doses are generally higher in OCD. Levels are not used, and no monitoring is generally required. All are oxidatively metabolized by the liver and renally excreted.

*Fluoxetine has an active metabolite (norfluoxetine) which has a mean half-life of 7–9 d.

Novel Agents: Serotonin Modulators

- Two new agents that have complex direct effects on the 7 individual serotonin receptor subtypes have been approved recently. They are considerably more expensive than existing agents and have limited head-to-head data compared with the traditional SSRIs
- **Vortioxetine (Trintellix):**
  Mechanism: SERT inhibition with 5-HT3 antagonism and 5-HT1A agonism
  Indications: MDD (may have greater improvements in depression-associated cognitive dysfunction than other agents)
- **Vilazodone (Viibryd):**
  Mechanism: SERT inhibition with partial 5-HT1A agonism (similar to an SSRI plus buspirone)
  Indications: MDD

Novel Serotonergic Antidepressants: Prescriber's Pharmacology (depression monotherapy)							
Medication	Metabolism	Half-Life (h)	Start (mg/d)	Goal (mg/d)	Freq	Titration	Level (µg/mL)
Vortioxetine	Liver (ox)	66	10	10–20	QD	+10 mg q7d	N/A
Vilazodone	Liver (ox)	25	10	20–40	QD	+10 mg q7d	N/A

ATYPICAL ANTIDEPRESSANTS

KETAMINE

General Facts
- A dissociative agent used as an anesthetic, a recreational drug, and a novel therapy for treatment-resistant depression (TRD)

Mechanism of Action
- NMDA receptor antagonists, also weak agonists of µ-opioid, κ-opioid, and D2 receptors; antidepressant effects thought to be driven by glutamate surge and prosynaptogenic activation

Indications
- *Treatment-resistant depression:* Multiple studies demonstrate a single infusion of ketamine producing rapid antidepressant response in >50% of patients but is usually transient (10–14 d). A 2016 double-blind, randomized, placebo-controlled, dose-frequency study found that IV ketamine (twice or thrice weekly dosing) had significantly greater antidepressant effect compared with placebo at 15-d, 30-d, and 4-wk follow-up (Am J Psychiatry. 2016;173(8):816-826)
- *Suicidal ideation:* Recent studies suggest greater improvement and resolution in suicidal ideation with ketamine infusions compared with placebo (Wilkinson ST, Ballard ED, et al. The effect of a single dose of intravenous ketamine on suicidal ideation: a systematic review and individual. J Clin Psychiatry. 2010;12:1605-1611). A recent meta-analysis showed rapid and clinically significant reduction in SI for 40 min to 10 d postinfusion (Am J Psychiatry. 2018;175(2):150-158)
- *Other disorders:* less data for PTSD, OCD, chronic neuropathic pain

Adverse Effects
- Nausea, dizziness; dissociative symptoms (transient, diminishes with repeated dosing); mild tachycardia and HTN; risk of bladder toxicity and drug abuse

Administration Route
- IV, IN, IM; poor absorption orally

Nota Bene (NB)

- Most ketamine treatments are conducted within research settings, although it is also sparsely available outside of research settings at academic centers and private clinics. An intranasal formulation of S-ketamine with a treatment-resistant depression indication may be approved soon

---

MIRTAZAPINE

General Facts

- Mirtazapine is a sedating atypical antidepressant that affects norepinephrine and serotonin. Its sedating and appetite stimulating properties make it particularly useful in palliative care and psycho-oncology. It is inexpensive and generally very well tolerated

Mechanism of Action

- Noradrenergic and specific serotonergic antidepressant (NaSSA) via central alpha-2 adrenergic antagonism (the opposite of clonidine) alongside potent 5-HT2, 5-HT3, and H1 antagonism

Indications

- MDD: A 2018 network meta-analysis of 21 unipolar antidepressants included 34 RCTs involving mirtazapine. It ranked as the 2nd-best agent in terms of efficacy (OR 1.89, 1.64–2.20) and average in terms of tolerability (OR 0.99, 0.85–1.15) compared with placebo (*Lancet.* 2018;391:1357)
- Appetite stimulation (off-label): In a meta-analysis of 116 antidepressant trials (19 of mirtazapine), it ranked among the worst offenders for weight gain at 1.74 kg (1.28, 2.20) in short-term studies (*J Clin Psychiatry.* 2010;71:1259)
- Secondary insomnia (off-label): No prospective evidence for primary insomnia, but small RCTs show efficacy for insomnia related to depression (*Pharmacol Rev.* 2018;70:197)

Adverse Effects

- GI upset (nausea, vomiting, constipation), dry mouth, dizziness, somnolence, increased appetite and weight gain, serotonin syndrome (especially in combination with an MAOI), case reports of fulminant hepatotoxicity, generally considered low risk in pregnancy

Monitoring

- None

Nota Bene (NB)

- Minimal sexual side effects compared with placebo and much less than SSRIs (*Ann Pharmacother.* 2002;36:1577)
- Mirtazapine and venlafaxine (synergistic activating effects on 5-HT and NE) combination used in level IV of STAR*D, but limited evidence otherwise (*Am J Psychiatry.* 2006;163:1531; *J Psychopharmacol.* 2007;21:161)
- May be more sedating at lower doses where antihistamine effects predominate, but robust clinical studies are lacking (*CNS Drug Rev.* 2001;7:249)

ATYPICAL 6-12

Mirtazapine: Prescriber's Pharmacology (depression monotherapy)						
Metabolism	Half-Life (h)	Start (mg/d)	Goal (mg/d)	Freq	Titration	Level (µg/mL)
Liver (ox)	20–40	15 (7.5 in geriatrics)	15–45	QHS	+15 mg q7d	N/A

TRAZODONE

Mechanism of Action
- Potent blockade of 5-HT2A/C receptors; less potent blockade of serotonin reuptake; alpha-1 blockade; antihistaminergic at low doses

Indications
- *Depression:* In a 2018 meta-analysis, trazodone was found to rank among the least effective antidepressants, as well as among the most poorly tolerated (*Lancet.* 2018;391:1357-1366)
- *Insomnia:* A 2018 meta-analysis found that while trazodone decreased the number of awakenings and improved perceived sleep quality, it did not improve sleep efficiency (*Sleep Med.* 2018;45:25-32). It is not recommended by the American Academy of Sleep Medicine for chronic (primary) insomnia, although it is commonly used in secondary insomnias (eg, depression, anxiety)
- *Anxiety/agitation:* Often used in minute doses (eg, 12.5–25 mg) multiple times per day as a nonnarcotic PRN for anxiety and agitation, especially in elderly patients for whom benzodiazepines and antipsychotics are undesirable (*AAFP.* 2000;61:1437-1446). One double-blind comparison study suggested favorability over haloperidol in repetitive verbal aggression and oppositional behaviors (*Am J Geriatr Psychiatry.* 1997;5:60-69)

Adverse Effects
- Sedation, orthostatic hypotension, headache, priapism (1 in 6000 men) (*Managing Side Effects of Psychotropic Medications, APA;* 2012:216), arrhythmia (rare); pregnancy risk category C

Monitoring
- None

Nota Bene (NB)
- May increase levels of digoxin and phenytoin via an unknown mechanism

Trazodone: Prescriber's Pharmacology (depression monotherapy)						
Metabolism	Half-Life (h)	Start (mg/d)	Goal (mg/d)	Freq	Titration	Level (µg/mL)
Liver (ox)	3–9	150	200–600	BID	+50 mg q3d	N/A

BUPROPION

General Facts

- Bupropion is an activating atypical antidepressant that affects norepinephrine and dopamine. Its relation to the stimulants gives it a unique side-effect profile including potential benefits for weight loss, smoking cessation, ADHD, and sexual function. It is inexpensive and generally well-tolerated, but it can lower the seizure threshold and may worsen anxiety

Mechanism of Action

- NDRI (norepinephrine dopamine reuptake inhibitor)

Indications

MDD: A 2018 network meta-analysis of 21 unipolar antidepressants included 33 RCTs involving bupropion. It ranked as average in terms of efficacy (OR 1.58, 1.35–1.86) and tolerability (OR 0.96, 0.81–1.14) compared with placebo (*Lancet.* 2018;391:1357)

Prevention of episodes of MDD with seasonal pattern (formerly seasonal affective disorder): A review of 3 RCTs (*n* = 1042) showed a 44% relative risk reduction of future depressive episodes (*Biol Psychiatry.* 2005;58:658)

Smoking cessation: A Cochrane review of 36 RCTs with 11,140 participants showed a risk ratio of long-term cessation of 1.69 (1.53–1.85) (*Cochrane Database Syst Rev.* 2007;1:1)

Weight loss: In combination with naltrexone, bupropion showed a 4–5 kg greater weight loss than placebo after 1 y in the 4 COR (Contrave Obesity Research) trials (*JAMA.* 2014;311:74)

ADHD (off-label): Often used as a noncontrolled stimulant alternative in adults (*Biol Psychiatry.* 2005;57:793)

SSRI-induced sexual dysfunction (off-label): Commonly used as an augmenting strategy to increase libido (*Ann Pharmacother.* 2002;36:1577)

Bipolar depression (off-label): Limited evidence of efficacy, but may have a lower risk of inducing mania than other unipolar antidepressants (*NEJM.* 2007;356:1711)

Contraindications

- Patients at high risks for seizures (eg, eating disorders, traumatic brain injury, epilepsy)

Formulations

- IR (immediate release, TID), SR (sustained release, BID), XL (extended release, QD)

Adverse Effects

- GI upset (nausea, vomiting, diarrhea), headache, dry mouth, diaphoresis, insomnia, weight loss, worsened anxiety, tachycardia, seizures (especially IR formulation), generally considered low risk in pregnancy

Monitoring

- None

Nota Bene (NB)

- Related to the stimulants by structure, mechanism of action, and side-effect profile but not addictive. Can cause false positives on the amphetamine drug screen (*J Med Toxicol.* 2011;7:105)

- Minimal sexual side effects compared with placebo and much less than those of SSRIs *(Ann Pharmacother. 2002;36:1577)*
- May worsen anxiety but NNH compared with SSRIs was relatively high at 17 in a review of 10 RCTs with 1275 patients with anxious depression *(J Clin Psychiatry. 2008;69:1287)*
- Carries the highest risk of morbidity and mortality among modern antidepressants due to seizures. In a review of nearly 1 million single agent exposures from the National Poison Control Centers, the mortality rate for every 10,000 overdoses was 37.5 for amitripty-line, 7.5 for bupropion, and 0.9 for sertraline and escitalopram *(Am J Psychiatry. 2017;174:438)*

Bupropion: Prescriber's Pharmacology (depression monotherapy)								
Formu-lation	Metabo-lism	Half-Life (h)	Time to [Peak] (Cmax, h)	Start (mg/d)	Total Goal (mg/d)	Freq	Titration	Level (µg/mL)
XL	Liver (ox)	21	5	150 QD	300–450	QD	+150 mg q3d	N/A
SR	Liver (ox)	21	3	150 QD	300–400*	BID	+150 mg q3d	N/A
IR	Liver (ox)	21	2	100 BID	300–450	TID	+100 mg q3d	N/A

*The FDA package insert recommends a maximum dose of 200 mg BID for the SR formulation.

ANXIOLYTICS

BENZODIAZEPINES

General Facts
- Anxiolytic, hypnotic, anticonvulsive, sedative, muscle relaxant, and/or amnesic properties

Mechanism of Action
- Potentiates GABA receptors (inhibitory neurotransmitter, most common neurotransmitter in the nervous system, particularly dense in the cortex and limbic systems) via positive allosteric modulation

Indications
- Commonly prescribed as needed for acute or chronic anxiety. Also used for insomnia, alcohol withdrawal, seizures, muscle spasms, para-somnias, and rapid tranquilization in psychosis, mania, or agitation. Psychoeducation and short-term use recommended, given risk of tolerance and dependence

Side Effects
- Sedation, lethargy, rebound anxiety, amnesia, disinhibition, psychomo-tor impairment. Overmedication can also lead to impaired thinking,

disorientation, confusion, and slurred speech. Delirium and falls; 50% increased risk of hip fracture in the elderly. Sometimes, a paradoxical effect can lead to worsened agitation or behavioral disinhibition (*PLoS One.* 2017;e0174730)

Metabolism

- Occurs mainly via hepatic cytochrome P450 system, then renally excreted. Patients with liver disease will experience longer half-life, particularly for diazepam and clonazepam (active metabolites). Exceptions: lorazepam, oxazepam, temazepam (no active metabolites, half-life remains stable in liver disease)

Adverse Effects

- Frequent or long-term use poses risk of tolerance, dependence, worsened depression, cognitive deficits, and abuse. Overdose can lead to respiratory depression, coma, or death. Withdrawal is notoriously uncomfortable (anxiety, dysphoria, tremor, hallucinations, psychosis, seizures) and can be fatal. Driving under the influence of BZDs can cause MVAs. Conflicted evidence regarding association with dementia (*Accid Anal Prev.* 2016;96:255-270; *Drugs R D.* 2017;17(4):493-507)

Discontinuation

- Tapering off benzodiazepines requires a slow progressive schedule with frequent monitoring for withdrawal or relapse with supportive therapy and adjuncts for symptomatic relief as needed. Systematic taper twice as effective than just advising the patient to stop. Inpatient level of care may be prudent when discontinuing from high doses (*Br J Psychiatry.* 2006;189(3):213-220)

Interactions

- Higher risk of overmedication, cardiopulmonary depression, and fatal overdose when used in combination with other depressants including alcohol, opiates, methadone, z-drugs (zolpidem, zopiclone, eszopiclone), and clozapine. Also higher risk in elderly because of age-related physiological changes in the liver and kidney leading to accumulation of metabolites. Drugs that potentiate or inhibit CYP450 enzymes will decrease or increase the half-life of BZDs, respectively

Route

- PO, IM (lorazepam), IV (lorazepam, diazepam, midazolam)

Nota Bene

- Benzos are one of the most widely prescribed medications in the US. In 2013, per CDC data, 5.6% of US adults filled a BZD prescription, and 31% of fatal overdoses involved BZDs (*Am J Public Health.* 2016;106(4):686-688)

Benzodiazepines			
Drug	Comparative Potency	Time to Peak (h)	Half-Life (h)
Lorazepam	1	1–6	10–20
Clonazepam	0.5	1–2	18–50

Benzodiazepines (continued)			
Drug	Comparative Potency	Time to Peak (h)	Half-Life (h)
Alprazolam	0.5	1–2	6–27
Diazepam	5	1–2	20–80
Chlordiazepoxide	10	0.5–4	5–30
Oxazepam	15	1–4	5–15
Ochsner J. 2013;13(2):214-223; Psychiatry Clin Neurosci. 2015;69(8):440-447; Aust Prescr. 2015;38:152-155			

BUSPIRONE

General Facts
- Buspirone is a serotonin agonist that is typically well tolerated and frequently used in anxiety disorders

Mechanism of Action
- High-affinity full agonist of presynaptic inhibitory 5-HT1A autoreceptors; high-affinity partial agonist of postsynaptic 5-HT1A. Weak-affinity D_{1-4} antagonist (at lower dose range → CNS ↑DA due to differential affinities for auto- vs postsynaptic receptors). No BZD/GABA activity (Brain Res. 2012;1461:111-118; Int J Neuropsychopharmacol. 2016;16:445-458)

Prescribing
- Starting: 10–15 mg/d divided, generally bid or tid dosing. Increase by 5 mg/d every 2–3 d. Max dose: 60 mg/d

Indications
- **FDA:** Treatment of anxiety disorders (approval based on ≤4 wk studies in the 1980s, w/ pts whose dx "roughly corresponds to" DSM-3 GAD; many w/ depression too)
- **Common off-label:** Maintenance tx for anxiety disorders; adjunct tx for anxiety d/o; adjunct tx for mixed depression/anxiety; adjunct or mono tx for MDD (Psychol Med. 2014;44:2255-2269)
- **Equivocal/limited evid:** Sexual dysfx 2/2 mood/anx and/or antidepr (Transl Androl Urol. 2016;5:576-591); panic d/o ± agoraphobia (Cochrane Database Syst Rev. 2014;9:CD010828); ADHD (Pharmacopsychiatry. 2016;49(3): 97-106); hostility, including pedi/geri (J Psychosoc Nurs Ment Health Serv. 2015;53(11):21-24); restricted/repetitive behaviors and irritability in ASD (J Pediatr. 2016;170:45-53.e1-e4; Pediatr Neurol. 2015;52:77-81)

Conditions without Evidence Base
- Cannabis use disorder (Drug Alcohol Depend. 2015;156:29-37); pediatric anxiety (J Child Adolesc Psychopharmacol. 2018;28:2-9)

Efficacy
- Onset within 0–3 wk (Drug Saf. 1997;16:118-132); anxiolytic effect likely inferior to pregabalin, BZDs, SSRIs, SNRIs, and antihistamines (J Psychopharmacol. 2007;21:864-872)

Cautions
- Hepatic or renal impairment → ↑↑↑ levels, though no specific dose adjustment available

Contraindications
- Metabolic acidosis; severe hepatic/renal disease

Adverse Effects
- **Common adverse effects:** Dizziness, mild/mod sedation (esp. >20 mg/d), HA, N/V; more likely if dosing inconsistent in timing or in relation to food.
  Little to no sexual dysfx, weight gain, or discontinuation syndrome
- **Serious adverse effects:** $\downarrow\downarrow$ DA (eg, akathisia (*J Clin Psychopharmacol.* 1988;8:296-297), EPS; very rare but described, esp. in overdose (*Clin Neuropharacol.* 1998;21:347-350)); serotonin syndrome (rare but described, esp. high dose or drug interaction (*Ann Pharmacother.* 2000;34:871-874)).
  No evidence for dependence potential or significant lethality in overdose

Kinetics
- Extensive 1st-pass via CYP3A4 (major) and CYP2D6 (minor); primarily renally excreted (*Drug Metab Dispos.* 2005;33:500-507)

Interactions
- $\uparrow$ **by:** 3A4 substrates and inhibitors (eg, many macrolides, azole antifungals, calcium-channel blockers, and antiretrovirals; omeprazole; cimetidine; nefazodone; grapefruit)
- $\downarrow$ **by:** 3A4 inducers (eg, carbamazepine, phenytoin, phenobarbital, St. John's wart, ritonavir) (*Clin Pharmacol Ther.* 1998;64:655-660; *Am Fam Physician.* 2007;76:391-396; *Proc (Bayl Univ Med Cent).* 2000;13:421-423)
- **May increase potency and $t_{1/2}$ of:** antipsychotics, BZDs, serotonergic agents (*Pharmacol Biochem Behav.* 1985;23:687-694; *J Clin Psychopharmacol.* 1991;11:193-197; *Am J Psychiatry.* 1997;154:1472-1473; *J Clin Pharm Ther.* 2012;37:610-613)

ANTIEPILEPTIC DRUGS (AEDs)

Background (*Epilepsy Behav.* 2015;52:267-274; *Epilepsia.* 2011;52:308-315)
- The following agents are used for neurologic, psychiatric, and general medical practice
- Their primary indication is for seizure disorders and therefore are referred to as AEDs
- Classically used in psychiatry as a mood stabilizer, though also can be used in other illness of behavioral dysregulation, impulsivity, and agitation
- See Seizure Disorders for more regarding treatment of epilepsy and comorbid psychiatric disorders

VALPROIC ACID (VPA)
General Facts
- **Names and Formulations:** Depakote (PO), Depakene (PO), Depacon (IV), Sprinkles (SOL)
- **MOA:** blocks voltage-gated sodium channels, increases GABAergic activity; for all indications, full activity may take days to weeks

- **Indications**
  - *Mood stabilization*: Efficacy in preventing mood episodes compared with placebo (RR 0.68) (*Cochrane Database Syst Rev. 2013;10:CD003196*); efficacy in treating acute mania (RR 0.62) (*Cochrane Database Syst Rev. 2003;1:CD004052*); may be less effective in treating and preventing depressive episodes
  - *Schizophrenia*: May be effective as an adjunct with antipsychotics (RR of response to treatment 1.31 compared with placebo), although data are limited; aggression was reduced (*Cochrane Database Syst Rev. 2016;11:CD004028*)
  - *Agitation and aggression*: A 2000 case series demonstrated a robust reduction in agitation in TBI patients over a follow-up period of 22 mo (*J Neuropsychiatry Clin Neurosci. 2000;12:395-397*). However, there is little high-quality evidence to support the use of VPA in aggression, in dementia, TBI, or otherwise, despite its occasional use in patients with parkinsonism when antipsychotics are contraindicated
  - *Other*: neuropathic pain, migraines, seizure disorders, and status epilepticus

Adverse Effects
- **Common side effects:** HA, GI upset, weight gain, sedation, alopecia, PCOS
- **Rare and serious side effects:** hepatotoxicity, hyperammonemia, delirium, suicidality, marrow suppression (most commonly resulting in thrombocytopenia), pancreatitis (more often with IV formulation)
- **Overdose:** characterized by altered mental status leading to sedation and coma, heart block, and possibly death
- **Discontinuation:** taper slowly, as abrupt discontinuation may precipitate seizures or relapse of psychiatric illness
- **Contraindications:** allergy, liver impairment, pancreatitis, urea cycle disorder, pregnancy
- **Significant interactions:** VPA inhibits metabolism of lamotrigine; therefore, reduce lamotrigine use by 50% when used in combination

Valproic Acid: Prescriber's Pharmacology						
Starting Dose (mg/d)	Goal/ Max Dose (mg/d)	Titration	Metabolism	Half-Life (h)	Before Starting	Monitoring
500	1000–2000	+500 mg q3d	CYP2C9 CYP2A6	8 (DR) 16 (ER)	LFTs, CBC, A1c, FLP, weight	Drug levels (with changes, after 3–4 doses): 60–120 LFTs and CBC @1, 2, 6, 12 mo, and then yearly. Ammonia as indicated. Weight at each visit.

(continued)

Valproic Acid: Prescriber's Pharmacology (continued)						
Starting Dose (mg/d)	Goal/ Max Dose (mg/d)	Titration	Metabolism	Half-Life (h)	Before Starting	Monitoring

Liver impairment: contraindicated
Renal impairment: no adjustments necessary
Pediatric: generally avoid, especially for younger children given reduced oxidative capacity
Geriatric: reduce dose and uptitrate slower
Pregnant/breastfeeding: Formerly designated category D (before FDA retired categories) due to risk of congenital malformations (eg, NTDs). Theoretical risk of side effects as above in breastfeeding, although no adverse effects have been reported.

LAMOTRIGINE (LTG)

General Facts
- **Names and formulations:** Lamictal (PO)
- **MOA:** blocks voltage-gated sodium channels in use-dependent manner, changing their conformation, and inhibits release of glutamate and aspartate; onset of action takes weeks due to slow uptitration to prevent adverse effects
- **Indications**

  Mood stabilization: Evidence of treatment for both unipolar and bipolar depression compared with placebo (RR of response to treatment 1.42) (CNS Spectr. 2016;21:403-418); it is also particularly effective in prolonging time to relapse of bipolar depression, although it is considered inferior to VPA (but superior to placebo) in preventing mania. Slow uptitration limits its efficacy in acute mania

  Borderline personality disorder: Low-quality data suggest lamotrigine may be effective in reducing mood symptoms, impulsivity, anger, and even substance use in patients with BPD (J Clin Med Res. 2012;4:301-308)

  Other: seizure disorders, neuropathic pain, MDD (adjunct), schizophrenia (adjunct)

Adverse Effects
- **Common side effects:** HA, GI upset, sedation/insomnia, tremor, ataxia/dizziness, benign rash (10%; resolve with discontinuation, can be rechallenged with slower titration)
- **Rare and serious side effects:** SJS/TEN (0.8/1000 with monotherapy), aseptic meningitis, bone marrow suppression, suicidality
- **Overdose:** characterized by confusion, ataxia, coma, arrhythmias, SJS/TEN, and in some cases death
- **Discontinuation:** slowly taper off over 2+ weeks; abrupt discontinuation may precipitate seizures or relapse
- **Contraindications:** allergy, SJS/TEN reaction previously with lamotrigine
- **Significant interactions:** levels are increased with concomitant use of VPA and other AEDs

Lamotrigine: Prescriber's Pharmacology						
Starting Dose (mg/d)	Goal/ Max Dose (mg/d)	Titration	Metabolism	Half-Life (h)	Before Starting	Monitoring
25	100–300	+25– 50 mg q1–2w	Liver (gluc), renal excr	25	Consider baseline CBC	Watch for rash; no drug levels

Liver impairment: dose reduce in severe impairment

Renal impairment: dose reduce due to renally excretion; pts on HD may need additional doses

Pediatric: useful in pediatric epilepsy, but monitor for increased risk of drug rash; pts <30 kg may require increased dosing due to increased clearance. Also increased risk of infection in this population

Geriatric: consider dose reduction

Pregnant/breastfeeding: formerly category C in pregnancy for risk of congenital malformation (cleft lip/palate). Lamotrigine is excreted in breast milk with some risk of sedation/irritability in infant

---

OXCARBAZEPINE (OXC)

General Facts

- **Names and formulations:** Trileptal (PO)
- **MOA:** blocks voltage-gated sodium channels in use-dependent manner, changing their conformation, and inhibits release of glutamate; onset of action takes weeks to months for mood stabilization
- **Indications:**

    Mood stabilization: Thought to be useful in acute mania, although a 2011 meta-analysis was unable to establish efficacy over placebo in acute affective episodes (*Cochrane Database Syst Rev.* 2011:CD004857). There are, however, ample low-quality data demonstrating its efficacy and tolerability in acute affective episodes (*J Affect Disord.* 2002:S23-S24). Similarly, there is little direct evidence that OXC is useful in the prophylaxis of affective episodes. It is, however, closely related to carbamazepine, which has been demonstrated to be useful in bipolar maintenance therapy. OXC is often used prior to carbamazepine due to its superior tolerability

    Agitation and aggression: A small-scale RCT of OXC use in impulsive aggression (secondary to any medical cause) demonstrated efficacy in reducing aggressive episodes over placebo (*J Clin Psychopharmacol.* 2005;25:575-579)

    Other: seizure disorders, neuropathic pain, trigeminal neuralgia

Adverse Effects

- **Common side effects:** sedation (less than carbamazepine), GI upset, ataxia/dizziness, weight gain, rash, SIADH; note: OXC is metabolized to 10-hydroxycarbazepine, which is related to the newer agent eslicarbazepine, which may have fewer adverse effects
- **Rare and serious side effects:** suicidality
- **Overdose:** no fatalities have been recorded; overdose generally benign but characterized by sedation and ataxia

- **Discontinuation:** taper slow to avoid recurrence of seizure or affective episode
- **Contraindications:** allergy (to TCA or oxcarbazepine), concurrent MAOI/TCA use (given structural similarity to TCAs)
- **Significant interactions:** CYP induction may reduce oxcarbazepine levels; oxcarbazepine may reduce levels of OCPs and calcium-channel blockers; it may increase substrates of CYP2C19, 3A4, and 3A5 via inhibition

Oxcarbazepine: Prescriber's Pharmacology						
Starting Dose (mg/d)	Goal/Max Dose (mg/d)	Titration	Metabolism	Half-Life (h)	Before Starting	Monitoring
300	600–1200	+300 mg q3d	Liver (ox) Renal excr	8–10	BMP	BMP to monitor for hyponatremia, especially when starting

Liver impairment: reduce dose for severe impairment
Renal impairment: reduce dose and slow uptitration for all impairment
Pediatric: may require increased dosing due to increased clearance
Geriatric: consider dose reduction
Pregnant/breastfeeding: Previously category C due to risk of NTDs; infants should be monitored for adverse effects while breastfeeding.

CARBAMAZEPINE (CBZ)

General Facts
- **Names and formulations:** Tegretol (PO), Carbatrol (PO)
- **MOA:** blocks voltage-gated sodium channels in use-dependent manner, changing their conformation, and inhibits release of glutamate; onset for all indications is usually within weeks
- **Indications:**
  Mood stabilization: A 2008 systematic review of multiple RCTs comparing lithium to carbamazepine demonstrated no difference in efficacy in treating acute manic episodes, and no difference in preventing affective episodes, although CBZ was found to be less tolerable (*Human Psychopharm Clin Exp.* 2008;24:19-28). This was consistent with a later meta-analysis of multiple treatments for acute mania demonstrating efficacy of CBZ over placebo and other AEDs but inferiority to most antipsychotics (*Lancet.* 2011;378:1306-1315)
  Agitation and aggression: Numerous case studies support its use in preventing agitation in patients with disinhibition following TBI (*Ann Phys Rehabil Med.* 2016;59:42-57)
  Other: seizure disorders, neuropathic pain, trigeminal neuralgia, schizophrenia (adjunct)

Adverse Effects
- **Common side effects:** sedation, GI upset, ataxia/dizziness, weight gain, SIADH

- **Rare and Serious Side Effects:** bone marrow suppression, SJS/TEN, intraventricular conduction delay, suicidality
- **Overdose:** may be fatal at doses as small as 2× the maximum dose; characterized by GI upset, tremor, arrhythmia, anticholinergic effects, and AMS
- **Discontinuation:** taper slowly and adjust interacting medications as necessary
- **Contraindications:** bone marrow suppression, allergy to CBZ and TCAs, HLAB1502 subtype
- **Significant Interactions:** potent CYP3A4 inducer resulting in many drug–drug interactions

Carbamazepine: Prescriber's Pharmacology						
Starting Dose (mg/d)	Goal/Max Dose (mg/d)	Titration	Metabolism	Half-Life (h)	Before Starting	Monitoring
400	800–1200	+200 mg qd	CYP3A4 Renal excr	Varies	CBC, LFTs, TSH, BMP	Drug levels frequently: 8–12 CBC q1mo for 2 mo; LFTs, TSH, BMP q6–12mo thereafter

Liver impairment: use with caution
Renal impairment: dose reduction with severe impairment
Pediatric: commonly used in epilepsy at the same drug levels
Geriatric: consider dose reduction
Pregnant/breastfeeding: formerly category D in pregnancy due to risk of congenital malformations. CBZ is found in breast milk, and side effects in infant should be monitored for if use is not discontinued or formula is used.
NOTE: CBZ induces its own metabolism, as well as that of other medications. The initial half-life of carbamazepine at start of therapy is 18–55 h but is substantially reduced to 5–20 h after successive dosing. Therefore, dose should be increased 2–3 wk after initiation to maintain blood levels. The XR formulation may be dosed BID, while all other formulations are dosed 3–4 times daily.

TOPIRAMATE

General Facts
- **Names and formulations:** Topamax (PO), Topamac (PO), Epitomax (PO), Trokendi XR (PO), Qsymia (PO)
- **MOA:** blocks voltage-gated sodium channels, inhibits glutamate, potentiates GABA, and inhibits carbonic anhydrase; onset is 2 wk for seizures, and weeks to months for mood stabilization
- **Indications:**
  Mood stabilization: Historically used for mood stabilization, although recent meta-analysis was unable to demonstrate efficacy in acute affective episodes (*Cochrane Database Syst Rev.* 2016;9:CD003384). There is little evidence to support maintenance monotherapy but may be useful as adjunct

Alcohol use disorder: Efficacy in reducing cravings, heavy drinking, and lengthening time to relapse, including an RCT increasing time to relapse by 6 wk over placebo (*BMC Psychiatry.* 2011;11:41)

Cocaine use disorder: A 2013 RCT demonstrated that topiramate reduced use, cravings, and lengthened time to relapse in patients with cocaine use disorder (*JAMA Psychiatry.* 2013;70:1338-1346)

Antipsychotic-associated weight gain: A 2014 meta-analysis demonstrated a statistically significant decrease in weight among patients prescribed SGAs by 2.83 kg more than placebo (*Hosp Pharm.* 2014;49:345-347)

Other uses: seizure disorders, migraines, mood lability, and impulsivity in BPD

Adverse Effects

- **Common side effects:** sedation, cognitive dysfunction (memory, language, slowing), weight loss and GI upset, ataxia
- **Rare and serious side effects:** metabolic acidosis, nephrolithiasis, suicidality, hyperthermia
- **Overdose:** no fatalities reported; characterized by AMS, GI upset, ataxia, and metabolic disturbances
- **Discontinuation:** taper to reduce risk of seizure or affective episode relapse
- **Contraindications:** metabolic acidosis
- **Significant interactions:** CYP3A4 inducer

Topiramate: Prescriber's Pharmacology						
Starting Dose (mg/d)	Goal/Max Dose (mg/d)	Titration	Metabolism	Half-Life (h)	Before Starting	Monitoring
50	200–400	+50 mg q1wk	Renal excr	20	BMP	Periodic BMP to monitor HCO_3^- levels

Liver impairment: use with caution
Renal impairment: dose reduce by half; removed by HD, so may need additional doses
Pediatric: may tolerate medication better than adults with fewer cognitive side effects
Geriatric: consider dose reduction
Pregnant/breastfeeding: Formerly category D in pregnancy due to risk of cleft lip/palate/hypospadia; monitor for adverse effects in infant when breastfeeding.

GABAPENTIN

General Facts

- **Names and formulations:** Neurontin (PO), Horizant (PO)
- **MOA:** as a leucine analogue, crosses BBB via leucine transport, and thereafter binds to voltage-gated calcium channels; despite its name, not known to be GABAergic; acts on the order of weeks

- **Indications:**
  NOTE: Not used in mood stabilization

  Anxiety: Effective in reducing symptoms of anxiety in SAD (Depress Anxiety. 2003;18:29-40); and panic disorder (J Clin Psychopharmacol. 2000;20:467-471). Also likely effective for other anxiety disorders such as GAD

  Alcohol use disorder: Efficacy in reducing heavy drinking and lengthening time to relapse (JAMA Intern Med. 2014;174:70-77)

  Other uses: seizure disorders, mood lability and impulsivity in BPD, neuropathic pain

Adverse Effects

- **Common side effects:** sedation, dizziness/ataxia, GI upset, blurry vision, peripheral edema
- **Rare and serious side effects:** suicidality
- **Overdose:** no fatalities reported; characterized by sedation and ataxia
- **Discontinuation:** taper for >1 wk to avoid relapse of epilepsy/ anxiety
- **Contraindications:** allergy to gabapentin/pregabalin
- **Significant interactions:** reduced bioavailability with antacids, increased levels with NSAIDs due to renal excretion

Gabapentin: Prescriber's Pharmacology						
Starting Dose (mg/d)	Goal/ Max Dose (mg/d)	Titration	Metabolism	Half-Life (h)	Before Starting	Monitoring
300	900–3600	+300 mg qd	Renal excr	5–7	None	Monitor for signs of abuse. Anecdotal reports of gabapentin abuse in combination with methadone, clonidine, and/or clonazepam may precipitate hypotension, bradycardia, and bradypnea.
Liver impairment: no adjustment						
Renal impairment: dose reduce						
Pediatric: used as adjunct in partial seizures						
Geriatric: consider dose reduction						
Pregnant/breastfeeding: formerly Category C, unknown risk profile; excreted in breast milk, so watching for sedation in infants is recommended during use.						

PREGABALIN

General Facts
- **Names and formulations:** Lyrica
- **MOA:** as a leucine analogue, crosses BBB via leucine transport, and thereafter binds to voltage-gated calcium channels; despite its name, not known to be GABAergic; acts on the order of weeks; structurally related to gabapentin
- **Indications:**
  NOTE: Not used in mood stabilization
  Anxiety: Effective in reducing symptoms of anxiety in GAD (*Can J Psychiatry.* 2011;56:558-566); also likely effective for other anxiety disorders
  Other uses: primary indication for fibromyalgia; also neuropathic pain, seizure disorders

Adverse Effects
- **Common side effects:** sedation, dizziness/ataxia, GI upset, peripheral edema
- **Rare and serious side effects:** suicidality
- **Overdose:** no fatalities reported; likely similar to gabapentin overdose features
- **Discontinuation:** taper over a week to minimize risk of relapse
- **Contraindications:** allergy
- **Significant interactions:** None known

Pregabalin: Prescriber's Pharmacology						
Starting Dose (mg/d)	Goal/ Max Dose (mg/d)	Titration	Metabolism	Half-Life (h)	Before Starting	Monitoring
150	150–600	+150–300 mg q1wk	Renal excr	5–7	None	None

Liver impairment: no adjustment
Renal impairment: dose reduce
Pediatric: unknown safety profile
Geriatric: consider dose reduction
Pregnant/breastfeeding: formerly category C, unknown risk profile; excreted in breast milk: watch for sedation if continuing.

AEDS IN NEUROLOGIC PRACTICE

These AEDs have no approved or off-label use in psychiatry but are commonly used in neurology and can have prominent neuropsychiatric side effects

Other Antiepileptic Agents			
Drug	Indication	Dosing	Comments
Levetiracetam (Keppra)	• Focal sz (± gen) • Primary generalized (off-label)	500– 1500 mg BID	• Higher rate of neuropsychiatric side effects than other AEDs (in some studies, 22% of patients developed depression, agitation, SI, or psychosis) • Levetiracetam is commonly used in both inpatient and outpatient setting due to its ease of dosing, IV/PO formulations, and no need for drug level monitoring
Zonisamide (Zonegran)	• Focal sz (± gen) • Primary generalized	100–300 mg BID	• High rate of neuropsychiatric side effects, although less than levetiracetam • May be useful in patients with migraine, binge eating, and Parkinson disease
Lacosamide (Vimpat)	• Focal sz (± gen)	100–200 mg BID	• Few neuropsychiatric side effects • Causes PR prolongation
Ethosuximide (Zarontin)	• Absence sz	250–750 mg BID	• May cause aggression, confusion, depression, and insomnia, although less severe than the Keppra
Phenytoin (Dilantin)	• Focal sz (± gen) • Primary generalized • Status epilepticus	Maintenance: 150– 200 mg BID SE: 15–20 mg/ kg IV, followed by 10 mg/ kg if no resp	• ER formulation can be dosed daily • Few neuropsychiatric side effects • Rare, serious adverse effects include arrhythmia, hepatotoxicity, marrow suppression, and SJS

(continued)

Other Antiepileptic Agents *(continued)*			
Drug	**Indication**	**Dosing**	**Comments**
Barbiturates (eg, phenobarbital)	• Focal sz (± gen) • Primary generalized	Maintenance: 60 mg BID-TID SE: 10–20 mg/kg q20min	• May be used in the management of severe alcohol withdrawal • Adverse effects include respiratory depression and sedation
Benzodiazepines (eg, clonazepam, clobazam)	• Lennox–Gastaut syndrome • Myoclonus	Clobazam: 10–20 mg BID Clonazepam: 0.5–5 mg TID	• Short-acting agents (eg, lorazepam, midazolam) 1st-line in status epilepticus and alcohol withdrawal • Adverse effects include respiratory depression and sedation

From *Epilepsy Behav Case Rep.* 2017;76:24-31. doi:10.1016/j.yebeh.2017.08.039

LITHIUM

General Facts
- **Formulations:** Tablet, capsule, extended release tablet, liquid

Indications (*J Psychopharmacol.* 2016;30:495-553; *World Psychiatry.* 2016;53-58; *Int J Bipolar Disord.* 2014;2:15; *AJP.* 2004;161(2):217-222, *J Clin Psychiatry.* 2006;688-695; *BMC Psychiatry.* 2017;17:231; *JAMA Psychiatry.* 2016;630-637; *Neuropsychobiology.* 2010;62:43-49; *Ther Adv Psychopharmacol.* 2016;6:33-38; *Br J Psychiatry.* 2009;194(5):464-465; *Biol Trace Elem Res.* 1990;25(2):105-113)

- **Bipolar mania:** FDA approved tx of acute mania and maintenance, *Acute mania*; days to 1 wk for effect; consider antipsychotic adjunct, *maintenance*; monotherapy effective/tolerated for longer duration compared with other mood stabilizers/antipsychotics
- **Bipolar depression:** Less effective for prevention, little data for acute episode
  - **Unipolar depression:** Used as an augmenting agent. + predictors: psychomotor retardation, weight loss, family hx MDD, >1 prior episode
  - **Suicidality:** ↓ suicide + all-cause mortality in BPAD/unipolar depression
  - **Aggression:** ↓ impulsive, aggressive, and self-mutilating behaviors in BPAD, ADHD, intellectually disability, conduct disorder, inmates w/ personality pathology
  - Evidence of ↓ suicidality/violence in communities w/ subtherapeutic levels of lithium in water
  Other: Lithium sometimes used to ↑ ANC for patients receiving clozapine

Mechanism of Action (Mol Psychiatry. 2015;661-670)

- Challenging to study due to similarity w/ Na+
- Distributes in CNS, thought to affect multiple 2nd messengers
- Likely promotes neurogenesis in hippocampus
- Variable evidence of ↓ NE and DA and ↑ 5-H-T and GABA

Prescribing						
Starting Dose	Goal/Max Dose	Titration	Metabolism	Half-Life	Before Starting	Monitoring
300 mg BID	Per level (maintenance: 0.6–0.8, mania: 0.6–1.2) or 2400 mg	+300–600 mg q5d	Renal	24 h	Renal fxn, EKG, TSH, wt, Ca, bHGC	Level q5d until therapeutic; Repeat level, renal fxn, TSH q6mo; Ca, wt qyear

Liver impairment: May need to ↑ dose if ascites (fluid shift)
Renal impairment: Contraindicated, used in CKD w/ HD + close monitoring of levels/toxicity
Children: Start 10–20 mg/kg, ↑ by 10 mg/kg q5d, usual monitoring
Geriatric: Start 150–300 mg, ↑ q5d as tolerated. Lower doses for therapeutic levels and half-life ↑ 28–36 h. > risk of toxicity w/ ↓ eGFR
Pregnant/breastfeeding: lowest necessary dose. Risk of cardiac defects in fetus (though much lower than previously thought). Check level q2wk; levels ↓ during pregnancy due to ↑ in eGFR; hold peri-delivery and ensure hydration
"Drugs for treatment of bipolar disorders" in *Handbook of Psychiatric Drug Therapy*; 2010; *Ann Gen Hosp Psych.* 2004;3:7; *Clin Appr in Bipol Disord.* 2007;6(2)54; *N Engl J Med.* 2017;376(23):2245; *AJP.* 2004;161(4):608-620; *Psychiatr Clin North Am.* 2010;33(2)273-293

Adverse Effects

Common Side Effects	
Side Effect	Details
Nausea/ diarrhea	Level-dependent, ↓ w/ chronic use; consider dosing multiple times IR formulation for initiation
Polyuria/ polydipsia	2/2 nephrogenic DI (polyuria → dehydration + thirst → polydipsia), risk ↑ w/chronic use + w/ toxicity; consider daily dosing, diuretic adjuncts, sugarless gum, or oral moisturizers for thirst
Tremor	Usually hands + symmetric/fine, presents anytime; tx by ↓ caffeine, antipsychotics, anxiety, EtOH, SSRIs, consider propranolol, primidone, BZD, vitamin B6
Weight gain	Common reason for discontinuation, dose-dependent, worst early in treatment; diet/exercise, ↓ high-calorie drinks (esp if polydipsia), ↓ add. causes (antipsychotics, hypothyroidism), consider topiramate
Cognitive impairment	Subjective slowness/loss of creativity, may be confounded by ↓ mania, level-dependent; consider ↓ dose + addressing confounders

(continued)

Common Side Effects (continued)	
Sexual dysfunction	Minor, relatively understudied; consider ASA or PD5 inhibitors
Acne/psoriasis	New onset or exacerbation, level-dependent; consider lowering dose or typical dermatological treatments (topical salicylic acid, inositol)
Serious Side Effects	
Lithium-associated nephropathy	Focal nephron atrophy + interstitial fibrosis, polyuria + gradual ↓ in renal fxn, usually irreversible, ↑ risk: dose, length of treatment, age, + prior episodes, consider discontinuation, amiloride to block Li from entering renal principal cells
Thyroid dysfunction	Inhibits thyroid hormone release, ↑ risk: +antithyroid Abs, ♀, older age, family hx hypothyroidism; treat w/ thyroxine, does not justify discontinuation
Hypercalcemia	↑ renal Ca^{2+} resorption + stimulates PTH release
Teratogenic	1st trimester exposure ↑ risk of cardiac malformations (classically Ebstein anomaly), absolute risk low w/ evidence risk historically overestimated

Mol Psychiatry. 2017;22(3):396; Int J Bipolar Disord. 2016;4:27; Intern Clin Psychopharmacol. 2013;28(6):287-296

Toxicity and Overdose (*Clin Toxicol. 2015;53(1):5; Clin J Am Soc Nephrol. 2015;10(5):875; Clin Neuropharmacol. 2005;28(1):38*)

- For patients with high risk of OD, note that lithium can be lethal
- Narrow therapeutic window:
  Level > 1.5: anorexia, nausea, vomiting, diarrhea, muscle weakness, drowsiness, confusion, ataxia, tremor
  Level > 2: AMS, ataxia, neuromuscular excitability, seizures, coma, death
- Risk factors: hyponatremia, low-salt diet, dehydration, drug interactions (diuretics, ACEis, NSAIDs), ↓ renal function, old age
- Treat acute toxicity w/ IVF, whole bowel irrigation w/ polyethylene glycol if awake and asymptomatic, HD if level >4, or if level <2.5 + AMS/szs, renal insufficiency, or comorbidity limiting IV hydration (CHF)
- **Syndrome of irreversible lithium-effectuated neurotoxicity (SILENT):** Long-term sequelae after Li is removed → cerebellar dysfunction, EPS, dementia

Interactions

Meds affecting renal Na+ metabolism: ACEi, thiazides, NSAIDs

Contraindications

Acute renal failure, severe cardiovascular or renal disease, severe dehydration, sodium depletion, diuretic use

Discontinuation

Dose reduction over >1 mo while monitoring levels to mitigate relapse of mania, → risk of relapse + suicidality w/ discontinuation (*Acta Psychiatr Scand. 2004;109:91-95*)

ATOMOXETINE

Atomoxetine (Strattera) (FDA; Ann Pharmacother. 2014;48(2):209)
• **Formulations:** immediate release oral capsule

Indications
• **ADHD.** Off-label uses include binge eating disorder, depression

Mechanism of Action
• Selectively inhibits reuptake of NE in the DLPFC, leading to increasing NE transmission. Because NET contributes to DA reuptake, atomoxetine increases intrasynaptic DA as well
• Thought to have minimal abuse potential because it does not act on key parts of the reward pathway and lag time of weeks for full effect

Prescribing						
Starting Dose	Goal/Max Dose	Titration	Metabolism	Half-Life	Before Starting	Monitoring
40 mg daily (qd or BID)	80–100 mg daily	20–40 mg weekly	CYP2D6	5.2 h	N/A	N/A

Liver impairment: Downward dose adjustment recommended in Child–Pugh class B or C liver failure
Renal impairment: No adjustment
Children: If <70 kg, 0.5 mg/kg per day initially, then after 3 d titrate to 1.2 mg/kg per day
Geriatric: Has not been studied in this population
Pregnant/breastfeeding: Pregnancy category C

Adverse Effects
Common side effects: dry mouth, ↓ appetite, nausea, insomnia
  Black box warning: SI in children/adolescents (J Am Acad Child Adolesc Psychiatry. 2007;46:7:894; J Child Adolesc Psychopharmcol. 2014;24(8):426)
  Overdose: No attributed deaths from overdose
  Discontinuation: No demonstrated discontinuation or withdrawal syndrome
  Contraindications: pheochromocytoma, narrow-angle glaucoma, and patients on MAOIs
  Significant interactions: levels can be significantly ↑ if patient is a CYP2D6 poor metabolizer (PM) or if taken with strong 2D6 inhibitors (fluoxetine, paroxetine, quinidine). MAOI (risk for serotonin syndrome, hypertensive urgency/emergency)

PSYCHOSTIMULANTS

Indications
ADHD, Narcolepsy, binge eating disorder (Vyvanse FDA-approved for BED)

Names and Formulations
Methylphenidate
- Short-acting:
  - *Methylphenidate* (brand *Ritalin IR*).
  - *Dexmethylphenidate* (brand *Focalin*)
- Intermediate long-acting:
  - *Ritalin LA* (releases medication in 2 sequential boluses, 1 immediately, followed by another 3–4 h later, referred to as a "double hump" mechanism)
  - *Metadate ER*—long-acting tablet form
- Long-acting:
  - *OROS MPH ER* (brand *Concerta*): tablet releases 22% of medication contained in outer coating immediately, then released slowly over ~12 h
  - *Daytrana TDS* (patch)—only approved for children
  - *Metadate CD*—capsules containing a mix 30% immediate release medication and 70% extended release beads
  - *Focalin XR* (d-MPH with a "double hump" release mechanism)
  - *Quillivant XR*—Oral suspension containing 20% immediate release and 80% extended release methylphenidate (must shake vigorously for 10 s prior to oral administration with a syringe)

Amphetamine
All contain 1 or both of the active enantiomers *dextroamphetamine* (D-amp) to reduce potential for abuse (cannot be snorted or injected) and *levoamphetamine* (L-amp).
- Short-acting:
  - *Amphetamine salts (*brand *Adderall)*—composed of 75% D-amp and 25% L-amp
  - *Pure D-amp,* brand *Dexedrine*
- Intermediate long-acting:
  - *D-amp XR* or *Dexedrine Spansules* ("double hump")
  - *Adderall XR* ("double hump")
- Longest acting (12 or more hours):
  - *Lisdexamfetamine* (brand *Vyvanse*), a prodrug metabolized to D-amp
  - *Mydayis:* an even more extended release version of amphetamine—"triple hump"

Mechanism of Action
Methylphenidate: Inhibits reuptake of both DA and NE via DAT/NET ↓ metabolism of DA/NE via inhibition of MAO

   Amphetamine: Same as above, plus ↑ release of DA and NE from presynaptic storage vesicles

Prescribing (*J Am Acad Child Adolesc Psychiatr.* 2007;46(7):894; *Prim Care Companion CNS Disord.* 2013;15(2): PCC.12f01472; *Ann Pharmacother.* 2014;48(2):209; *FDA*)
- ≥70% response rate to at least 1 stimulant
- Some respond to only AMP or only MPH, reasons for this are not understood
- Effect observed <1 wk of use, allowing for faster titration
- Long-acting formulations preferred in those with concern for misuse or diversion

- A "booster" dose of short-/medium-acting medication in the afternoon may be required to cover full work/school day
- "Drug holidays" : Breaks from medication on weekends or vacations controversial but in select cases may be appropriate

Methylphenidate						
Name	**Starting Dose**	**Goal/ Max Dose**	**Titration**	**Duration of Action (h)**	**Before Starting**	**Monitoring**
Ritalin, Methylin (MPH IR) *Strengths (mg):* Tabs: 5, 10, 20 Chew: 2.5, 5, 10 PO Soln: 5 mg/mL, 10 mg/ mL	5–10 BID-TID	20–60	5–10	3–4	Baseline BP/HR; screen for FHx SCD or structural heart disease	BP/HR until dose stabilized; tox screens, PMP checks per state laws
Ritalin LA (MPH ER capsules) *Strengths (mg):* 10, 20, 30, 40	10–20	10–60	10	8–10		
Concerta (OROS MPH ER tablet) *Strengths (mg):* 18, 27, 36, 54	18	18–72	9–18	10–12		
Metadate CD (MPH ER capsules) *Strengths (mg):* 10, 20, 30, 40, 50, 60	20	10–60	10–20	8		

(continued)

Methylphenidate (continued)						
Name	Starting Dose	Goal/ Max Dose	Titra- tion	Duration of Action (h)	Before Starting	Monito- ring
*Daytrana (MPH TDS) Strengths (mg/9 h): 10, 15, 20, 30	10 mg/9 h	10–30	5 mg/ 9 h per day	Wear time + ~3 h		
*Quillivant XR (MPH XR powder for oral suspen- sion) Strengths: 25 mg /5 mL	20	20–60	10–20	12		
Focalin (d-MPH IR tablets) Strengths (mg): 2.5, 5, 10	2.5 BID	5–20	2.5–5	6		
Focalin XR (d-MPH XR capsules) Strengths (mg): 5, 10, 15, 20, 25, 30, 35, 40	5	5–30	5	12		

Liver impairment: No specific guidance
Renal impairment: No adjustment needed
Children: Should not be used in children <6
Geriatric: Not studied in patients >65
Pregnant/breastfeeding:
• Pregnancy: No human controlled studies. In rabbits, teratogenic effects seen in offsprings of those fed ~40× max daily human dose, but not in those given 11× max. In rats, ↑ fetal skeletal variations seen when doses of 7× max given to pregnant rats and decreased offspring body weight gain at 4× max. No teratogenic or other significant effects observed when pregnant/lactating rats given 1× max dose. Careful cost–benefit analysis recommended.
• Breastfeeding: unknown if secreted in breast milk Nursing not recommended.

*No generic formulation available.

Amphetamine						
Name	**Starting Dose**	**Goal/ Max Dose**	**Titra- tion**	**Duration of Action (h)**	**Before Starting**	**Monito- ring**
Adderall (MAS IR—75% d-AMP/ 25% l-AMP) *Strengths (mg):* 5, 7.5, 10, 12.5, 15, 20, 30	5qDay-BID	5–40	5	4–6	Baseline BP/HR; screen for FHx SCD or structural heart disease	BP/HR until dose stabilized; tox screens, PMP checks per state laws
Adderall XR (MAS XR) *Strengths (mg):* 5, 10, 15, 20, 25, 30	5–10	30	5–10	8–12		
Dexedrine (d-AMP) *Strengths (mg):* IR tabs: 5, 10 XR capsules: 5, 10, 15	5–10	60	5	IR: 4–5 XR: 8–12		
*Vyvanse (Lisdexamfetamine) *Strengths (mg):* 20, 30, 40, 50, 60, 70	20–30	30–70	10–20	12		

Liver impairment: No specific guidance
Renal impairment: For Vyvanse—severe CKD: max 50 mg/d; ESRD:max 30 mg/d
Children: Should not be used in children <6
Geriatric: Not studied in patients >65
Pregnant/breastfeeding:
• Pregnancy: No human controlled studies. In pregnant rats fed 0.8–4 times max recommended adolescent human dose (20 mg/d) from gestation day 6 to lactation day 20, evidence of ↓ pup survival, ↓ weight gain, hyperactivity at all doses. Effects on pup body weight and subsequent fertility noted at higher doses
• Breastfeeding: Contraindicated while breastfeeding. Amphetamines excreted in breast milk

*No generic formulation available.

Adverse Effects (FDA, https://www.accessdata.fda.gov/scripts/cder/daf/)
Common Side Effects
• Appetite suppression, insomnia, restlessness, anxiety, dry mouth, constipation, ↑ BP (avg 2–4 points), ↑ HR (3–6 bpm), mania, psychosis
• Physical AEs thought to be mediated by increased peripheral sympathetic activity
• Risk of psychosis thought to be mediated by increased central DAergic signaling

Rare and Serious Side Effects
- SCD: Increased risk in pts congenital or structural heart disease, SCD family hx

Overdose
- Manifestations (similar in both amphetamines and Ritalin)
  - CNS overactivation
    - Restlessness/agitation, confusion, panic, assaultiveness, hallucinations, hyperreflexia, tremor. Reports of SS-/NMS-like syndrome
    - Posthyperactivation phase: severe fatigue, depressed mood
    - Rarely seizures → coma → death
  - Other effects:
    - Constitutional (fever, rhabdomyolysis), cardiovascular (HTN or hypotension/shock, arrhythmias), GI (n/v/d/abdominal cramps)

Discontinuation
- No known harmful discontinuation/withdrawal syndrome. May cause temporary fatigue, depressed mood

Contraindications
- Do not give during while the patient is taking MAOIs (or for 14 d thereafter). Risk of HTN crisis, SS-/NMS-like syndrome
- Other absolute: Glaucoma, known hypersensitivity
- Relative: anxiety, Tic d/o or Tourette syndrome

Pharmacokinetics
- Tmax, Cmax, and duration of actions vary by formulation
- Elimination half-life
- Clearance faster on average in children and adolescents
- MPH: typically 2–5 h
- D-AMP: mean 9–11h, l-AMP: mean 11–14 h

ANTIPSYCHOTICS

Background (Stahl. 2011;2013; Schiz Bull. 36(1):94-103; Am J Psychiatry. 161(2):1-56; N Engl J Med. 353(12):1209-1223)
- All with similar efficacy and tolerability; aside from olanzapine + clozapine (see below)
- Dosing > FDA recommended doses ≠ improved symptom control & ↑ risk SE
- All metabolized through the liver, aside from paliperidone
- Black box warning for elderly pts with dementia—↑risk of stroke, MI, + death

Side Effects (Psychopharmacology (Berl). 2017;234(17):2563; J Clin Psychiatry. 2009;70(5):627-643; Curr Treat Options Psychiatry. 2016;3:133-150; PLoS One. 2015;10(10):e0139717

- **Side effects below can occur across all antipsychotics though generally the principals below apply:**
  - 1st gen ↑ risk EPS, TD, + prolactin change 2/2 D2 blockade outside mesolimbic system
  - 2nd gen ↓ risk EPS, ↑ antihistaminergic, anticholinergic + antiadrenergic SE (below), + insulin resistance/metabolic syndrome

Nigrostriatal D2 Blockade → EPS		

Acute (Time of onset varies—PO forms: 50% rxns within 48 h, 90% within 5 d; IM/IV—most reactions within 1–48 h)

Dystonic reaction	• Painful muscle spasms usually of extremities, neck (torticollis, retrocollis), back (opisthotonos), ± ocular muscles (oculogyric crisis). Laryngospasm is life-threatening. Highest risk if antipsychotic naïve • Tx: Acute—IM/IV benztropine or diphenhydramine • Prophylactic (ie, if administering IM haloperidol)—PO/IM benztropine or diphenhydramine • Long-term—↓ dose, switch to low-potency antipsychotic, low-dose BZD or beta-blocker
Akathisia	• Intense restlessness, urge to move lower extremities. Include on differential for agitated patient. ↑ risk at high doses • Tx: ↓ dose or switch to agent w/ ↓ EPS risk; beta-blocker (propranolol), benztropine, BZD

Delayed (Typically during 1st several weeks)

Parkinsonism	• Tremor, bradykinesia, masked facies, festinating gait, cogwheeling rigidity. ↑ risk in elderly, high doses • Tx: ↓ dose or switch to agent w/ ↓ EPS risk; benztropine, amantadine
Tardive dyskinesia	• Involuntary choreoathetoid movements of face, neck, trunk, and extremities. 5% per year, ↑ risk in elderly, patients with h/o acute EPS, longer duration of exposure • AIMS (Abnormal Involuntary Movement Scale) to assess • Tx: Risk/benefit psychiatric stability/need for medication with movements/burden—consider quetiapine/olanzapine
NMS	• Life-threatening condition: fever, autonomic instability, muscle rigidity, delirium → NMS chapter for more detail

---

Mesocortical D2 Blockade → Cognitive Impairment + neg sx

• Avolition, anhedonia, amotivation, poverty of speech, isolation
• Tx: limited. Consider switch to atypical agent, utilize lowest dose that controls positive symptoms; consider antidepressant, CBT

Tuberoinfundibular D2 Blockade → stimulates prolactin secretion

• Elevated plasma prolactin—> ♀—galactorrhea, amenorrhea, sexual dysfunction, ♂—gynecomastia, sexual dysfunction. Most common with 1st generation antipsychotics, risperidone, asenapine, and paliperidone
• Tx: switch to alternate agent—quetiapine (will not increase prolactin levels) or aripiprazole (can lower prolactin levels)

Alpha-1 Adrenergic Blockade → dizziness, sedation, hypotension

Histaminergic Blockade → weight gain, drowsiness

Cholinergic Blockade → dry mouth, constipation, blurry vision, urinary retention, confusion

Other Side Effects
Metabolic Syndrome: obtain prior to start then monitor: weight/BMI, fasting glucose, lipid panel, A1C, BP
Alteration of temperature regulation and setpoint → *poikilothermia*—body temperature varies with the environment
QT Prolongation → ↑ risk for torsade de pointes + lethal arrhythmias

1ST GENERATION ANTIPSYCHOTICS: "TYPICALS"

Further classified by binding affinity with D2 receptor: low, medium, or high potency

High Potency = High Affinity for D2 Receptors; Higher Rates of EPS	
Haloperidol (Haldol)	
PO/IM/IV	2.5–30 mg/d orally; Half-life 12–38 h IM immediate release injection—2–5 mg each dose. Often used in emergency settings Coadminister with diphenhydramine or benztropine to prevent EPS
LAI (dec.)	Q4wk—10–20× daily dose of oral. Overlap PO ×2–3 wk 100 mg is limit for 1st dose. If >100 mg 1st dose required, administer remainder 3–7 d later Half-life ~3 wk. Reaches steady-state after 3–4 injections
Fluphenazine (Prolixin)	
PO/IM	1–20 mg/d; Half-life 15 h IM immediate release—1.25 mg initial dose. 2.5–10 mg/d q6–8h. Max dose usually 10 mg/d
LAI (dec.)	1st dose 12.5–25 mg q3wk. Onset of action 24–72 h after injection (overlap PO ×3 d). Subsequent dose determined by response, generally no >50 mg Q3wk Standard conversion: 10 mg PO daily = 12.5 mg IM q3wk
Other: pimozide (Orap), thiothixene (Navane), trifluoperazine (Stelazine).	

Mid Potency	
Perphenazine (Trilafon)	
PO/IM	Dose: typically 4–8 mg TID or 8–16 mg BID-4×/d. Max 64 mg/d. Half-life 9.5 h IM immediate release injection—5 mg D2, histamine (H1) and cholinergic (M1) blockade (may reduce nausea and vomiting)

Mid Potency *(continued)*	
Loxapine	
PO/IM/IV	PO: Start 10 mg BID, titrate over 1 wk, 60–100 mg/d in divided doses. Max 250 mg/d. Half-life 4 h Oral liquid—25 mg/mL Injection 25–50 mg/mL, can be used for emergency, onset of action w/in 60 min. Half-life 12 h Though classified as typical, potent serotonin 2A antagonist (most relevant at low doses) Can ↑ efficacy in clozapine partial responders when given together Weight gain < other antipsychotics, ± weight loss

Other: molindone (Moban).

Low Potency = Low Affinity for D2 Receptors; Less Likely to Cause EPS	
Antiautonomic (Hypotensive), Sedating, Anticholinergic Effects	
Chlorpromazine (Thorazine)	
PO/IM/IV	Dose: 50–600 mg/d IM formulation—50 mg IM, often used for agitation. Caution with repeated IM administrations, as rapid absorption can lead to respiratory and/or vasomotor collapse, sudden apnea Highly sedating with significant hypotension and anticholinergic effects

Other: mesoridazine (Serentil), thioridazine (Mellaril—brand name discontinued 2/2 risk of severe arrhythmias).

2ND GENERATION ANTIPSYCHOTICS: "ATYPICALS"

Background *(Stahl. 2011;2013; Schiz Bull. 36(1):94-103; Am J Psychiatry. 161(2):1-56; N Engl J Med. 353(12):1209-1223)*

- Serotonin (5-HT2) antagonism >dopamine (D2) antagonism
- ↑ mesocortical, nigrostriatal, + tuberoinfundibular DA → improve cognition, neg sx, mood
- DA usually suppressed by 5H-T; atypicals *block 5H-T + enhance DA* in these tracts

Atypical Antipsychotics	
Aripiprazole (Abilify)	
PO, LAI	Dose: 10–30 mg single dose (half-life 75 h) **Partial D2 receptor *agonism* with high-potency 5-HT2A antagonism** Acts as D2 antagonist in areas of relative dopamine excess, acts as agonist in hypodopaminergic regions
LAI (Maintena)	Starting dose 400 mg IM, q4wk, Consider dose reduction to 300 mg if adverse effects. PO overlap ×2 wk. Level peaks at 4–7 d, half-life 46.5 d SE: Akathisia

(continued)

Atypical Antipsychotics *(continued)*	
Asenapine (Saphris)	
PO	Dose: 10–20 mg (BID dosing) Multiple receptors: serotonin, adrenergic, dopaminergic, histaminergic, muscarinic acetylcholine SE: Akathisia
Clozaril (Clozapine) Am J Psychiatry. 153(12):1579-1584	
PO	Dosing: Initial 25 mg daily, ↑ 25–50 mg QD, target dose ~300–450 mg QD. Max dose—900 mg Check levels to guide dosing: Target level range: 200–300 ng/mL [50–150 ng/mL often ineffective, can push to 300–450 ng/mL if continued sx]. Dose >450 mg QD or combined levels cloz & norcloz >1000 ng/mL associated with increased seizure risk. Slow titration 2/2 risk seizure, syncope, sedation Linear pharmacokinetics—double dose = double blood level Metabolite—norclozapine (10% activity of clozapine). Levels in literature refer to only clozapine Need to titrate given risk for: seizure, syncope, sedation Requires ANC of at least 1500/mm^3 for routine prescribing; https://www.clozapinerems.com/CpmgClozapineUI/rems/pdf/resources/ANC_Table.pdf All prescribers and patients must be registered in Clozapine REMS; patients entered into database—www.clozapinerems.com Decreased suicidality and "gold standard" for efficacy in schizophrenia Wide antagonism at 5HT2A, D1, D2, D4, H1, muscarinic, and alpha-1 receptors Metabolized by CYP1A2 and 3A4—*fluvoxamine* blocks 1A2, *cigarette smoking* induces SE: • Sedation, orthostatic hypotension • *Substantial weight gain*, metabolic problems • *Constipation*—can result in Ogilvie syndrome • Hypersalivation. Tx with glycopyrrolate • Increased risk for seizure (at higher doses, fast titrations) • **5 black box warnings**: agranulocytosis (0.8%—highest risk during 1st 6 mo, increases with age), seizure, myocarditis, orthostatic hypotension with syncope or cardiorespiratory arrest, increased mortality in elderly patients with dementia-related psychosis
Iloperidone (Fanapt)	
PO	Dose: 8–32 mg/d, half-life 12–15 h SE: Orthostatic hypotension—titrate slowly, QT prolongation
LAI	Q1mo—still under development, not yet approved
Lurasidone (Latuda)	
PO	Dose: 40–160 mg Some agonist activity at 5-HT1A SE: Akathisia, parkinsonism, sedation. Not as much weight gain, few metabolic abnormalities

Atypical Antipsychotics (continued)	
Olanzapine (Zyprexa)	
PO/ODT/IM	Dose: 5–20 mg/d. 21–54 h half-life Wide antagonism at 5HT2A, D1, D2, D4, H1, muscarinic, alpha-1 (similar to clozapine) Most efficacious antipsychotic in CATIE trial (aside from clozapine) *SE: Significant weight gain and metabolic side effects*; hyperglycemia, hyperlipidemia (affects insulin sensitivity)
LAI	*Zyprexa Relprevv*—q2–4wk—**black box warning**: postinjection delirium/sedation syndrome. Must be administered in health care facility and monitored ×3 h • 10 mg PO = 210 mg q2wk or 405 mg q4wk. Maintenance after 8 wk = 150 mg q2wk or 300 mg q4wk Relprevv • 15 mg PO = 300 mg q2wk Relprevv. Maintenance Relprevv = 210 mg q2wk or 405 mg q4wk • 20 mg PO = 300 mg q2wk Relprevv. Maintenance Relprevv = 300 mg q2wk
Paliperidone (Invega)	
PO	9-OH metabolite of risperidone (half-life 21 h) Dose 3–12 mg PO
LAI	*Invega Sustenna*—q4wk. No PO overlap required. Monthly max dose—234 mg • Release of drug starts day 1, lasts up to 126 d. Half-life 25–49 d. Levels peak after 13 d • 3 mg PO = 78 mg LAI; 6 mg PO = 117 mg LAI; 12 mg PO = 234 mg LAI *Invega Trinza*—q3mo. Start only after adequate tx with Sustenna ×4 mo • Release of drug starts at day 1, lasts up to 18 mo. Half-life 84–95 d. Levels peak at day 30–33 78 mg Sustenna = 273 mg Trinza; 117 mg S = 410 mg T; 156 mg S = 546 mg T; 234 mg S = 819 mg
Quetiapine (Seroquel)	
PO	Dose: 25–50–400–800 mg Antagonist at 5HT2A, D2, alpha-1,2, H1, short-term anxiolytic *SE: moderate weight gain, orthostatic hypotension*
Risperidone (Risperdal)	
PO/ODT	Dose: start 1–2 mg/d, final 4–6 mg/d. Half-life 3 h + disintegrating tab + liquid available *SE: less likely to cause weight gain than olanzapine or clozapine, more likely to cause EPS and increase prolactin levels than other atypicals (dose-dependent)*
LAI (consta)	LAI: 25–50 mg q2wk. Increase dose in 12.5 mg intervals, with increases 4 wk apart. PO overlap ×3 wk. Main release during 3–6 wk, subsides by week 7

(continued)

Atypical Antipsychotics *(continued)*
Ziprasidone (Geodon)
PO/IM	Dose: 40–160 mg (given BID—half-life 4–10 h), take with meals Antagonist at 5HT1A + 2A, D2, D3, monoamine (NE, 5HT, DA) reuptake pumps *SE:* QT prolongation (20–25 ms)

ACAMPROSATE

Trade Name
Campral

Indications (Am J Psychiatry. 2018;175(1):86-90; National Library of Medicine. 2017a, O'Shea et al. 2010)

- Moderate to severe AUD; particularly in pts seeking abstinence w/ hepatic impairment because of renal metabolism

Mechanism of Action (Stahls et al. Essential Psychopharmacology; Am Fam Physician. 2006;74(4):645)

- Exact mechanism unknown, thought to promote abstinence by attenuating withdrawal sx, ↓ early abstinence cravings, ↓ reinforcement of drinking
- Analogue of GABA and ↓ activity of glutamate at NMDA receptors, may also affect CNS Ca^{2+} channels

Prescribing (Am J Psychiatry. 2018;175(1):86-90; Aliment Pharmacol Ther. 2017;45:865-882; Stahls et al. Essential Psychopharmacology)

- Begin treatment ASAP after achieving abstinence, continue even if pt relapses
- Do not crush or chew tablets
- Take with meals to help with compliance

Dosing						
Starting Dose (mg)	Goal/ Max Dose (mg)	Titration	Metabolism	Half-Life (h)	Before Starting	Monitoring
666 PO TID weight >60 kg 666 PO BID weight <60 kg	999– 1998	N/A	Not metabolized; excreted unchanged through the kidneys	20–33	Cr, depression/SI screen	renal fxn

Liver impairment: generally, no contraindication or dose adjustment needed
Renal impairment: It should not be used 1st-line in mild–moderate impairment (CrCl 30–50 mL/min). For CrCl 30–50 mL/min; initial dosage 333 mg TID. For CrCl ≤30 mL/min; use is contraindicated
Children: Safety and efficacy have not been established
Geriatric: Caution and lower doses → renal fxn ↓ in age
Pregnant/breastfeeding: Not recommended for use during pregnancy. Unknown if acamprosate is secreted in breast milk but recommended to discontinue drug or bottle feed

Effectiveness (*Rosner et al. Cochrane Database System Rev. 2010;9; Eur Neuropsychopharmacol. 2007;17:558-566; J Psychopharmacol. 2003;17:397-402*)
- ↑Chance of abstinence after detox by ~15%
- Head-to-head comparison naltrexone versus acamprosate → naltrexone ↓ subjective craving > acamprosate, acamprosate ↓ tachycardia a/w craving
- Acamprosate ↓heavy drinking in those who relapse

Adverse Effects (*Aliment Pharmacol Ther. 2017;45:865-882; Am Fam Physician. 2006;74(4):645*)
- **Common side effects:** CNS: insomnia, dizziness, paresthesia; GI: diarrhea, nausea, flatulence; skin: pruritus, diaphoresis
- **Rare and serious side effects/black box warning:** ↑ adverse events related to suicide (SI, suicide attempts, and completed suicides)
- **Overdose:** Usually limited to diarrhea (*Aliment Pharmacol Ther. 2017;45:865-882*)
- **Significant interactions:** Only known interaction is tetracyclines, which may be partially inactivated by the calcium component (*Labbate et al. Handbook of Psychiatric Drug Therapy*)

Discontinuation
Taper not necessary

BUPRENORPHINE

General Facts (*JAMA. 2015;313:1636; Am J Public Health. 2013;103:917*)
- DEA schedule III medication
- Buprenorphine can only be prescribed by: (1) physicians w/ active DEA + 8 h suboxone certification training w/ x license, (2) PA/NP w/ DEA registration + additional 24 h training with x license (CARA Legislation)
- Initiation in acute setting leads to ↑ addiction tx engagement; ↓ mortality a/w OUD; ↓ HIV/HCV; ↓ criminality; ↑ sobriety; ↓illicit use; and ↓ inpatient addiction services
- Buprenorphine >20× more potent than morphine
- **Acute pain in opioid dependent patients: See OUD**
- **Indications:** OUD and mitigation of opioid withdrawal (See OUD), chronic pain management: (often TID dosing)

Formulations					
Buprenorphine			**Buprenorphine + Naloxone**		
Name	Administration	Indications	Name	Administration	Indications
Subutex	Sublingual tablet	OUD	Suboxone	Sublingual film	OUD
Belbuca	Buccal film	Pain	Bunavail	Buccal film	OUD
Buprenex	IV, IM	Pain	Zubsolv	Sublingual tablets	OUD
Butrans	Transdermal patch	Pain			

(continued)

Formulations *(continued)*					
Buprenorphine			**Buprenorphine + Naloxone**		
Name	Administration	Indications	Name	Administration	Indications
Sublocade	Extended-release injection	OUD			
Probuphine	Implant	OUD			

Mechanism of Action *(Curr Neuropharmacol. 2004;2(4):395-402)*
- Partial mu agonist and weak kappa antagonist; partial agonism = ceiling effect at moderate doses → ↓ OD risk; compared w/ full agonist → ↓ SE and abuse potential, analgesic effects may plateau
- High affinity to opioid receptors → displace full agonists → precipitate withdrawal
- If combined w/ **naloxone** (antagonist); inactive if taken as prescribed → ↓ IV abuse as IV use of crushed/dissolved drug → active = acute withdrawal

Adverse Effects *(J Subst Abuse Treat. 2015;52:48-57; J Sex Med. 2012;9(12):3198-3204; Buprenorphine: Drug Information. In: UpToDate. Accessed 11 October 2018)*
Common side effects: headache, dizziness, drowsiness, sleep issues, nausea, constipation, decreased libido
Rare and serious side effects/black box warning: physical dependence, neonatal opioid w/d syndrome; additional sedation/respiratory depression a/w concomitant use of BZD, CNS depressants; GI obstruction; hypersensitivity
Overdose sx: respiratory depression, sedation, slowed breathing, HoTN
Discontinuation: withdrawal sx and risk of relapse when abruptly d/c'd
Significant interactions: concurrent BZD or other sedative use, meds metabolized by P450, opioid antagonists, long QTc 2/2 any cause

Prescribing *(Reckitt Benckiser Pharma. 2011;2010; Endo Pharma. 2015; Indivior. 2017; Purdue Pharma. 2014; Braeburn Pharma. 2016; BioDelivery Sci. 2014; Orexo. 2013)*
- DO NOT give until pt shows opioid w/d or may precipitate w/d. Consider half-life of opioid (heroin, oxycodone, vicodin vs methadone)
- **All primarily metabolized by liver CYP450**
- Monitor: toxicology, LFTs; respiratory depression esp w/in 24–72 h of initiating therapy and dosage increases; diversion, monitor signs of hypogonadism or hypoadrenalism (no specific screening indicated unless suspected)
- **Sample induction protocol:** can be in-office, at home, or at hospital
  - Consider toxicology screen ± pain management profile + discussion of use to guide anticipated time to start → as can precipitate withdrawal pt should already demonstrate sx to prevent this → in-house: can score COWS to guide→start when >8 (see OUD for COWS), use pt input the best time to initiate (at home, discuss sx to watch for)

- Common induction pathway:
  - Day 1: Once adequate withdrawal noted → buprenorphine 4 mg ×1 → If well tolerated, repeat q6h ×2 more, target dose = 12 mg; If sx well managed at lower dose, instruct pt they can adjust amount taken accordingly
  - Day 2: If no issues noted day 1 (withdrawal/oversedation), generally can aim for 16 mg/d; for most → target dose (see OUD)
  - Always offer "comfort meds" through the process, including clonidine, bentyl, NSAIDs/Tylenol; once on stabile dose can be DC'd

Buprenorphine					
Name	**Starting Dose**	**Max Dose**	**Titration**	**Half-Life**	**Before Starting**
Subutex	4 mg	32 mg/d	• 2–4 mg/d • Can give + 4 mg 30 min after the 1st dose for continued w/d sx	24–60 h	
Belbuca	• If 30–89 mg MME, start 150 mcg q12h • If 90–160 mg MME, start 300 µg q12h • If >160 mg MME, consider alternative analgesic	900 µg q12h	↑ by 150 µg q4–8d PRN	27.6 h	• Taper current opioid dose to ≤30 mg MME QD • Not indicated as PRN analgesic
Buprenex	• 0.3 mg/mL	Max single dose: 0.6 mg IM (not IV) adults	• Repeat ×1 (up to 0.3 mg) if required, 30–60 m after initial dosage—thereafter only PRN	1.2–7.2 h	• Can be used in children ≥2 y old
Butrans	• Opioid naïve or <30 mg MME: 5 µg/h, q7d • If 30–80 mg MME: • 10 µg/h q7d • If >80 mg MME: 20 µg/h, consider alternative analgesi.	20 µg/h	Every 3 d, can increase by 5, 7.5 or 10 µg increments by no more than 2 total patches	26 h	• Taper current opioid dose • Not indicated as PRN analgesic • Has not been evaluated in pts with severe hepatic impairment

(continued)

Buprenorphine *(continued)*					
Name	**Starting Dose**	**Max Dose**	**Titration**	**Half-Life**	**Before Starting**
Sublocade	• 300 mg monthly for the 1st 2 mo	300 mg for induction and maintenance	Maintenance 100 mg monthly	43–60 d	• Baseline LFT • Must have initiated tx on transmucosal buprenorphine-containing product delivering equivalent of 8–24 mg/d ≥7 d
Propbuphine	80 mg/implant every 6 mo			24–48 h	• For pts requiring ≤8 mg/d of buprenorphine • Capable of wound healing

Liver impairment: Can worsen transaminitis. May not be appropriate in moderate impairment. Not recommended in patients with severe impairment

Renal impairment: Effects unknown

Children: Safety and effectiveness have not been established in pediatric patients, except for buprenex

Geriatric: Cachectic or debilitated patients: monitor for respiratory depression and sedation

Pregnant: In pregnancy use, buprenorphine without naloxone is preferred. A risk for neonatal w/d syndrome

Breastfeeding: Buprenorphine passes into mother's milk

Buprenorphine + Naloxone				
Name	**Starting Dose**	**Goal/Max Dose**	**Titration**	**Half-Life (h)**
Suboxone	Up to 8 mg/2 mg in divided doses	• Maintenance tx:16 mg/4 mg QD • Max is 24 mg/6 mg QD (32 mg/8 mg can be used in practice)	↑ or ↓ 2 mg/0.5 mg or 4 mg/1 mg	• Buprenorphine 24–42 • Naloxone 2–12
Bunavail	Up to 4.2 mg/0.7 mg in divided doses	• Maintenance tx: target is 8.4 mg/1.4 mg QD • Max is 12.6 mg/2.1 mg QD	↑ or ↓ 2.1 mg/0.3 mg	• Buprenorphine 16.4–27.5 • Naloxone 1.9–2.4
Zubsolv	Up to 5.7 mg/1.4 mg divided doses	• Maintenance tx: target is 11.4 mg/2.9 mg QD • Max is 17.2/4.2 mg QD	↑ or ↓ 2.9 mg/0.71 mg	• Buprenorphine 24–42 • Naloxone 2–12

Liver impairment: Can worsen transaminitis. May not be appropriate in moderate impairment. Not recommended in severe impairment

Renal impairment: Effects unknown

Children: Safety and effectiveness have not been established in pediatric patients

Geriatric: Cachectic or debilitated patients: monitor for respiratory depression and sedation

Pregnant: In pregnancy use, buprenorphine without naloxone is preferred. Risk for neonatal w/d syndrome

Breastfeeding: Buprenorphine passes into mother's milk

DISULFIRAM

Trade Name
Antabuse

Indications *(Am J Psychiatry. 2018;175(1):86-90; Aliment Pharmacol Ther. 2017;45:865-882; Addiction. 2000;95:1335-1349)*
- Moderate to severe AUD who intend total abstinence
- Given potential interaction with EtOH + inferior efficacy versus naltrexone/acamprosate, not generally a 1st-line therapy
- Other use: cocaine addiction particularly w/ comorbid AUD

Mechanism of Action *(Aliment Pharmacol Ther. 2017;45:865-882; Stahls et al. Essential Psychopharmacology)*
- Irreversibly blocks ALDH (2nd step of EtOH metabolism) → toxic levels of acetaldehyde w/ EtOH ingestion → disulfiram rxn (flushing, nausea, vomiting, tachycardia, HoTN, dyspnea, dizziness, headache), onset 5–15 min s/p EtOH consumption + lasts 30 min–h
- Toxic metabolites are diethyldithiocarbamate (DDC) + carbon disulfide (CS2)

Prescribing *(Am J Psychiatry. 2018;175(1):86-90; Aliment Pharmacol Ther. 2017;45:865-882; J Pharm Pharmacol. 2015;6:86-93; Am Fam Physician. 2005;72(9):1775-1780; Annu Rev Pharmacol Toxicol. 1981;21:575-596; U.S. Department of Health and Human Services. 2007)*
- Do not start until at least 12 h after last drink; adverse reactions w/ EtOH can occur 14 d after last dose; use caution w/ certain food, mouthwashes, + cold remedies that have EtOH
- Advise to carry a wallet card, noting on disulfiram
- Effectiveness data limited, compliance generally poor, → most effective when monitored *(Addiction. 2004;99(1):21-24; Alcohol Clin Exp Res. 1992;16(6):1035-1041)*

Dosing						
Starting Dose	Goal/ Max Dose (mg/d)	Titration	Metabolism	Half-Life (h)	Before Starting	Monitoring
PO: 250 mg/d for 1–2 wk	250–500 mg/d	N/A	Metabolized by liver, toxic + nontoxic metabolites	Parent drug 60–120 DDC 13.9 CS2 8.9	LFTs, cardiac fxn, inform pt of disulfiram rxn (above)	LFTs 10–14 d CBC, BMP

Liver impairment: Use with extreme caution
Renal impairment: Not recommended in chronic renal failure d/2 direct toxic effects on kidneys
Cardiac impairment: Contraindicated
Children: Safety and efficacy have not been established
Geriatric: Not recommended >60 y.o
Pregnant/breastfeeding: Not recommended during pregnancy, esp 1st trimester; unknown if disulfiram is secreted in human breast milk; recommended either to discontinue drug or bottle feed
Other: Not recommended for severely impulsive, psychotic, or suicidal patients

Adverse Effects
- **Common side effects:** CNS: peripheral neuropathy, drowsiness, dizziness, fatigue, headache, tremors; GU: impotence; Skin: acne, allergic dermatitis, skin rash, body odor; GI: metallic/bitter taste, halitosis (may improve if ↓ dose)
- **Rare and serious side effects:** hepatotoxicity, neuropathies, psychosis, catatonic-like rxn

Significant Interactions (Am J Psychiatry. 2018;175(1):86-90)
- Sertraline (contains 12% EtOH), ritonavir (43% EtOH)
- May ↑ blood levels of phenytoin, ↑ prothrombin time (monitor w/ anticoagulant)
- ↑ CNS toxicity of isoniazid + metronidazole
- MAOIs, α/β adrenergic antagonists, TCA, antipsychotics worsen disulfiram rxn

Overdose
- GI upset/vomiting, sedation → coma + abnormal EEG, hallucinations, incoordination
- Tx w/ gastric aspiration/lavage + supportive therapy
- Tx of disulfiram rxn = supportive, monitor arrhythmias + severe hypotension

Discontinuation
- Taper not necessary

NALTREXONE

Trade Names
ReVia: oral form; **Vivitrol:** intramuscular (IM) form

Indications (Stahl's Essential Psychopharm. 5th ed; 2014; Expert Opin Pharmacother. 2016;17:835; Iran J Psychiatry. 2017;12:142)
- Alcohol use disorder (AUD)
- Opioid use disorder (OUD)
- Off-label: impulse control disorders (kleptomania, compulsive gambling), self-injurious behavior

Mechanism of Action (J Med Toxicol. 2016;12:71; Minn Med. 2006;89:44; Iran J Psychiatry. 2017;12:142)
- **AUD:** alcohol → activation of the mesolimbic dopamine (reward) pathway through increased release of endogenous opioid peptides; naltrexone blocks the effects of endogenous opioids → ↓ euphoria with alcohol consumption
- **OUD:** naltrexone blocks the effects of exogenous opioids through direct antagonism of opioid receptors, with highest affinity for mu receptors
- **Off-label:** unclear, but suspected to be similar to mechanism in AUD. Hepatically metabolized and excreted by kidneys

Dosing					
Starting Dose	**Goal/Max Dose**	**Titration**	**Half-Life**	**Before Starting**	**Monito-ring**
AUD (oral): 50 mg daily	50 mg daily or 100 mg on M, W, and 150 mg on Fri	N/A	13 h	Baseline LFTs, urine tox, 7–10 d opioid-free (incl trama-dol), take w/ food to ↓GI side effects	Consider periodic LFTs given risk of transami-nitis
OUD (oral): 25 mg daily	50 mg daily	↑ if no signs of withdrawal			
AUD/OUD (intramus-cular): 380 mg q4wk	380 mg q4wk	N/A, pretreat-ment w/ oral naltrexone not required	5–10 d		

Dose adjustments:
Liver impairment: Mild–moderate, no adjustment; severe— use with caution in people with compensated cirrhosis, *contraindicated* in people with acute hepatitis or liver failure
Renal impairment: Mild–no adjustment; moderate–severe—use with caution
Children: Safety and efficacy have not been established
Geriatric: Safety and efficacy have not been established, may tolerate lower doses
Pregnant/breastfeeding: Recommend *discontinuation*, with possible switch to buprenorphine or methadone in women with OUD and high risk of relapse

NALTREX. 6-49

Effectiveness

- More effective for treatment of alcohol use disorder than opioid use disorder
  Alcohol use disorder: a large meta-analysis revealed a 17% (95% CI 10–24%) reduction in heavy drinking with oral form (Rösner et al. Cochrane Database Syst Rev. 2010); a large randomized control trial (RCT) revealed a 25% (95% CI 6–40%) reduction in heavy drinking with IM form (JAMA. 2005;293:1617)
  Opioid use disorder: a large meta-analysis revealed no difference in opioid use between treatment and control arm (Minozzi, et al. Cochrane Database Syst Rev. 2010)
- Limited effectiveness in opioid use disorder may reflect the risk of precipitated withdrawal leading to poor adherence
- Recent noninferiority RCT comparing IM naltrexone and oral buprenorphine-naloxone for treatment of opioid use disorder over a 12-wk study period revealed equal effectiveness between the 2 treatments (JAMA Psychiatry. 2017;74:1197)

Adverse Effects

- **Common side effects:**
  CNS: headache, insomnia, anxiety, fatigue

GI: nausea, vomiting, decreased appetite, diarrhea, transaminitis
  Skin: injection site reaction (bruising, pain, itching, swelling)
  Musculoskeletal: increased creatine phosphokinase, arthralgias, myalgias
  Respiratory: pharyngitis
- **Rare and serious side effects/black box warning:**
  Hepatocellular injury (at >5× recommended dose)
  Eosinophilic pneumonia
  Severe injection site reaction requiring surgery (for IM form)

Significant Interactions
- **Opioid analgesics:** naltrexone may diminish their effect and precipitate withdrawal
- **Peripherally acting mu-opioid antagonists:** eg, methylnaltrexone, naldemedine, naloxegol; naltrexone may enhance their adverse/toxic effects and precipitate withdrawal
- **Lofexidine:** may ↓ the serum concentration of naltrexone

Overdose
- Signs/symptoms: Nausea, abdominal pain, sedation, dizziness, injection site reactions
- Treatment: activated charcoal, gastric lavage, IV fluids, laxatives, and possible HD

Discontinuation
- Taper not necessary

TOBACCO CESSATION

Smoking = Major Contributor to Mortality in Mental Illness
(*JAMA Psychiatry.* 2015;72(12):1172-1181; *J Psych Res.* 2014;48(1):102-110; *BMJ.* 2014;348:g1151)
- Quitting smoking by age 50 cuts mortality in half
- Half of pts with prior psychiatric hospitalization for SCZ, BPAD, or MDD will die tobacco related illness
- **28-y** mortality gap for individuals with SCZ compared with gen population
- Smoking cessation significantly improves psychiatric symptoms (depression, anxiety, stress) and quality of life

Counseling Patients on Cessation
(*Lancet.* 2016;387(10037):2507-2520; *Curr Psych.* 17(2):28,33)
- Clinicians need to prioritize efforts in smoking cessation at each visit, emphasize to patients this is *the most important thing they can do to improve their health*
- Smoking cessation can save a patient over $4000 a year
- Pharmacotherapeutics are 1st-line tx
  - Medication more than doubles pt chance of quitting smoking (5× more likely with varenicline in SMI population)
  - Medications reduce cravings and withdrawal, are not addictive, and are *less dangerous* than continuing to smoke

Nicotine Withdrawal
- Peak at *4 d*, duration 2–3 wk for worst sx, should then improve
- Anxiety, awakening during sleep, depression, difficulty concentrating, impatience, irritability/anger, restlessness, decreased heart rate, increased appetite

Antipsychotic Interactions
- Tobacco smoke ↑ activity of cytochrome P450 1A2, metabolizes several antipsychotics
- Concentrations of **clozapine, fluphenazine, haloperidol,** and **olanzapine** may ↑ following cessation—dose ↓ may be warranted.
- Conversely, if patients resume smoking (ie, after a hospitalization), doses of these medications may need to be ↑.

MEDICATION MANAGEMENT OF CESSATION

Varenicline (*Lancet.* 2016;387(10037):2507-2520)
- EAGLES Trial—black box suicidality warning removed. **NO increased risk of neuropsychiatric side effects or risk for suicidality** compared with placebo
- **Method of action:**
  Non-nicotine
  High affinity for nicotinic acetylcholine receptor
  Results in reduced nicotine cravings and reduced pleasure from nicotine use
- Half-life, 24 h; minimal metabolism, 92% excreted in urine. No absolute contraindications
- **Side effects:** nausea (take with food), vivid dreams (take PM dose earlier, decrease PM dose, eliminate PM dose)
- **Prescribing:**
  Start 1 wk before proposed quit date in gen pop., 4 wk in those with SMI.
  Starter pack = 0.5 mg daily ×3d, 0.5 mg BID ×4d, then 1 mg BID for 12 wk
  Consider maintenance therapy—1 y maintenance tx tripled abstinence rates (60%) at 1 y in smokers with SMI.

Bupropion (*Lancet.* 2016;387(10037):2507-2520)
- **Method of action:**
  Non-nicotine
  Norepinephrine dopamine reuptake inhibitor (NDRI), noncompetitive antagonist at nicotinic acetylcholine receptor
  Results in reduced nicotine cravings and reduced pleasure from nicotine use
- Half-life 21 h, metabolized in liver. Contraindicated in pts with seizure disorder, eating disorder, or if abruptly discontinuing EtOH, benzo, barbiturates, or antiepileptics
- **Side effects:** insomnia (take PM dose earlier), agitation/anxiety (reduce dose)
- **Prescribing:**
  Start 1 wk before quit attempt
  150 mg daily ×3 d, then 150 mg BID after. Usually tx ×12 wk.

Nicotine Patch (*Lancet*. 2016;387(10037):2507-2520)
- **Method of action:**
  Nicotine-containing patch, body absorbs through skin, provides release of nicotine throughout day
- Half-life 15–20 h
- **Side effects:** vivid dreams (take patch off before bed), rash (rotate site), nicotine tox—nausea, dizziness, palp (sign that dose is too high)
- **Prescribing:**
  Start patch 30 d before quit date, continue for 12 wk after quitting. Place new patch every AM.
  >10 cigarettes/d: 21 mg/d patch
  <10 cigarettes/d: 14 mg/d patch
  After 6–8 wk step down to lower dose, 2–4 wk later step down to next lower dose (7 mg to off)

PRN Nicotine Replacement (*Lancet*. 2016;387(10037):2507-2520)
- Gum, lozenge, inhaler
- Recommended to use along with nicotine patch. Do not eat or drink within 15 min of below therapies
- **Side effects:** hiccups/moth sores (spit), nicotine tox (lower dose)
- **Prescribing:**
  If >20 cigarettes, 4 mg gum or lozenge; otherwise 2 mg q2h. Gradually increase time between uses, number of uses, and/or reduce dose
- **Gum**—"chew and park"—chew 10× then park btw teeth and cheek
- **Lozenge**—do not chew. Park in cheek, move from 1 side of mouth to the other
- **Inhaler**—1 cartridge = 4 mg nicotine = 80 inhalations over about 20 min. Avg = 10 cartridges/d. Recommend puffing continuously ×20 min

NUTRACEUTICALS

Background (*Focus*. 2018;16:2-11; *Am J Psychiatry*. 2016;173:575-587; *J Clin Psychopharmacol*. 2013;33:643-648; *J Affect Disord*. 2010)
- **Definitions:** Pharmaceutical grade nutrients that augment activity of a medication or provide a range of biological effects
  - The FDA monitors safety not efficacy, treated like dietary supplements
  - There isn't any monitoring prior to market
  - Different preparations by different companies may vary in potency
- **Epidemiology:** A 2007 National Health Interview Survey found that 38% of adults and 12% of children had used "complementary" or "alternative" medicine (CAM) practices and products in the past year
- **Pros:** Can work for mild illness, may be good adjuncts to medications, may work for patients who haven't responded to standard pharmaceuticals or are not amenable to other treatments, may have fewer side effects
- **Cons:** More expensive, evidence remains limited, especially in pregnancy

Nutraceuticals for Depression		
Nutraceutical	**Studied Dosing**	**Notes**
5-HTP		Derivative of tryptophan, an essential monoamine precursor required for the synthesis of 5-HT; has been shown to be superior to placebo for depression (Alino et al., 1976), and equal in efficacy to imipramine and fluvoxamine (Angst et al., 1977; Poldinger et al., 1991)
Methylfolate and folinic acid		Active forms of folate involved in the methylation processes of monoamines which are implicated in mood. Methylfolate is a patented derivative, and there is some concern that trials are biased toward positive results
Omega-3 fatty acids (EPA)	1000– 2000 mg/d	Stabilizes neuronal membrane and modulates NE, DA, and 5-HT reuptake, synthesis, degradation, and receptor binding. Has anti-inflammatory properties and can be used for augmentation. Increased risk of bleeding and cycling in bipolar disorder at high doses. DHA formula may not be effective
S-Adenosyl methionine (SAMe)	200– 3200 mg/d	Intermediate in the metabolism of folate and B12. Enhances methylation of catecholamines and increased 5-HT turnover, reuptake inhibition of NE, and enhanced DA activity. Has anti-inflammatory properties
St. John's Wort (*Hypericum perforatum*)	300– 1800 mg/d BID-TID	Interacts with HPA axis to reduce cytokine and cortisol production. Better than placebo, about equal effects to TCAs and SSRIs for mild–moderate depression (Linde et al., 2008). Has MAOI activity and can cause serotonin syndrome and cycling into mania. Do not combine with SSRIs or other serotonergic agents. Induces CYP-3A4, so will decrease effectiveness of warfarin and oral contraceptive pills
Vitamin D		Increases the expression of genes encoding for tyrosine hydroxylase, the precursor of DA and NE. Vitamin D receptors are identified in the prefrontal cortex, hypothalamus, and substantia nigra, areas involved with depression

Nutraceuticals for Anxiety		
Nutraceutical	**Studied Dosing**	**Notes**
Kava kava (*Piper methysticum*)		Inhibits excitatory neurotransmitter release by blockade of voltage-gated Na and Ca ion channels, enhances ligand binding to GABA-A receptors, and inhibits MAO-B; can cause hepatotoxicity
Melatonin	0.1–10 mg/d	Hormone that interacts with the suprachiasmatic nucleus and resets circadian rhythm; has a direct sedative effect
Rhodiola rosea		Enhances catecholaminergic system by inhibiting the activity of enzymes responsible for monoamine degradation and facilitation of neurotransmitter transport; may also induce opioid peptide biosynthesis
Valerian (*Valeriana officinalis*)	450–600 mg before bedtime	Sedative and mild hypnotic that contains GABAergic compounds. Some studies suggest equivalence to BZDs, with fewer side effects and no tolerance (*Mischoulon*, 2002). Powerful smell can be a limitation. Needs 1–2 wk to work.

Nutraceuticals for Dementia		
Nutraceutical	**Studied Dosing**	**Notes**
Ginkgo biloba	120–240 mg/d, BID-TID	Stabilizes neuronal membranes and scavenges free radicals; may slow cognitive decline in dementia but no preventive effect (*Andrade et al.,* 2009). Minimum 8-wk course recommended

COMMON SIDE EFFECTS

EXTRAPYRAMIDAL SYMPTOMS

Definition and Etiology (*Drug Saf.* 2005;28:190)

Extrapyramidal system (as distinct from the pyramidal tracts, which go through the pyramids of the medulla) regulates involuntary skeletal muscle tone and posture

Any drug which affects CNS dopamine has the potential to cause EPS, particularly antipsychotics and certain antinausea agents (eg, metoclopramide)

Acute Dystonia

- **Definition:** Sustained muscle contraction affecting face and trunk >> limbs

  Torticollis: sustained neck muscle contraction resulting in forced twisted posture; painful

  Opisothotonos: hyperextension of the neck or back from axial muscle contraction

  Laryngeal spasm: closure of the vocal cords resulting in stridor, and if severe, airway blockage

- **Epidemiology:** young males (may relate to increased muscle mass) and persons with a history of dystonia are most commonly affected

  Can occur after the 1st dose of medication, mostly within 48 h of dose

  Less common with SGA versus FGA

- **Treatment:** anticholinergic medication (eg, diphenhydramine, benztropine), parenteral administration preferred for more rapid resolution and in case of laryngeal spasm

  Dose reduction or change in medication recommended following acute dystonic reaction

  Can coadminister anticholinergic with medication for prophylaxis (recommended especially for antipsychotic naïve individuals receiving IM eg, for a restraint)

  In case of depot injection of an antipsychotic, symptoms may persist for weeks depending on the kinetics of the depot, and so anticholinergic may need to be continued for prolonged period

Akathisia

- **Definition:** Motor restlessness with a strong urge to move and inability to sit still; may be difficult to distinguish from pacing resulting from agitation. In patients who have received IM antipsychotics and paradoxically become more activated, consider akathisia as cause
- **Epidemiology:** Most common form of EPS, rates up to 31% after 2 wk of treatment with FGA; lower incidence rate with SGA
- **Treatment:** 1st-line therapies include propranolol; 2nd-line agents are benzodiazepines, or benztropine

  Acute akathisia is self-limiting with discontinuation of the causative medication

Parkinsonism

- **Definition:** syndrome of bradykinesia (slowed movements), tremor, rigidity, and postural instability. Hypophonia and masked facies may also be present. Drug-induced (secondary) parkinsonism may be clinically indistinguishable from primary (idiopathic) Parkinson disease, but some studies indicate it is more likely to be symmetrical versus asymmetric tremor in idiopathic Parkinson disease
- **Epidemiology:** More common in the elderly and females. Occurs with all antipsychotics, more frequently with higher potency D2 blockers and with lower rates with clozapine and quetiapine
- **Treatment:** Dose reduction or elimination of offending agent if clinically possible is the mainstay of treatment; parkinsonism is generally reversible with discontinuation

If medication must be continued, addition of benztropine or amantadine may be helpful

Levodopa or dopamine agonists generally are not helpful

Extrapyramidal Symptoms, Timecourse, and Management			
Movement	Description	Onset	Treatment
Dystonia	Sustained muscle contraction	Hours to days	IM or IV anticholinergic
Akathisia	Subjective feeling of restlessness	Hours to days	Propranolol Benzodiazepines Anticholinergics
Parkinsonism	Bradykinesia, tremor, rigidity	Weeks to months	Benztropine Amantadine
Tardive dyskinesia	Late-onset hyperkinetic movements	Months to years	Quetiapine, clozapine VMAT2 inhibitors Benzodiazepines

TARDIVE DYSKINESIA

Definitions (J Neurol Sci. 2018;389:67)

Tardive dyskinesia: Delayed-onset, iatrogenic movement disorder caused by exposure to dopamine-blocking medications, and continuing at least 1 month after discontinuation of the offending medication

Tardive dystonia: prolonged contracture of muscle groups resulting in sustained twisting motions or abnormal limb movements

Etiology

- Mechanism is not clear but possibly involves excitotoxicity-mediated cellular changes in the basal ganglia in dopaminergic and GABA neurons, resulting in an overall hyperkinetic state

Epidemiology

- TD most correlated to age and duration of treatment with dopamine-blocking agents. Elderly and females are at higher risk. Patients who suffered EPS are more likely to develop TD

  With FGA, rates of TD are ~5–6%/y, with 5- and 10-y prevalence of 25% and 50%, respectively

  SGA have lower TD rates by ~25% relative to FGA, or 4%/y. Clozapine, quetiapine, and pimavanserin have lower rates of TD

Diagnosis

- TD is a clinical diagnosis based on classic hyperkinetic movements

  Oral–buccal–lingual movements >> limbs, trunk, and respiratory muscles. Movements are suppressible and disappear during sleep

  Patients are often unaware of their symptoms in early stages and are frequently unbothered by them

- Patients on antipsychotics should have regular monitoring for TD with a clinical scale such as the Abnormal Involuntary Movements Scale (AIMS)
- Presence of focal neurological signs other than dyskinesia or dystonia points to a likely alternative diagnosis or underlying neurologic condition

Treatment
- Discontinuation of offending medication, if clinically feasible, at the 1st signs of TD is best; if not possible, switching to SGA (particularly quetiapine, clozapine) may be helpful
  Increasing the dose may temporarily mask symptoms but risks worsening the TD in the long term
  VMAT2 inhibitors tetrabenazine, deutetrabenazine, or valbenazine have been shown to reduce TD symptoms in the short term, but long-term studies are lacking (Am J Psychiatry. 1999;156:8)
- Deutetrabenazine and Valbenazine are FDA Approved for TD
  Benzodiazepines, particularly clonazepam, may reduce TD movements and the anxiety associated with them
  Moderate evidence supports *Ginkgo biloba*, and some limited evidence supports vitamin E and vitamin B6 in reducing TD symptoms (Arch Gen Psychiatry. 1999;56:9)
    Refractory cases may benefit from deep brain stimulation
  Tardive dystonia may benefit from focal botulinum toxin injections

---

QTc PROLONGATION

Introduction (Psychosomatics. 2013;54:1; Am J Psychiatry. 2001;158:1774)
- The QTc is a corrected ECG interval corresponding to ventricular depolarization and repolarization
- Prolongation with most medications is produced by blocking cardiac delayed rectifier potassium channels (IKr); a minority of medications block depolarization through effect on sodium channels (eg, TCAs)
- Serves as a surrogate marker for risk of sudden cardiac death, as it is associated with torsades de pointes (TdP, "twisting of the points"), a polymorphic ventricular tachycardia that can degenerate into ventricular fibrillation
- Leading cause of drug withdrawal during phase IV postmarketing drug surveillance
- Risk is continuous, although often arbitrarily dichotomized. Population normal values in men are <430 ms and in women <450 ms
- Many clinicians use 500 ms (or an increase >60 ms) as the cut off for significant concern (risk of cardiac event 1.66 fold at 500 ms compared with 400 ms). The absolute risk remains very low at less than 1 in 4000 even at a QTc of 600 ms (Psychosomatics. 2018;59:105)
- Correlation between prolongation and risk of torsades is imperfect and likely involves mechanisms beyond simple magnitude of prolongation (eg, myocardial dispersion)

- Associated with many nonpsychiatric drugs (eg, macrolides, fluoro-quinolones, conazole antifungals, antiarrhythmics, methadone)
- The Arizona Center for Education and Research on Therapeutics (AzCERT) maintains an updated database of drugs at www.QTdrugs.org (aka. www.crediblemeds.org). Caution is advised, as this database stratifies meds into broad categories that have large differences in risk

Common Risk Factors *(Psychosomatics. 2018;59:105)*
- Bradycardia
- Hypokalemia/magnesemia
- Female sex
- Preexisting cardiac disease
- Illicit drug use

Measurement *(J Electrocardiol. 2004;37:81; Am J Cardiol. 1988;61:83)*
- Machines average all leads, but manual measurements often use V2 or V3
- Eyeball method: Likely prolonged if it appears longer than ½ the RR interval
- **Bazett formula:** $QTc = QT/(RR\ interval)^{(1/2)} = QT/(60/HR)^{(1/2)}$

   Used by most ECG machines but only accurate between 60 and 80 bpm so not preferred

   Overestimates QTc for tachycardia and underestimates QTc for bradycardia
- **Fridericia formula:** $QTc = QT/(RR\ interval)^{(1/3)} = QT/(60/HR)^{(1/3)}$

   Similar to Bazett's but with a cubed root
- **Framingham formula:** $QTc = QT + 0.154\ (1-RR\ interval)$

   Alongside Fridericia's, showed the best evidence for predicting 1-y mortality in a cohort of 6609 patients *(J Am Heart Assoc. 2016;5:6)*
- **Hodge formula:** $QTc = QT + 1.75(HR-60)$

   Least impacted by heart rate and easy to calculate

Measurement in the Presence of QRS Prolongation *(Circulation. 2003;108:1985)*
- A prolonged QRS (>120 ms, eg, bundle branch blocks, paced rhythms) can artificially prolong the QTc
- There is no consensus on the best way to calculate a QTc equivalent in this scenario, and there is limited evidence to support any particular method.
- The JT Index (JTI) is one proposed formula *(Psychosomatics. 2013;54:502)*.
   JT = QT−QRS
   JTI = JT(HR+100)/518
   A normal JTI is <112 ms
- Method of estimation involves using a QTc adjusted for a normal QRS of 100 ms which is then compared against the standard 500 ms cut-off *(Psychosomatics. 2018;59:105; J Am Coll Cardiol. 2009;23:982)*
   QTc (wide QRS adjusted) = QTc−(QRS−100)

Citalopram and the FDA Warning on QTc Prolongation
- In an RCT commissioned by the FDA, citalopram clearly caused dose-dependent QTc prolongation (18.5 ms at 60 mg, 12.6 ms at

40 mg, 8.5 ms at 20 mg). As the 60 mg dose was no more effective than 40 mg in multiple trials, the FDA advised against doses above 40 mg in 2011 and against doses above 20 mg for adults >60 yo in 2012.

- Following these warnings doses were rapidly reduced across the country, but the impact has been controversial
- In 2013 the VA compared 618,450 patients on citalopram to 365,898 patients on sertraline and examined dose relationships with arrhythmias and all-cause mortality. They actually observed a decrease in risk for doses of citalopram over 40 mg QD (Am J Psychiatry. 2013;170:642)
- In 2016 the VA reviewed the impact of this warning on 35,848 patients on citalopram (mean dose before warning 64 mg QD, 180 d after 60% had dropped below 40 mg QD). This study found a subsequent increase in all-cause deaths and hospitalizations (HR 4.5, CI 4.1–5.0) (Am J Psychiatry. 2016;173:896)
- Citalopram at higher doses may increase the QTc slightly, but not enough to meaningfully impact the risk of TdP
- Although the FDA did not extend the warning to escitalopram, the same RCT found that it also prolonged the QTc at about half the rate (4.5 ms at 10 mg, 6.6 ms at 20 mg, 10.7 at 30 mg)

Antipsychotics and Sudden Cardiac Death
- A retrospective cohort study of Tennessee Medicaid enrollees (n = 279,000) demonstrated an increased risk of sudden cardiac death among users of typical (adjusted incidence rate ratio 1.99, CI 1.68–2.34) and atypical (2.26, CI 1.88–2.72) antipsychotics with a dose response. The same relationship was demonstrated in cohort members with only mood disorders, making it unlikely that the risk was due to schizophrenia alone (NEJM. 2009;360:225)
- This risk should be balanced against other cohort evidence suggesting reductions in all-cause mortality when patients with schizophrenia are treated with antipsychotics (Lancet. 2009;374:620).

Monitoring Guidelines (J Psychiatr Pract. 2014;20:196)
- There is limited consensus on the best practice for monitoring the QTc when a patient is on psychiatric medications. The NNS is unclear but likely high.
- A 2011 review of guidelines on screening for cardiovascular risk factors in schizophrenia found an even split between those that recommended for and against ECG monitoring (Br J Psychiatry. 2011;199:99).
- Routine ECG monitoring (eg, at drug initiation and dose increases) is acceptable but probably unnecessary except for high-risk drugs or high-risk patients (eg, personal history of heart disease, family history of sudden cardiac death, congenital long QT syndrome)
- IV haloperidol is alleged to cause more severe QTc prolongation than the IM or PO routes. This has never been shown definitively, and the evidence is at least partially confounded by medical illness. In 2007, the FDA recommended routine QTc monitoring when given IV (either with daily EKGs or continuous telemetry). They

also issued a reminder that haloperidol lactate is only approved for IM use and IV administration is considered off-label (*J Hosp Med.* 2010;5:E8). When IV haloperidol is administered, electrolytes should probably be monitored daily and repleted to a K of 4 and a Mg of 2

QTc Prolonging Psychotropic Medications		
Class	**High Risk**	**Relatively Low Risk**
Antipsychotics	Ziprasidone Iloperidone IV haloperidol Thioridazine Mesoridazine Droperidol	Aripiprazole Lurasidone
Antidepressants	Citalopram TCAs	Sertraline, fluoxetine, paroxetine, fluvoxamine SNRIs Bupropion Mirtazapine Trazodone
Others	Methadone	Valproate Lamotrigine Carbamazepine Benzodiazepines Amphetamines Methamphetamines

Lancet. 2013;382:951; *Psychosomatics.* 2013;54:1; *Dtsch Arztebl Int.* 2011;108:687

LANDMARK STUDIES IN PSYCHOPHARMACOLOGY

Alcohol Use Disorder: COMBINE
- *Name:* Effect of Combined Pharmacotherapies and Behavioral Interventions
- *Funding:* National Institute on Alcohol Abuse and Alcoholism (NIAAA)
- *Design:* Double-blind, multicenter, placebo-controlled RCT
- *Sample size:* 1383 patients
- *Inclusion/exclusion criteria:* >18 yo, DSM-IV dx of AUD at least 14 drinks/wk (women) or 21 drinks/wk (men) with 2+ days heavy drinking in last 90 d, abstinence for 4–21 d prior to randomization, no other substance use except cannabis/nicotine, no psychiatric disorder requiring medication, LFTs not >3 times upper limit of normal, not pregnant/breastfeeding
- *Follow-up:* 1 y

- *Arms:* Factorial design with 9 arms = acamprosate/placebo × naltrexone/placebo × CBT/medication management + CBT with no pills
- *Primary outcome:* Percent days abstinent, time to 1st heavy drinking day
- *Primary finding:* Naltrexone (80% of days abstinent on average) and CBT (called "CBI" in this study, 79.8%) separated from placebo (73.8%). Acamprosate did not
- *Secondary findings:* Difficult to interpret clinical significance of results but NNT = 5–6 for secondary "good clinical outcome" composite score for naltrexone and CBT. Used high doses of naltrexone (mean 88 mg QD)
- *Limitations:* Strict inclusion/exclusion criteria, used higher dose of naltrexone than routinely prescribed, very complicated statistical analyses made findings difficult to interpret
- *Why it matters:* Largest study on MAT for AUD, helped to establish naltrexone as the 1st-line medication
- *Representative paper:* JAMA. 2006;295:2003
- *See also:* Project MATCH (Alcohol Clin Exp Res. 1988;22:1300), VA Naltrexone Cooperative Study (NEJM. 2001;345:1734)

Bipolar Affective Disorder, Depression: STEP-BD
Psychopharm
- *Name:* Systematic Treatment Enhancement Program for Bipolar Disorder
- *Funding:* National Institute of Mental Health (NIMH)
- *Design:* Double-blind, multicenter, placebo-controlled RCT
- *Sample size:* 366 patients
- *Inclusion/exclusion criteria:* >18 yo, DSM-IV dx of bipolar I or II depression, no prior intolerance to study drugs, no need for new antipsychotic medication or acute treatment of a substance use disorder
- *Follow-up:* 26 wk
- *Arms:* Bupropion, paroxetine, and placebo (1:1:2) all atop any FDA-approved mood stabilizer
- *Primary outcome:* Percentage obtaining durable recovery (8 wk euthymic)
- *Primary finding:* Antidepressants did not separate from placebo (23.5% vs 27.3% achieving recovery)
- *Secondary findings:* No difference in switching to mania between antidepressants and placebo
- *Limitations:* Low recruitment rate, short definition of recovery, coexisting psychosocial study with high utilization of psychotherapy limits generalizability
- *Why it matters:* Studied the 2 antidepressants previously thought safest and most effective in bipolar disorder with null results, demonstrated that bipolar and unipolar depression should be conceptualized as distinct entities
- *Representative paper:* NEJM. 2007;356:1711
- *See also:* STEP-BD Psychosocial (Arch Gen Psychiatry. 2007;64:419), EMBOLDEN I and II (J Clin Psychiatry. 2010;71:150; J Clin Psychiatry. 2010;71:163), BALANCE (Lancet. 2010;375:385), CHOICE (J Clin Psychiatry. 2016;77:90)

Electroconvulsive Therapy: CORE-II

- *Name:* Consortium for Research in ECT
- *Funding:* National Institute of Mental Health (NIMH)
- *Design:* Double-blind, multicenter RCT (no placebo/sham arm)
- *Sample size:* 230 patients
- *Inclusion/exclusion criteria:* >18 yo, DSM-IV dx of MDD or bipolar depression, MMSE>21, judged to need ECT by study physician, no ECT within past 6 mo, no schizoaffective disorder, no intellectual disability or dementia, no OCD or anxiety disorder diagnosed within 1 y, no active substance use disorders
- *Follow-up:* 2–4 mo
- *Arms:* Bifrontal, bitemporal, and right unilateral electrode placement
- *Primary outcome:* remission defined as ≥60% decrease from baseline in HDRS–24 total score with HDRS–24 ≤ 10 on 2 consecutive ratings
- *Primary finding:* Remission rates equivalent (55% RUL, 61% BF, 64% BT) after 5–6 treatments on average (2 wk)
- *Secondary findings:* BT electrode placement resulted in more rapid response. RUL required a much higher stimulus dose (6 times seizure threshold vs 1.5 times) to achieve equal efficacy. No differences in cognitive side effects when RUL used higher dose to achieve same effect. Bipolar and unipolar depression responded equally
- *Limitations:* Vague inclusion criteria with strict exclusion criteria, no placebo (sham) arm, only powered for superiority
- *Why it matters:* One of the largest RCTs on ECT, demonstrated rapid remission
- *Representative paper:* Br J Psychiatry. 2010;196:226
- *See also:* CORE-I (Arch Gen Psychiatry. 2006;63:1337); CUC (JAMA. 2001;285:1299)

Major Depressive Disorder: STAR*D

- *Name:* Sequenced Treatment Alternatives to Relieve Depression
- *Funding:* National Institute of Mental Health (NIMH)
- *Design:* Open-label, multicenter semirandomized controlled trial with 4 sequential "levels" (no placebo arm)
- *Sample size:* 4041 (initial size in level 1) to 123 (final size by level 4)
- *Inclusion/exclusion criteria:* 18–75 yo, DSM-IV dx of nonpsychotic MDD with HDRS≥14, outpatients (not actively suicidal or needing inpatient detox), no bipolar or schizophrenia, no primary dx of OCD or eating disorders, not pregnant/breastfeeding, never treated with any treatment in Levels 1 or 2
- *Follow-up:* 16–24 mo depending on phase remission achieved (each level lasted 12–14 wk)
- *Arms:*
  Level 1: Citalopram
  Level 2: Buspirone (augment), bupropion SR (switch or augment), CBT (switch or augment), sertraline, venlafaxine XR
  Level 3: Mirtazapine, nortriptyline, Li (augment), T3 (augment)
  Level 4: Tranylcypromine, venlafaxine XR with mirtazapine
- *Primary outcome:* Remission defined by ≤5 on the Quick Inventory of Depressive Symptomatology-Self-Report (QIDS-SR16)

- *Primary finding:* All agents were equivalent (including augmentation and switching strategies)
- *Secondary findings:* The chance of remission decreased with successive drug trials with a sharp drop (inflection point) after level 2 (36.8%, 30.6%, 13.7%, 13.0%). Relapse also increased for those that took more levels to respond. Overall 67% of participants obtained remission
- *Limitations:* Substantial dropout rates complicate interpretation of response, primary outcome was changed from HDRS to QIDS, no placebo or ECT arms, open-label, only powered for superiority
- *Why it matters:* Largest RCT on MDD, suggested that all antidepressants were equally effective (including switch vs augmentation strategies)
- *Representative paper:* Am J Psychiatry. 2006;11:1905
- *See also:* STAR*D Level 1 (*Am J Psychiatry.* 2006;163:28); Level 2 (*NEJM.* 2006;354:1231; *NEJM.* 2006;354:1243), Level 3 (*Am J Psychiatry.* 2006;163:1161; *Am J Psychiatry.* 2006;163:1519), Level 4 (*Am J Psychiatry.* 2006;163:1531), TADS (*JAMA.* 2004;292:807), TORDIA (*JAMA.* 2008;299:901), NIMH Depression Collaborative Research Program (*Arch Gen Psychiatry.* 1989;46:971), EsDEPACS (*JAMA.* 2018;320:350)

Schizophrenia, Chronic: CATIE Phase 1

- *Name:* Clinical Antipsychotic Trials of Intervention Effectiveness Phase 1
- *Funding:* National Institute of Mental Health (NIMH)
- *Design:* Double-blind, multicenter RCT (no placebo arm)
- *Sample size:* 1493 patients with schizophrenia (only powered for superiority)
- *Inclusion/exclusion criteria:* 18–65 yo, DSM-IV dx of schizophrenia, no prior intolerance to treatments, not 1st episode of psychosis, no schizoaffective disorder, no intellectual disability or dementia, not pregnant/breastfeeding
- *Follow-up:* 18 mo
- *Arms:* Risperidone, olanzapine, quetiapine, ziprasidone (added half-way through), and perphenazine (1st generation)
- *Primary outcome:* Time to all-cause medication discontinuation
- *Primary finding:* No difference between 1st and 2nd generation agents
- *Secondary findings:* 74% of patients discontinued their medication. Olanzapine showed some advantages with fewer hospitalizations (NNT = 10–20) and almost twice the time to all-cause discontinuation (mean 9.2 mo vs 5 mo), but it also caused significant weight gain (1–2 lbs/mo)
- *Limitations:* Choice of primary outcome widely criticized, differences in dose equivalencies complicates results (olanzapine > quetiapine), only powered for superiority, no placebo arm
- *Why it matters:* Largest RCT on schizophrenia, demonstrated that 2nd and 1st generations were more similar than previously thought, confirmed side effect differences of individual drugs
- *Representative paper:* NEJM. 2005;353:1209
- *See also:* Phase 1B (*Am J Psychiatry.* 2006;163:611), Phase 2E (*Am J Psychiatry.* 2006;163:600), Phase 2T (*Am J Psychiatry.* 2007;164:415), CATIE-AD (*NEJM.*

2006;355:1525), CUtLASS I (Arch Gen Psychiatry. 2006;63:1079), SOHO (CNS Drugs. 2006;20:293), FIN11 (Lancet. 2009;374:620), InterSePT (Arch Gen Psychiatry. 2003;60:82)

Schizophrenia, 1st Episode Psychosis: CAFE

- *Name:* Comparison of Atypicals in 1st Episode
- *Funding:* AstraZeneca Pharmaceuticals
- *Design:* Double-blind, multicenter RCT (no placebo arm)
- *Sample size:* 400 patients with 1st episode psychosis
- *Inclusion/exclusion criteria:* 16–40 yo, DSM-IV dx of schizophreniform/ schizophrenia/schizoaffective disorders with symptoms for 1–60 mo and no recovery >3 mo, no prior treatment with antipsychotics for >16 wk, no serious risk of suicide, not pregnant/breastfeeding
- *Follow-up:* 52 wk
- *Arms:* Risperidone, olanzapine, quetiapine
- *Primary outcome:* Time to all-cause medication discontinuation
- *Primary finding:* All agents equivalent
- *Secondary findings:* 70% of patients discontinued their medication. Quetiapine performed worse on positive symptoms. Patients in their 1st episode responded to about half the doses used in chronic schizophrenia in CATIE
- *Limitations:* Choice of primary outcome widely criticized, industry sponsored
- *Why it matters:* Replicated the findings of CATIE for 1st episode psychosis but adequately powered for noninferiority
- *Representative paper:* Am J Psychiatry. 2007;164:1050
- *See also:* EUFEST (Lancet. 2008;371:1085)

Landmark Network Meta-Analyses in Psychiatry				
Condition	Year	RCTs (n)	Findings	Reference
Adult MDD	2018	522 (116,477)	Analyzed 21 drugs with small differences in efficacy/ tolerability evident	Lancet. 2018;391:1357
Adult MDD	2009	117 (25,928)	Analyzed 12 drugs with sertraline and escitalopram ranking best for efficacy and tolerability	Lancet. 2009;373:746

Landmark Network Meta-Analyses in Psychiatry *(continued)*				
Condition	**Year**	**RCTs (n)**	**Findings**	**Reference**
Pediatric MDD	2016	34 (5260)	Analyzed 14 drugs with only fluoxetine separating from placebo	*Lancet.* 2016;388:881
Bipolar maintenance	2014	33 (6846)	Analyzed 17 drugs with lithium recommended as the 1st-line treatment	*Lancet Psych.* 2014;1:351
Bipolar mania	2011	68 (16,073)	Analyzed 13 drugs with antipsychotics being more effective than mood stabilizers	*Lancet.* 2011;378:1306
Schizophrenia	2013	212 (43,049)	Analyzed 15 drugs with clozapine, olanzapine, and risperidone ranking as most efficacious	*Lancet.* 2013;382:951

MEDICAL CLEARANCE

Overview

- **Definition:** The process by which neurologic, general medical, and substance-induced causes of emergency psychiatric presentations are identified or ruled out and/or the stabilization of acute or ongoing general medical conditions that would preclude safe discharge or transfer to a psychiatric facility. Ideally, medical clearance also includes recommendations regarding foreseeable medical needs after discharge or transfer

- **Disposition:** In patients for whom psychiatric admission is indicated, the threshold for medical clearance may vary depending on the medical resources available to the receiving facility. A medical-psychiatric unit in a general hospital has greater capacity for care of patients with active medical problems than a free-standing psychiatric facility

  Example 1. A stable patient with low-acuity bacterial pneumonia who is appropriate for PO antibiotics (ie, low 30-d risk of death) may be transferred to *most* psychiatric facilities depending on their policies

  Example 2. A patient who requires IV antibiotics but is otherwise stable may be cleared for admission to a med-psych unit, but likely not a free-standing psychiatric hospital

  Example 3. A patient with EKG changes and metabolic abnormalities from an ingestion will generally require prolonged observation in the ED or stabilization as a medical inpatient prior to transfer to a psychiatric unit

  Example 4. A patient presenting for co-occurring depression and alcohol use disorder may be admitted to an inpatient detoxification unit, general inpatient psychiatric unit, medical-psychiatric unit, or general hospital inpatient unit depending on the severity of their current and prior withdrawals (eg, persistent vital sign changes despite adequate medication administration in the ED and prior ICU stays for withdrawal would likely preclude transfer to free-standing psychiatric hospitals until further stabilized)

- **There is no evidence-based, standardized process to guide medical clearance of the emergency psychiatric patient and no agreed-upon panel laboratory tests and/or imaging required**

  The two main bodies issuing guidelines are the American Association for Emergency Psychiatry Task Force on Medical Clearance of Adult Psychiatric Patients' 2017 publication and the Clinical Policy Committee of the American College of Emergency Physicians' 2006 policy proposal (*West J Emerg Med.* 2017;18:235-242, 640-646; *Ann Emerg Med.* 2006;47:79-99)

  Most studies support the use of a thorough history and physical by ED staff only, in addition to complaint-based workup. Controversy exists largely because of the inability to standardize H&P components

  A 2012 study found that only one of 502 patients who received routine labs on admission to psychiatric hospital would have had their disposition changed, had these labs been drawn in the ED setting (*J Emerg Med.* 2012;43:866-870)

A 2009 study found that of 375 psychiatric patients, only 56 had non-substance-induced laboratory abnormalities; 42 of those had abnormal history or physical to indicate lab draws; 10 had normal H&Ps and insignificant laboratory abnormalities; the remaining 4 with normal H&Ps had abnormal UAs, which were considered to affect neither presentation nor disposition (West J Emerg Med. 2009;10:97-100)

However, at least one study in patients with new psychiatric symptoms found that H&P alone was insufficient to rule out coexisting general medical condition in half of patients (Ann Emerg Med. 1994;24:672-677)

- **The best evidence supports the following practices on presentation to the ED:**

   An appropriate history, including a thorough review of systems by ED staff

   An appropriate physical exam, including vital signs and a robust neurological exam (paying special attention to cognitive functioning) by ED staff

   Laboratory tests and imaging as indicated by the findings of the above

   Special attention paid to the following groups: (1) the elderly; (2) those with known prior medical conditions; (3) those with medical complaints or abnormal vital signs; (4) substance users; (5) first psychiatric presentation, especially if outside the usual range or with atypical or rapid onset of symptoms; (6) confused or cognitively impaired patients

Labs, Imaging, and More

- Despite the lack of evidence for routine screening, many psychiatric facilities will require some laboratory workup prior to transfer, often owing to the lack of robust medical backup available. Labs and imaging should be ordered as clinically indicated by ED providers or as determined by requesting facilities

- Common studies ordered prior to inpatient psychiatric admission include the following:

   BMP: Useful in the workup for AMS (metabolic delirium); patients with CKD; and those taking Li or anti-epileptic drugs (AEDs)

   CBC: Useful in the workup of AMS (infection); in patients with substance use disorders; and in patients taking AEDs or clozapine

   LFTs: Useful in the workup of AMS (acute hepatitis); in patients with acute ingestion or alcohol intoxication; and in those taking AEDs

   PT/INR: Useful in those with chronic liver disease, in patients on anticoagulation, and in those with concerns for acute hepatitis

   TSH: Usually part of the standard workup for most initial psychiatric presentations (most notably depression and mania)

   Urine toxicology: Useful in most patients with psychiatric presentations

   Urine pregnancy test: Indicated for nearly all psychiatric presentations of women of child-bearing age

   UA and urine culture: Useful in elderly patients with AMS (infection)

   Drug levels: Useful for patients taking AEDs (for mood stabilization or seizures) for which there are clinically relevant drug levels to determine adherence and rule out toxicity. Clozapine levels take several days to return; if they are sent in the ED setting, they should be followed up by the admitting inpatient team. In patients presenting for ingestion, levels of salicylates, acetaminophen, and TCAs are also useful

Serum ethanol level: Useful in suspected intoxication

EKG: Generally obtain for elderly patients, those with known cardiac disease, chest pain or abnormal vitals signs, and those postingestion

- Less common and rarely ordered studies:

Ca, Mg, Phos: Useful in patients with known arrhythmias or prolonged QTc; in patients with anorexia; and in those with AMS

Serum osm: Useful in patients with ingestion, anion gap, and/or kidney dysfunction

RPR/syphilis screen: Useful in first presentation of most neuropsychiatric complaints to rule out neurosyphilis

Vitamins (thiamine, B12, folate, D3): May be useful in some patients depending on history (eg, those living at high latitudes, alcohol use disorders, restrictive eating), although unlikely to fully explain most psychiatric presentations

Serum copper and ceruloplasmin: Once considered routine part of first-break psychosis workup; now no longer required and only sent when otherwise clinically indicated

Heavy metal screen: Rarely indicated

Paraneoplastic and encephalitis panels: Routine use is not recommended given low diagnostic yield. The clinical picture should fit a larger pattern than a single psychiatric presentation alone (eg, acute/subacute mental status change, additional changes in neurological exam, history of fevers of unknown origin, weight loss)

A1c and fasting lipid panel: Not useful for medical clearance from an emergency department

CT head: May be useful in elderly or grossly intoxicated patients presenting after a fall, patients with atypical psychiatric presentations, acute personality change, or focal neurologic (including cognitive) deficits in addition to psychiatric symptoms

MRI brain: See above. May be useful in those with cognitive deficits, although unlikely to be useful in the emergency department

EEG: May be useful in select patients, but often difficult to obtain in the ED; yield of scalp leads may be lower in psychiatric presentations of epilepsy (eg, TLE, FLE)

SUICIDE AND RISK ASSESSMENT

Background (Lancet. 2016;288(10053):1450; Am J Epidemiol. 2008;167:1155; J Affect Disord. 2013;150(2):540-545; JAMA Intern Med. 2018;179(5):692)

- Although completed suicide is relatively uncommon, suicide is the 10th leading cause of death in the US and 14th leading cause globally
- Risk factors:
  - Modifiable: active psychiatric symptoms, substance use, living alone, homelessness, acute stressors, posthospitalization, active suicidal ideation

- Nonmodifiable: prior suicide attempt, suicidality or self-injury, family history, multiple psychiatric dx, male, lack of social supports, no children, older age, adolescent age, Caucasian, living in rural setting, LGBTQ identification
- Protective factors: social connectedness, dependent children, pregnancy, good relationship with outpatient treaters, coping skills and flexibility, religion, meaningful employment, additional factors identified by patient
- In the US, most common means of completed suicide: firearms > suffocation/hanging > poisoning/overdose

Suicide Risk Assessment (*Psychol Med.* 2014;44(16):3361; *Am J Psychiatry.* 2003;160(11 suppl):1; *Am J Psychiatry.* 2015;172(8):798-802)

How to Start? Ask About:	
Psychiatric symptoms	Depressive symptoms (worthlessness, hopelessness), psychotic symptoms (some command hallucinations, paranoia, persecutory delusions), impulsivity, agitation, severe anxiety, intoxication
Prior history	Prior suicidal ideation or attempts, circumstances, consequences; prior hospitalizations, treatment, comorbid dx, outpatient treaters/strength of alliance
Suicidal ideation	Active ("I want to kill myself") vs passive ("I would be better off dead"), acute versus chronic, duration, frequency, precipitants, coping skills, ambivalence, change in severity or quality compared with prior or baseline
Suicidal plan	How developed is the plan, means, access to guns or toxic meds, lethality, risk:rescue ratio
Suicidal intent	**Preparation or rehearsal, what has stopped patient thus far**
Other details	Medical comorbidities and associated demoralization, substance use history, support system, living situation, employment, religion, acute stressors

- Asking about suicide does NOT increase suicide risk and can be protective; many patients are ambivalent about suicidal thoughts and are relieved to talk about them

Management of the Suicidal Patient (*Am J Psychiatry.* 2003;160(11 suppl):1; *N Engl J Med.* 2007;356(23):2343; *Am J Psychiatry.* 2007;164(12):1786)
- Acute
  - Use least restrictive means necessary to ensure safety; when in doubt, err on the side of caution
  - Do not leave the patient alone once an acute risk has been established
  - Direct observation while determining patient safety—in the community and hospital setting
  - Consult outpatient treaters and/or support system if possible
  - Depending on acuity (both medical and psychiatric), consider: hospitalization, locked versus unlocked unit, residential, partial hospitalization program, intensified outpatient care

- Once safety is ensured, address acute psychiatric symptoms and precipitating events with medication, counseling, and support system
- When transitioning to lower level of care, arrange follow-up plan with enhanced outpatient supports given high risk posthospitalization
- Chronic
  - Collaborate with inpatient providers, outpatient providers, and patient support system/family to develop personalized safety plan, including warning signs, coping strategies, who to call, resources, and threshold to activate higher level of care
  - Discuss elevated risk with family/support system
  - Limit access to potential means (eg, remove firearms, lock medications)
  - Although frequently done, no evidence that "contracting for safety" reduces risk, though an inability to "contract for safety" is an indicator of risk
- Treat psychiatric morbidity with appropriate medication with counseling and monitoring
  - No clear evidence that antidepressant use increases risk of suicidality. Limited data suggest mild increased risk just after starting medication in young adults, likely attributed to activation of goal-directed behavior associated with treatment of depression. On the other hand, clear risk that depressive syndromes significantly increase risk of suicidality

VIOLENCE RISK ASSESSMENT

Background (Curr Psychiatr. 2018;17(5):27)
- Psychiatrists are often asked to assess probability, means, and ability that an individual pt may commit a violent act and devise plan to mitigate risk
- Mental illness plays small role in total violence enacted across the general population—only 4% of violence in the US is attributed to serious mental illness, and risk factors for violent recidivism are similar for those with and without mental disorders
- **Patients with HI and intent for violence are at ↑ risk for suicide. Violence risk assessment should also include suicide risk assessment**

Violence Subtypes (Int J Law Psychiatry. 2009;32(4):209)
- **Affective violence:** occurs in response to provocation, real or imagined; often ego-dystonic; often marked by state of increased emotional arousal
- **Predatory violence:** planned; low level of arousal; generally marked by lack of remorse unless perpetrator was unsuccessful in violent act or act resulted in negative consequences for perpetrator

Risk Factors for Violence (Curr Psychiatr. 2018;17(5):27; Hosp Community Psychiatry. 1990;42(9):954; Am J Psychiatry. 2002;159:1973; Med Clin North Am. 2010;94:1089; J Clin Psychol. 2016;72:329)

- **Static risk factors:** stable, not easily changeable, rarely amenable to clinical intervention
- **Dynamic risk factors:** can change over time, amenable to intervention
- Risk factors can be identified through clinical interview, available records, collateral information, observation of behaviors and assessment tools

Risk Factors for Violence	
Static Risk Factors	**Dynamic Risk Factors**
• History of violent behavior (best predictor of risk of future violence) • Age of first violent act (before adolescence ↑ risk) • Witnessing/experiencing abuse as juvenile • Male gender • Age (age 15–24 at highest risk) • Low socioeconomic status • Antisocial personality disorder (particularly raised with traits associated with psychopathy— lacking empathy and close relationships, behaving impulsively, superficially charming, primarily interested in self-gratification) • Low IQ • Prior arrest • History of head injury	• Untreated, active psychiatric symptoms (see below) • Substance use (SUD ↑ risk 12–16×) • Stressful life events • Access to weapons • Unemployment • Anger • Impulsivity • Similar circumstances to prior violence (eg, if prior violent acts have occurred primarily in the setting of new homelessness and substance relapse, presence of those features again should raise concern)

Mental Illness as a Risk Factor (J Clin Psychol. 2016;72:329)

- Studies suggest indirect link between mental illness and violence; individuals with mental illness are more likely to have other modifiable risk factors
- Risk of violence in mental illness is related to specific symptoms rather than diagnosis, eg, hostility, suspiciousness, hallucinations, grandiosity, delusions accompanied by anger, threat/control override delusions ↑ risk; neg sx of SCZ decrease risk; general delusions without anger and disorganization have no effect on violence risk
- Pt's impressions about mental health tx modify risk; risk for violence lower when pts see need for tx, adhere to tx, and endorse positive perceptions about tx effectiveness

Approach to Assessment (*Curr Psychiatr.* 2018;17(5):27; *Med Clin North Am.* 2010;94:1089; *Am J Psychiatry.* 2012;169:3)
- **There is no evidence showing that asking patients about violent/homicidal ideas will increase the risk of violence**

Psychiatrists can take any of 3 general approaches in assessing risk:
- **Unaided clinical judgment:** psychiatrist estimates violence risk based on his own experience and judgment, with knowledge of risk factors but without use of structured tool. Most commonly used but least accurate method
- **Actuarial tools:** statistical models that use formulas to show relationships between risk factors and violence. VRAG is a commonly used actuarial tool. VRAG scoring sheets are available for free through the VRAG website (http://www.vrag-r.org/)
- **Structured professional judgment (SPJ):** hybrid of actuarial methods and unaided judgment. SPJ tools help evaluators identify risk factors, which are then combined with clinical judgment to assess risk. Most commonly used SPJ tool is HCR-20. HCR-20 scoring sheets are available for free through HCR-20 website (http://hcr-20.com/). HCR-20 is additionally often combined with SAPROF, which assists in assessment of protective factors. SAPROF coding sheets are available for free on the SAPROF website (http://www.saprof.com/)

Managing Violence Risk (*Curr Psychiatr.* 2018;17(5):27)
- Interventions should be directed at mitigating dynamic risk factors—may include changing level of care, medication changes, initiation of substance use treatment, efforts to eliminate firearm access
- If there is explicit threat toward identifiable victim, clinician has duty to warn/protect that victim (see "Tarasoff" section)

AGITATION

Overview (*J Clin Psych.* 2006;67(suppl 10):13-21)
- Agitation has been defined by FDA as "exceeding restlessness associated with mental distress" and by Project BETA as "an extreme form of arousal that is associated with increased verbal and motor activity." Other features include irritability, heightened response to stimuli, and semipurposeful motor activity (*World J Bio Psych.* 2016;17:86-128; *West J Emerg Med.* 2012;13(1):3-10)
- Not defined by violence or aggression but may progress to them
- Up to 10% of emergency psychiatric visits involve agitation; up to 50% of visits involve patients at risk of becoming agitated (*World J Bio Psych.* 2016;17:86-128)
- Neurobiology: Poorly understood, likely multifactorial, depends on associated condition (*J Clin Psych.* 2006;67(suppl 10):5-12)
  Primary psychotic disorders: reduced GABAergic inputs, increased DA and NE

Manic and psychotic agitation associated with reduced frontal lobe inhibition, linked with progression to violence

Agitation in dementia → often expression of distress; worsening frontal and temporal lobe function is associated with agitation

- Associated syndromes: Mania, schizophrenia, dementias, personality disorders (primarily ASPD, BPD); general medical conditions affecting the CNS (eg, meningitis, delirium, hyperthyroidism), intoxication/withdrawal syndromes
- May warrant medical evaluation, esp if findings suggest medical etiology (eg, atypical or new psychiatric presentation, abnormal VS or PE, altered LOC/decreased attention, neurologic sx or dx), and absence of known/causal psychiatric diagnosis
- Agitated pt requires urgent psychiatric assessment—even brief MSE; definitive psychiatric evaluation can wait until the pt is calmer

Approaching the Agitated Patient (Nonpharmacologic Interventions) (*J Clin Psych.* 2006;67(suppl 10):13-21; *West J Emerg Med.* 2012;13(1):17)

- **Modify the environment for safety:**

  Ensure pt is physically comfortable

  Minimize provocative stimulation (eg, remove aggravating individuals, move pt to a quieter area)

  Remove dangerous objects (eg, weapons, sharps, heavy objects, moveable furniture)

  Interview should be private but not isolated; open areas better than unsafe rooms

  Be aware of panic buttons, means of egress; there should be no barriers between the interviewer and exit

  Consider security presence, either in/out of pt eyesight, depending on context

  Maintain distance, out of range of pt grasp

- **Verbal de-escalation:**

  Approach pt in a polite, nonthreatening manner while appearing in control

  Calm, soothing tone of voice; honest, straightforward manner

  Communicate a respectful, caring attitude; convey empathy; use active listening; try to understand pt's wants; agree and offer choices when possible; be concise and repetitive about what you're asking

  Avoid direct confrontation, threatening body language, eye contact

  Reassure that pt is safe from harm

  Build trust and comfort (eg, offer chair/blanket, NRT, pain relief, snack)

  Calm limit setting (eg, "I can help you with your problem, but I cannot allow you to continue threatening the staff")

  Ask about agitation and violence directly (eg, "You look angry. Do you feel like hurting someone?")

  Supportive statements (eg, "You're doing a great job keeping your anger under control")

- If threat of assault to self or others becomes concern, ensure safety of patient and others (eg, exit room, chemical/physical restraint)

Pharmacologic Interventions (West J Emerg Med. 2012;13(1):26-34; J Clin Psych. 2006;67(suppl 10):13-21)
- **Goal:** Calm pt, ensure safety, enable pt to participate in assessment and tx plan
- **Principles of pharmacologic management:**
  Always have a working diagnosis to guide medication choice
  Consider underlying etiology of agitation, co-occurring medical conditions, and currently prescribed agents. Eg, neuroleptics preferable to lorazepam in acute alcohol intoxication, as BZDs will potentiate intoxication; in contrast, anticholinergic-induced agitation (ie, hallucinogens) may be better treated with BZDs, given anticholinergic side effects of SGAs
  Employ nonpharmacologic interventions as above
  Offer medications early along with nonpharm intervention, ask pt preference (both type and route); offering oral meds may avoid traumatic restraint
  SL, liquid, and rapidly dissolving formulations can reduce risk of "cheeking" medications, not significantly faster onset than tablets
  Use IM/IV formulations as last resort, for imminent risk of harm to self or others
  Generally administer medications immediately following a physical restraint, as goal is to discontinue physical restraint as agitation decreases/resolves
  Monitor VS and mental status frequently after med administration and restraint

Common Medications for Agitation			
Agent	**Dose (mg)**	**Onset (min)**	**Considerations**
Lorazepam*	0.5–2	60 (SL), 60–360 (PO), 60–90 (IM), <10 (IV)	May result in respiratory depression or delirium; therefore, avoid in respiratory disease and in elderly
Haloperidol*	1–10	– (SL), 120–360 (PO), 30–60 (IM), 15–30 (IV)	IM haloperidol has the highest risk of EPS if given without anticholinergic IV haloperidol has the highest risk of QTc prolongation (ensure electrolytes are repleted)

(continued)

Common Medications for Agitation (continued)			
Agent	**Dose (mg)**	**Onset (min)**	**Considerations**
Chlorpromazine*	25–50	– (SL), 60–240 (PO), 15–30 (IM), – (IV)	IM formulation associated with local site reaction and sterile abscess formation May result in severe hypotension
Olanzapine*	2.5–5	360 – (SL), 360 (PO), 15–45 (IM), – (IV)	Do not coadminister IM with lorazepam or other sedatives within 4 h: high risk of respiratory depression
Ziprasidone*	10–20	– (SL), 360–480 (PO), 60 (IM), – (IV)	Use is limited by severity of QTc prolongation
Risperidone	0.5–2	60 (SL), 60 (PO), – (IM), – (IV)	Considered as effective as haloperidol, especially in combination with lorazepam
Quetiapine	12.5–100	– (SL), 90 (PO), – (IM), – (IV)	May result in hypotension Reports of abuse potential
Diphenhydramine*	12.5–50	– (SL), 60–180 (PO), <10 (IM), <10 (IV)	Often used in combination with haloperidol and lorazepam for acute physical aggression ("5-2-50") May ameliorate risk of EPS from IM haloperidol Avoid in elderly because of anticholinergic effects
Hydroxyzine	12.5–50	(SL), 15–30 (PO), – (IM), – (IV)	Commonly prescribed as a nonnarcotic anxiolytic because of its rapid absorption
Trazodone	12.5–50	(SL), 60–120 (PO), – (IM), – (IV)	May be beneficial in geriatric patients in whom BZDs carry a risk of delirium and antipsychotics carry cardiac risks May result in hypotension

Common Medications for Agitation (continued)			
Agent	Dose (mg)	Onset (min)	Considerations
Clonidine	0.05–0.3	(SL), 180–300 (PO), − (IM), − (IV)	Commonly prescribed in pediatric agitation May result in hypotension Patch formulation available to moderate agitation over several hours

Adapted from *J Clin Psych*. 2006;67(suppl 10):13-21 and manufacturer prescribing information. For more details about the above medications, please see dedicated sections elsewhere in this text.

*IM/IV available.

Other Medications
- Ketamine (IM, IV, NAS), though not commonly used, can be useful for acute agitation. In an ED study, ketamine controlled agitation faster than standard agents (*Am J Emerg Med*. 2017;35:1000-1004). Carries small risk of dissociation → may worsen agitation, psychosis in pts primary psychotic disorders
- IM aripiprazole (9.75 mg) has similar efficacy to haloperidol and other antipsychotics in reducing agitation; may reduce incidence of multiple antipsychotic prescriptions and transition to PO aripiprazole (*Curr Med Res and Opin*. 2013;29:241-250); IM ziprasidone also available with similar considerations
- 2018 multicenter RCT compared inhaled loxapine (first-generation antipsychotic) with IM aripiprazole, demonstrated faster response time with no difference in safety profile (*Eur Neuropsychopharm*. 2018;28:710-728)

Restraints (*West J Emerg Med*. 2012;13:35-40)
- Defined as any method of physically constraining the patient to immobilize the patient and their limbs; methods include staff physically holding the patient, mechanical devices (such as leather straps, often used as "four-point" restraints holding limbs), restraint chairs, and medications when they are used to limit the patient's freedom
- Consider using physical restraints when pt's safety is threatened, when others are threatened, or when pts are interfering with medical treatment *and* lack capacity to refuse care; risks → medical complications, psychological trauma, serious physical harm to pt
- Consider using seclusion as a form of de-escalation if agitated pt is not an immediate threat to self or others; use of seclusion rooms declining in the US because of regulatory concerns and complications (escape from seclusion, staff/pt injury, increased harmful behavior). Pts in seclusion should be closely monitored to assess response and prevent complications

- Physical restraints are last resort interventions, should be accompanied by medication to prevent injury and minimize restraint time; after restraint, pt should be reevaluated w/in 1 h
- Adverse effects (usually due to excess/inappropriate force): asphyxia, blunt chest trauma, physiological exertion and catecholamine surge, rhabdomyolysis, thrombosis, adverse effects of medications, psychological trauma, and possibly death (Can J Psychiatry. 2003;48:330-337); VS must be monitored frequently after restraint

Special Populations

Pediatric Patients (Pediatr Drugs. 2011;3:1-10)

- Pediatric presentations to EDs for agitation are increasing, as is restraint use (Curr Psych Rep. 2016;18:41); pediatric pts are uniquely at risk of adverse effects
- Assess for organic causes of agitation as pediatric pts may have difficulty expressing discomfort, become agitated because of untreated sx
- Always consider drugs of abuse and prescription meds as potential causes
- Pediatric agitation assoc w/ the following psychiatric conditions: ADHD, ASD and developmental disorders, bipolar disorder, ODD and conduct disorder, PTSD
- **Pharmacologic considerations:**
  FGAs are avoided in the pediatric population because of the risk of adverse effects, particularly EPS (more common in children, even in SGAs) (JAACAP. 2008;47:9-20). *Olanzapine 2.5 mg ODT or IM is the generally preferred antipsychotic for emergency use in pediatric agitation*
  BZDs more often assoc w/ paradoxical reaction in children than in adults (Am J Nurs. 2001;101:34-39), especially in children w/preexisting impulse control difficulties → disinhibition; antihistamines may also cause paradoxical reaction. The preferred benzodiazepine is *lorazepam 0.05–0.1 mg/kg PO or IM (max 2 mg)*; the preferred antihistamine is *diphenhydramine 1 mg/kg PO or IM (max 50 mg)*
  Also, *clonidine 0.05–0.1 mg PO* is commonly used
  Preferable to use single agent in children rather than the multiple concurrent agents used in adults (ie, "5-2-50")

Geriatric Patients (Mt Sinai J Med. 2006;73:976-984)

- Agitation in elderly patients is highly multifactorial (primary psychiatric conditions, neurologic [such as dementias], general medical conditions)
- General medical causes must be ruled out, including delirium (see *Delirium* chapter in this text for more details)
- **Pharmacologic considerations:**
  Antipsychotics should be used with caution. A 2018 meta-analysis found that elderly pts and pts w/ dementia are at increased risk of short-term mortality from all causes when prescribed antipsychotics (Lancet Psychiatry. 2018;5:653-663). Avoid FGAs in pts with Parkinson's disease and assoc syndromes because of risk of worsening parkinsonism; SGAs (eg, quetiapine owing to low D2 affinity) can be used at low doses with caution. *Olanzapine 2.5 mg ODT or IM is the preferred emergency antipsychotic*

BZDs are associated with increased risk of falls and respiratory depression in the elderly, should be used cautiously (*Mt Sinai J Med.* 2006;73:976-984). BZDs may worsen agitation associated with delirium, to be avoided when possible

Anticholinergic agents (eg, diphenhydramine) can be deliriogenic, should be avoided

Trazodone may be beneficial in controlling agitation if pt accepts PO medication (*Am J Geri Psych.* 1997;5:60-69)

Minority Patients
- Black, Asian, and Latinx patients more likely to be perceived by health care providers as dangerous when agitated than are white patients, leading to disproportionate use of seclusion/restraint (*J Am Acad Psychiatry Law.* 2004;32:163-168)
- Following restraint, minority patients less likely to follow-up w/ outpatient care than white counterparts (*J Psychiatr Pract.* 2011;17:387-393)
- Some studies have suggested that Asian and Latinx patients may require lower doses of antipsychotics because of genetic variations in drug metabolism (*Psychiatr Serv.* 2005;56:31-33). Black patients are more likely to be prescribed FGAs and at higher doses than white patients → higher risk of EPS (*Psychiatr Serv.* 2005;55:677-684)
- For these reasons, it is important for providers to consider historical and cultural contexts when managing agitation in ethnic minority patients

TOXIDROMES

APPROACH TO TOXIDROMES

(*Chest.* 2011;123:795-798; *Emerg Med Clin North Am.* 2007;25:252; *Crit Care Clin.* 2017;33:523; *Emerg Med Clin North Am.* 2010;28:665)

Definition
- Clinical syndromes associated with drug action on major neurotransmitter systems

Common Scenarios
- Evaluation of accidental or intentional overdose, iatrogenic drug toxicity in inpatient or outpatient setting, altered mental status and delirium

History
- In emergent cases, acute stabilization may take priority
- Toxin(s) ingested, time of ingestion, amount, vomiting (may ameliorate toxicity, can also suggest aspiration risk)
- Intent, help-seeking behaviors if any, psychiatric history (hospitalizations, suicide attempts), substance use history
- Current medications/supplements, preexisting end-organ vulnerabilities
- Vitals and symptoms prior to intervention (ie, EMS field reports), progression of symptoms

Physical Exam

- **Vitals** (hyperdynamic or depressed), **Arousal** (alertness, psycho-motor activity), **HEENT** (pupil size and reactivity, nystagmus, wet or dry mucous membranes, burns, breath odor, airway patency), **CV** (regular or irregular, rate, peripheral pulses), **Pulmonary** (rate, depth, wheezing, crackles), **GI** (pain, bowel activity), **Extremities** (color changes, temperature, signs of IV drug use, bullae, edema from prolonged immobility, transdermal patches), **Neuromuscular** (tone, tremor, abnormal movements, reflexes, clonus, Babinski, gait), and **Psychiatric** (paranoia, hallucinations)

Toxidrome	Activity/ Rigidity	HR/BP	T	Pupil Size	RR	Bowel Sound	Sweat
Sympathomimetic	↑	↑	↑	↑	↑	↑	↑
Anticholinergic	↑	↑	↑	↑	=	↓	↓
Serotonergic	↑	↑	↑	↑	↑	↑	↑
NMS	↑	↑	↑	=	↑	=	↑
Cholinergic	↓	Variable	=	↓	Variable	↑	↑
Opioid	↓	↓	↓	↓	↓	↓	↓
Sedative-hypnotic	↓	↓	↓	=	↓	↓	↓

Labs/Studies

- EKG: QT prolongation, QRS widening, arrhythmias
- Finger stick blood glucose, electrolytes + serum osmolarity, CBC, liver function tests, lactate, coagulation labs, troponin, CPK, ABG/VBG, urine pregnancy test
- Serum tox to rule out other ingestions, urine tox (but care with interpretation), drug levels
- CXR (aspiration, edema), KUB XR (drug packets), CT head (to screen out acute intracranial pathology)
- Consider LP (often performed in hyperthermic delirium), brain MRI, EEG

Management

- Consists of supportive care (ABCs, decontamination, expedited elimination, agitation treatment), antidotal treatment if available and indicated; dextrose, oxygen, naloxone, thiamine are low-risk interventions in undifferentiated altered mental status

  Resources: medical toxicology consultation, regional poison control center, NIH TOXNET database of drug toxicities

---

SYMPATHOMIMETIC

(Crit Care Clin. 2017;33:532; J Med Toxicol. 2008;4:87; Prim Care Companion CNS Disord. 2013;15:13; Emerg Med Clin North Am. 2010;28:667-671)

Causes

- Cocaine, amphetamines and derivatives (methamphetamine, bath salts, MDMA, ephedrine), hallucinogens (psychedelics, PCP, ketamine),

OTC decongestants (eg, pseudoephedrine), B2-agonists (asthma medication), caffeine, stimulant weight loss supplements (yohimbine, clenbuterol, citrus aurantium)

Syndrome
- Agitated delirium (ranges from anxiety to agitation with paranoia, hallucinations to seizures, coma)
- Psychomotor agitation (restlessness, tremor, hyperreflexia)
- Extreme elevations in HR, BP, also elevated T and RR
- Mydriasis, diaphoresis, piloerection

Complications
- MI, arrhythmias, hypertensive emergency (encephalopathy, acute renal failure, cardiac ischemia), PRES, vascular catastrophes (intracranial hemorrhage, arterial dissection), ARDS, rhabdomyolysis (associated with cocaine); cocaine also proarrhythmic sodium channel blocker

Differential
- Sedative-hypnotic withdrawal and hypoglycemia can present similarly. Mixed serotonin syndrome can occur with MDMA, bath salts; anticholinergic (nondiaphoretic), NMS/hyperthermia, and salicylate toxicity also cause hyperthermic delirium. Medical differential includes catatonia, CNS infection, hyperdynamic sepsis, adrenal storm (pheochromocytoma), thyrotoxicosis, and post-TBI autonomic dysfunction

Management
- Benzodiazepines for agitation management, can moderate vitals, suppress seizures; barbiturates, dexmedetomidine, propofol for severe, refractory cases. Postacute persistent paranoia and hallucinations may respond to antipsychotics. Supportive care: rapid-acting blood pressure control (avoid beta-blockers in cocaine intoxication), vigorous hydration (particularly if rhabdomyolysis), and external cooling

---

ANTICHOLINERGIC

(Br J Clin Pharmacol. 2016;81:517-519; Prim Care Companion CNS Disord. 2013;15:8-9)

Causes
- "Pure" anticholinergics: Plant-based (*Datura*/Jimson weed, angel's trumpet), scopolamine, antidystonics (benztropine, trihexyphenidyl), oxybutynin, antidiarrheals (Lomotil)
- Mixed anticholinergics: first-generation antihistamines (diphenhydramine, hydroxyzine), atypical and low-potency antipsychotics, TCAs, cyclobenzaprine, heroin adulterant (scopolamine)

Syndrome
- Agitated delirium (visual hallucinations, stereotypic picking behaviors, dysarthric mumbling)
- Mydriasis
- Decreased glandular and peristaltic activity (hot sweatless skin, dry mouth, ileus, urinary retention)
- Often increased HR/BP, hyperthermia

Complications

- Injuries from agitation and falls, mental status progression to seizures, coma in severe cases. Mixed toxidromes common: antihistamines (sedation, seizures), antipsychotics (QT prolongation, antihistaminic, sympatholytic syndromes), TCAs (sodium channel blocker—seizures, arrhythmias heralded by QRS widening, also sympatholytic)

Differential

- Toxidromes with agitated delirium and hyperthermia include sympathomimetic overdose, serotonin syndrome, NMS, malignant hyperthermia, salicylate toxicity, and sedative-hypnotic withdrawal. Medical ddx includes heat stroke, hyperdynamic "warm" sepsis, CNS infection, thyrotoxicosis, and catatonia

Management

- Agitation and seizures managed with benzodiazepines; neuroleptics risk worsening hyperthermia. Physostigmine given in severe cases with expert guidance, risk of arrhythmia with TCAs, QT prolongers. Supportive care: activated charcoal, hydration, external cooling, address other drug effects (sympatholysis, sodium channel blockade)

SEROTONIN SYNDROME AND NMS

(NEJM. 2005;352:1114; Br J Anesth. 2000;85:131)

- See chapters on Serotonin Syndrome and NMS for more information about causative agents and management

Syndromes

- Hyperthermic delirium with gross neuromuscular abnormalities, see Hunter and Sternbach criteria for characteristic signs of serotonin syndrome; classic NMS characterized by fever, autonomic instability (labile BP), and muscle rigidity. Rhabdomyolysis, renal failure, metabolic derangement, and end-organ failure can occur

Differential

Serotonin syndrome can be dominated by muscle rigidity, misdiagnosis common w/ NMS; consider other hyperthermic toxidromes and medical causes of agitated delirium

---

CHOLINERGIC

(Lancet. 2008;371:598; Schizophr Bull. 1996;22:593; Ann Pharmacother. 2007;41:1634-1635; Semin Neurol. 2004;24:199-200)

Causes

- Organophosphate and carbamate pesticides in suicide attempts and accidental exposures; overdose on anticholinesterase inhibitors, muscarinic (eg, pilocarpine), or nicotinic agonists

Syndrome

- Muscarinic: N/V/D/abdominal pain, miosis, productive cough, bronchospasm, bradycardia, salivation, lacrimation, urinary incontinence, CNS depression

- Nicotinic: weakness, cramping, and fasciculations are characteristic; can precipitate arrhythmias, seizures, and respiratory failure; if nicotinic effects are prominent, tachycardia, mydriasis, and hypertension can develop

Complications
- Life-threatening arrhythmias and multifactorial respiratory compromise (paralysis, bronchospasm, edema, aspiration); electrolyte imbalances from GI losses. "Intermediate syndrome" of proximal muscle weakness, respiratory failure can occur after acute toxidrome resolves. Delayed-onset polyneuropathy (1–2 wk) progressing to lower extremity paralysis has been described

Differential
- Altered mental status with miosis can occur with opioids, sympatholytics, and pontine infarction. Respiratory compromise and weakness in neuromuscular disease (myasthenic crisis, GBS, botulism). Severe acid–base disturbances (DKA, salicylate poisoning) and acute abdomen can present with altered mental status and GI distress

Management
- Benzodiazepines are first-line for agitation given benefit for seizures. Specific management includes early initiation of atropine and pralidoxime (can mitigate acetylcholine block). Supportive care includes volume resuscitation and cardiorespiratory stabilization, decontamination in cases of pesticide exposure

---

OPIOID

(NEJM. 2012;367:150; Addict Med. 2017;11:257; Criti Care Clin. 2017;33:531; Crit Care Clin. 2012;28:483-484)

Causes
- Heroin, newer synthetics (eg, fentanyl analogs), medical opioids (hydrocodone, hydromorphone, codeine, morphine, oxycodone, fentanyl, tramadol, meperidine), long-acting opioids (oxymorphone, methadone, buprenorphine, transdermal fentanyl, oxycodone ER)

Syndrome
- Stupor
- Respiratory depression (shallow, RR < 12/min)
- Miosis
- Hypotension, bradycardia, hypothermia

Complications
- Rhabdomyolysis, compartment syndrome from prolonged immobility; noncardiogenic pulmonary edema, hypoxic encephalopathy. Frequently co-ingested with acetaminophen, sedative-hypnotics, sympatholytics (clonidine), and stimulants. Tramadol, meperidine can produce mixed serotonergic toxidrome (with mydriasis, seizures); contaminants can alter presentation

Differential
- Sedative-hypnotic, sympatholytic intoxication (tricyclic antidepressants, clonidine, antipsychotics); consider differential for stupor

including hypoglycemia, hepatic encephalopathy, hyponatremia, CO poisoning, CNS pathology (CVA, infection, etc)

Management
- Naloxone administration to restore RR to lower end of normal, minimize withdrawal state. May require repeat or continuous naloxone dosing to maintain respiratory stability; supportive care includes volume and blood pressure support, postnaloxone monitoring for long-acting opioids at least 24 h

SEDATIVE-HYPNOTIC

(*Crit Care Clin.* 2017;33:529; *Chest.* 2011;140:1079; *Emerg Med Clin North Am.* 2007;25:257-258)

Causes
- Benzodiazepines, nonbenzodiazepines (ie, zolpidem), barbiturates, muscle relaxants (tizanidine, cyclobenzaprine, baclofen, carisoprodol, meprobamate, methocarbamol), GHB, alcohol

Syndrome
- Decreased level of consciousness (drowsiness to coma, persistent delirium can occur)
- Ataxia, slurred speech, gaze-evoked nystagmus (pupils often normal size)
- Hyporeflexia, hypotonia
- Respiratory depression (more typical of barbiturate, poly-sedative ingestion)

Complications
- Life-threatening respiratory depression with polydrug ingestions, common coadministrants: opioids, other sedative-hypnotics, and sympatholytics (may have miosis). Anion gap metabolic acidosis may suggest toxic alcohol ingestion or starvation state

Differential
- Sedating intoxicants including opioids, antihistamines, sympatholytics (including antipsychotics, tricyclics), lithium, AEDs, and inhalants. Medical differential includes hepatic encephalopathy, postictal state, CVA, head trauma, CO poisoning, hypoglycemia, and other causes of toxic-metabolic delirium

Management
- Supportive care: maintain respiratory and hemodynamic stability, prevent aspiration, shorten delirium, and monitor for withdrawal. GI decontamination may be desirable but aspiration risk. Flumazenil can be used to reverse severe benzodiazepine intoxication, but ineffective for barbiturates and can precipitate seizure or arrhythmia in polydrug ingestion (eg, TCAs, sympathomimetics) or patients with epilepsy

INVOLUNTARY TREATMENT

- Tx of those deemed lacking capacity and/or competency in medical setting (see Capacity Assessment chapter)

Types of Involuntary Holds
Emergency Hold (Psychiatr Serv. 2016;67(5):529-535)
- Brief involuntary detention of person w/ presumed mental illness; intent to determine if meets criteria for involuntary civil commitment
- Justification varies by state—common reasons: threat to self/others due to mental illness, gravely disabled/unable to protect self in community
- Duration 24–72 h by state; longer periods require court hearing
- 1975 Supreme Court decision in *O'Connor v. Donaldson*: mental illness alone = insufficient for involuntary hold

Civil Commitment (Psychiatry (Edgmont). 2010;7(1):30; Intl J Law Psychiatry. 1995;18(3):249-263)
- **The state/government role:** 2 main principles guiding government interest in civil commitment:
  1. *Parens patriae*: "parent of the country": government's duty to intervene on behalf of residents unable to act in own best interest
  2. Government's duty to protect society at large, even if restricting liberties of individuals; uses *dangerousness* criteria of civil commitment, AKA the police state model
- All states have a legal process for hold and commitment; laws vary by state
- Criteria for commitment determined by state, *not psychiatrists*, similar to criteria for emergency hold

Outpatient Civil Commitment
- Rarely practiced means of isolating mentally ill person from society within community, eg, locked in home, requires monitoring resources
- Sanctioned in most states, limits arrests and hospitalizations, can prompt inpatient hospitalization earlier if relapse of sx

Types of Involuntary Treatment
Overview (Am J Psychiatry. 1984;141(2):202-205)
- **In those lacking capacity:** Based on whether the treatment is deemed *low versus high risk*, state dependent
- Not limited to the setting of psychiatry
- Consent of family members or a guardian or based on previously existing advance directives

Emergency Forced Medications
- Used if "emergency" → when failure to treat could result in serious or irreversible deterioration of pt's condition, or imminent danger to pt or others, finite, right to treat without consent ends upon stabilization
- Refusal of tx prior to emergent situations can override the lawfulness of emergent forced medication, based on capacity

- **Right to refusal of medications:** In some states based on involuntary confinement versus other states based on risk of pt endangering self/other independent of confinement status
- Often regards administration of antipsychotics given side effect profiles

Special Populations (Testa M, West SG. Civil commitment in the United States. Psychiatry (Edgmont). 2010;7(10):30)
- Persons who break the law and found **not guilty by reason of insanity—**see "Legal Standards of Competency"
- **Prisoners:** varies by state re: involuntary treatment, most permit tx over objection through review committee (*Washington v. Harper 1990, US Supreme Court*), some require judicial review or transfer to state psychiatric hospital; solitary confinement or restraint often substitute for meds in ill-equipped facilities
- **Sexually violent predator:** laws allow civil commitment if convicted of sexually violent crimes related to mental illness
- **Eating disorders:** often overlooked as having serious mental illness, despite high mortality rate, often related to difficulty around capacity and imminence of harm (*Am J Psychiatry. 2000;157:1806-1810*)
- **SUD:** Most states w/ statutes allowing involuntary civil commitment; many states distinguish between mental health and SUD, requirements of dangerousness +/− grave incapacitation apply. Time of initial detention range 8 h–5 d, involuntary tx can ↑ employment retention + intervention success (NIDA. *Principles of Drug Addiction Treatment: A Research-Based Guide*. Rockville, MD: NIH; 2012)

TARASOFF REPORTING

Background (*Tarasoff v. Regents of the University of California 1976; 17 Cal 3d 425; Psychiatr Clin North Am. 1999;22:49; Am J Psychiatry Resid J. 2018;13:6*)
- **Definition:** Clinician duty to "to use reasonable care to protect" all known or suspected potential and readily identifiable victims directly +/− through law enforcement of any explicit threats of violence made by patients assigned to their care
- **Principle:** Ethically permissible to breach confidentiality if necessary to protect pt/3rd party
- **Legal precedent:** 1974 suit brought against University of CA after murder of a student, it was revealed killer disclosed to therapist intention to obtain a gun and kill peer he was enamored with. Therapist had warned campus police of threat, but victim was not warned
- **Implementation:** laws vary by state (duty to warn vs protect, mandatory vs permissive)

Indications for Warning (*J Am Acad Psychiatry Law Online. 2006;34:338; Am J Psychiatry. 2012;169:3*)
- **Serious and probable risk of violence** based on clinical assessment, even if no verbal threat. Consider use of violence risk assessment tool (HCR-20, VRAG)
- *Explicited/stated threat of violence* against an identified individual

- **Request by would-be victim** who has been previously attacked, threatened or feels endangered by pt. Usually prior to release from jail, hospital, or prison

Assessment (Adapted with permission from *Psychiatr Clin North Am.* 1999;22(1):49)

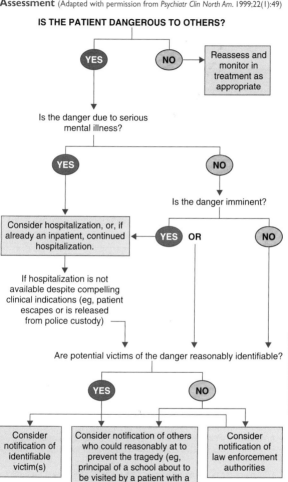

IS THE PATIENT DANGEROUS TO OTHERS?

YES / NO → Reassess and monitor in treatment as appropriate

Is the danger due to serious mental illness?

YES / NO

NO → Is the danger imminent?

YES OR / NO

Consider hospitalization, or, if already an inpatient, continued hospitalization.

If hospitalization is not available despite compelling clinical indications (eg, patient escapes or is released from police custody)

Are potential victims of the danger reasonably identifiable?

YES / NO

Consider notification of identifiable victim(s)

Consider notification of others who could reasonably at to prevent the tragedy (eg, principal of a school about to be visited by a patient with a semiautomatic)

Consider notification of law enforcement authorities

Procedure for Notification (*LA County DMH.* 2005; Policy 202.2; *SB County DBH* 2007; *Tarasoff Procedure*)

- Discuss with clinical supervisor, document decision and clinical reason in health record; consider inpt hospitalization as above
- Discuss with available hospital/clinic/institution legal counsel

- Make reasonable effort to contact intended victim(s) via telephone, in-person visitation, or mailed letter; document attempts in health record, incl. date and time
- Notify police (may be done via hospital security); minimize released info; name + address, threat, whether pt. is hospitalized, obtain report #
- Document Tarasoff warning, police report #, police officer who took report

LEGAL STANDARDS OF COMPETENCY AND SANITY

Overview
- The mental state of a defendant may be evaluated multiple times over the course of a criminal proceeding
- Determinations are made regarding **competency** to participate in the judicial process and **criminal responsibility** for the crime(s) in question
- **Epidemiology:** the insanity plea is raised in **less than 1% of felony trials** and leads to acquittal in about 26% of attempts; successful pleas usually involve defendants with prior known mental illness (Bull Am Acad Psyc Law. 1991;19:331)

COMPETENCY IN THE LEGAL SYSTEM

Competency to Proceed (Dusky v. U.S. [1960]; Drope v. Missouri [1975]; Cooper v. Oklahoma [1996]; Saddler v. U.S. [2nd Cir, 1976]; Chavez v. U.S. [9th Cir, 1981]; Godinez v. Moran [1993]; Indiana v. Edwards [2008])
- **Eg, enter a plea, stand trial, be sentenced**
- Determined by a judge +/− psychiatric assessment
- Based on defendant's **state of mind at the time of trial/proceedings**
- To meet, a defendant must be able to:
  1. Understand the factual basis for the alleged crime
  2. Understand the pending charges and legal consequences
  3. Consult with a lawyer (**Competency to waive counsel** based on defendant's understanding of decision + potential consequences, separate from competency to stand trial)

If found **incompetent to proceed** (Sell v. U.S., 2003).
- Voluntary treatment w/ medication +/− other treatment
- +/− involuntarily civil commitment to forensic hospital to restore competency
- Involuntary tx w/ antipsychotics only permissible when medically indicated, unlikely to have SE undermining fair trial, and necessary to further a compelling government interest

Competency to be Executed (Ford v. Wainwright. 1986; Louisiana v. Perry. 1992)
- Executing a prisoner who is incompetent violates the cruel and unusual punishment clause
- States differ on whether antipsychotics may be used to restore competency for the purpose of execution

CRIMINAL RESPONSIBILITY

Insanity Defense (*J Am Acad Psychiatry Law.* 2014;42:S3)

- Defense plea of not guilty by reason of insanity
- Valid in most court jurisdictions, the federal court system, and all but 4 (ID, KS, MT, UT) US states
- Based on defendant's **state of mind at the time of the crime**
- **If found not guilty by reason of insanity**: defendant may be committed to a psychiatric facility until determined safe for release
- Legal definitions and criteria differ by jurisdiction

  Most courts allow for a **cognitive test** (*M'Nghten test*)

  Some permit alternative **volitional test** (*Irresistible Impulse Test*)

  Standard encompassing both is the **ALI test**

Tests to Establish Insanity Defense		
Test	**Accepted**	**The Law**
M'Naghten test	Federal courts + most US states	"To establish a defense on the ground of insanity, it must be clearly proved that, at the time of committing the act, the party accused was laboring under such a defect of reason, from disease of the mind, as: • **not to know the nature and quality of the act he was doing;** or • if he did know it, that he **did not know what he was doing was wrong.**" **(UK House of Lords, 1843)**
Irresistible impulse test **(volitional test)**	Some US states	Not criminally responsible if: • his **disease deprived him of the ability to choose right from wrong** (conform his conduct to the law; resist an impulse) • and the **crime was the sole product of this mental disease.** **(Alabama v. Parson, 1887)**
"ALI test" (American Legal Institute Moral Penal Code test)	Some US states	Not criminally responsible if: • "as a result of mental disease or defect he **lacks substantial capacity either to appreciate the criminality of his conduct or to conform his conduct to the requirements of the law**" Unlike others, this standard specifically excludes "abnormality manifested only by repeated criminal or otherwise antisocial conduct" **(ALI, 1962)**

Caveats to Insanity Plea (*J Am Acad Psychiatry Law.* 2009;37:182; *U.S. v. Burnim* [1978]; *U.S. v. Garcia* [1996]; *J Am Acad Psychiatry Law.* 2007;35:172)
- **Insanity defense CANNOT be claimed for:**
  Mental illness only of **repeated criminal/antisocial behavior** (eg, pedophilia, pyromania, antisocial PD), though little precedent/controversial
  Voluntary intoxication (however, may because for "diminished capacity" → ⇓ charges/sentence)
- Unexpected reactions to drugs, nonvoluntary intoxication, or long-term sequalae 2/2 substance abuse ("**settled insanity**") may be grounds for insanity defense
- **Burden of proof:** Most states, burden placed on defense to establish a preponderance of evidence (*In a minority of states, placed on prosecution to establish sanity beyond a reasonable doubt*)

MANDATED REPORTING

Child Abuse and Neglect (*U.S. Department of Health & Human Services, Child Maltreatment.* 2016; *JAAPL.* 2010;38(1):49)
Types of abuse: physical, sexual, psychological, neglect (most common)

Prevalence
Estimated to occur at a rate of 9.1 per 1000 children
  In 2016: 1750 children died as result of maltreatment
- Risk highest in the 1st year of life (24.8 per 1000 children ≤1 y)
- American Indian, Alaska Native, and African American kids at highest risk

Mandated Reporting of Child Abuse
- All 50 states + DC have statutes mandating certain professionals report suspected child abuse/neglect to social service agencies
- States vary on who must report (and who is exempt) and process of reporting
- Obligation to report requires only suspicion, not evidence
- System heavily weighted toward protection of minors—immunity from liability for people who report abuse/neglect in good faith, failure to report when mandated can result in criminal and civil action

Elder Abuse and Neglect (*NEJM.* 2015;373:1947)
Types of abuse: physical, sexual, psychological, financial, neglect
Prevalence: Estimated to be 10%
Risk factors: female gender, living w/ caregiver, lower income, isolation/lack of social support, dementia (specifically financial exploitation), functional impairment, poor physical health

Mandated Reporting of Elder Abuse
- 49 states (NY is exception) have laws that require mandated reporting of suspicion of abuse
- All states have state specific mechanisms for reporting suspected abuse in nursing homes or long-term care facilities

Disabled Persons Abuse (*Lancet.* 2012;379:1561)
- Adults with disabilities are more likely to experience violence than nondisabled adults; individuals with severe and persistent mental illness are particularly vulnerable
- Many states require certain professionals to report abuse of adults w/ mental or physical disability
- Laws regarding mandated reporting and process of reporting vary state by state

CAPACITY

Terminology (*Prim Care Companion J Clin Psychiatry.* 1999;1(5):131; *N Engl J Med.* 1988;319:1635)
- **Competency**—legal term that refers to a person's ability to carry out legally recognized acts (eg, enter a contract, prepare a will, make medical decisions) in rational manner
  - Determination of **incompetence** made in court; presumed until deemed incompetent by a judge
  - If found incompetent after court assessment he/she will have a court assigned guardian to make decisions on his/her behalf
  - Determined in task-specific manner to give as much autonomy as possible (eg, incompetent to execute a will but competent to make treatment decisions); can be deemed generally incompetent (eg, vegetative state, severe dementia)
- **Capacity**—medical term that refers to a person's ability to make informed, rational decisions with appreciation of risks/benefits and treatment options regarding medical care
  - Determined by a physician; presumed until determined to be lacking
  - If found to not have capacity, surrogate decision-maker appointed
  - Intent is surrogate makes decision based on previously expressed pt pref
  - Specific to proposed procedure/treatment, not general
  Note: Ability of minors to consent to certain types of treatment varies state to state

Assessing Decision-Making Capacity (*Prim Care Companion J Clin Psychiatry.* 1999;1(5):131; *NEJM.* 2007;357:1834; *NEJM.* 1988;319:1635; *Am Fam Physician.* 2001;64(2):299)
- Any physician can assess capacity; psychiatrist may assist in difficult cases
- Cannot be assessed unless pt has been adequately informed: pt should receive sufficient info on nature of d/o, proposed interventions, likely benefits, risks, possible alternatives including no tx, risks and benefits of alternative/no tx
- Evaluate understanding of a question/set of questions. Patients can have capacity to make some decisions and not others, stringency of standards varies w/ the seriousness of consequences of decision— referred to as a **sliding scale approach** (eg, likely consequences of refusing MVI < likely consequences of refusing abx for systemic infection; thus, ↑standards for capacity to refuse abx than to refuse MVI)

- Evaluated in the moment as it can change w/ time
- **One should demonstrate ability in 4 domains, as below:**

Ability	Assessment
Make a consistent choice	Ask for pt's choice regarding proposed intervention Assess stability of choice by rephrasing the question later in the interview (however, pts can change their mind; they should provide reasonable justification for changing choice) Example questions: Have you decided whether you'd like to follow the recommendation for treatment? What is your decision?
Understand relevant info	Ask pt to describe their understanding of proposed intervention/procedure Example questions: Can you tell me what is the problem with your health right now? What is the proposed tx? What are risks/benefits of tx? What alternative options are there? What are the risks/benefits of alternative tx (or no tx)?
Appreciate situation and its implications	Assess whether individual understands what having illness means, likely course and outcomes Assess pt's understanding of likely consequences of agreeing to tx or refusing tx Example questions: What do you believe is wrong with your health? What do you think tx would do for you? What do you think would happen w/o tx? Why do you think your doctor recommends tx?
Rationally manipulate information	Assess if a decision is made through a rational thought process, regardless of what decision is made Example questions: How did you come to your decision? What makes your decision better than alternative?

After the Determination of Incapacity (NEJM. 2007;357:1834)
- If not emergent, identify any potential causes contributing to lack of capacity (eg, psychosis, delirium) and remedy these
- If urgent or pt lacks capacity despite remedy of reversible etiologies, surrogate decision-maker should be sought
- If emergent, physician can provide care under the assumption that a reasonable person would accept treatment. However, if advanced directives or surrogate decision maker are readily available, those should be consulted

Surrogate Decision-Makers (NEJM. 2017;376(15):1478; JAMA Intern Med. 2015;175(10):1687)
- **Alternate decision-maker:** person who takes part in decision-making for a patient regardless of how their decision-making ability came about; required attributes of alternate decision-makers vary state to state (eg, whether the decision-maker needs to be willing to serve, have familiarity with pt preferences, availability)

- **Advanced directive:** legal document that records pt's tx preferences and/or designates durable power of attorney for health care
- **Guardian:** surrogate decision-maker appointed by judge; at times is an organization or paid official w/ no relationship to/knowledge of the pt prior to appointment—this is called a **professional guardian**
- **Default surrogate:** someone w/ decisional authority without court appointment or advance indication by pt (eg, HCP)—the hierarchy of default surrogate and how chosen varies state to state
- Surrogate decision-makers should make decisions using **substituted judgment**—using pt's values (not personal values) to determine care; if substituted judgment is not possible (particularly relevant w/ professional guardian), surrogate decision-makers should use a **best interests standard**—weighing options and making decisions based on perspective of generic, reasonable person

General Considerations for Treatment of Psychiatric Illness During Pregnancy
- Up to 1/5 of women suffer from psych illness during pregnancy
- Recs on how to treat psych illness during pregnancy must be individualized and made on a case-by-case basis
- Recs for tx should weigh the risks of the proposed tx vs the risks of untreated maternal psych illness for both mother and infant

General Considerations for Use of Psychotropic Medication in Pregnancy
- Consider medication when the risk of untreated maternal psychiatric illness > the risk of exposure to psychotropic medication for the infant
- The previous FDA risk classification system for the reproductive safety of medications (class A, B, C, D and X) was discontinued in 2015. The New Pregnancy and Lactation Labeling Rule provides more thorough descriptions regarding medication and reproductive safety
- The available pregnancy safety data on psych medications are limited by lack of RCTs, lack of long-term follow-up, existence of few studies on polypharmacy in pregnancy

---

UNIPOLAR DEPRESSION IN PREGNANCY

Epidemiology (*JAMA.* 2006;295:499; *Arch Gen Psychiatry.* 2008;65:805)
- Approx 10% of pregnant women suffer from a depressive d/o; age < 25, being single, hx of trauma associated with ↑ risk of illness
- In women who discontinued their antidepressant before becoming pregnant, approx. 2/3 had a relapse of depression while pregnant
- Even in women who continued their antidepressant for pregnancy, about 1/4 had a relapse of depression while pregnant
- Women who are depressed during pregnancy are less likely to engage in prenatal care, have ↑ rates of preterm birth, ↑ risk for LBW infants, and their neonates more often require tx in NICU

Clinical Presentation and Diagnosis
- Same DSM-5 criteria as a major depressive episode, use qualifier "with peripartum onset" when episode occurs during pregnancy
- Anxiety sx frequently present in depression during pregnancy
- Assess suicide risk closely—suicide is a leading cause of death in perinatal women (*Br J Psychiatry.* 2003;279)

Pharmacologic Treatment
- **SSRIs** (*Am J Psychiatry.* 2008;165:749; *NEJM.* 2014;370:2397)

  Most commonly used class of antidepressant in pregnancy. Fluoxetine, sertraline, citalopram are the best studied

  Risk of malformations: Numerous studies performed: overall, there appears to be no ↑ risk for congenital malformations with SSRI use in 1st tri. If there is ↑ risk, it is expected to be quite small. Earlier studies raised concern that paroxetine may be associated with ↑ risk of cardiac defects, although more recent data suggest no ↑ risk

  Neonatal adaptation syndrome: Occurs in ~1/4 cases where the neonate is exposed to antidepressant in late pregnancy. Characterized by increased irritability, tremor, restlessness, tachypnea in 1–4 d postdelivery. Self-resolving and transient; no specific tx required. Not an indication to discontinue SSRI prior to delivery; may increase mother's risk of PPD

Persistent pulmonary hypertension of the newborn (PPHN): Inconsistent data regarding ↑ risk with SSRI; more recent data suggest no ↑ risk. If ↑ risk does exist, likely very low

Long-term effects on children: Growing and mixed data; continues to require more investigation; consider role of maternal illness as confounder. Reassuring study of preschoolers showed no diff in global IQ, behavioral development, or language development in children with in utero fluoxetine exposure vs unexposed children (*NEJM.* 1997;336:258)

- **Bupropion** (*Pharmacoepidemiol Drug Saf.* 2014;23:1066)

  Risk of malformations: Some mixed data regarding risk of cardiac defects (ie, VSD) with 1st tri risk exposure; if there is ↑ risk of defects, likely low

  Neonatal adaptation syndrome: Described above; should monitor neonates after use of bupropion during pregnancy

  Long-term effects on children: More data needed

- **SNRIs** (*Basic Clin Pharmacol Toxicol.* 2016;118:32)

  SNRIs less well studied compared with SSRIs. More data on venlafaxine than duloxetine; minimal data on other SNRIs

  Risk of malformations: Available data suggest no ↑ risk of congenital malformations with use of venlafaxine, duloxetine

  Neonatal adaptation syndrome: Described above; should monitor neonates after use of SNRI during pregnancy

  Long-term effects on children: More data needed

- **TCAs** (*Am J Psychiatry.* 1996;153:592)

  Prefer the lesser anticholinergic TCAs for pregnancy (ie, nortriptyline) to avoid orthostatic hypotension

  Risk of malformations: Available data suggest no ↑ risk of congenital malformations

  Neonatal adaptation syndrome: Described above; should monitor neonates after use of TCAs during pregnancy

  Long-term effects on children: Study of preschoolers showed no diff in global IQ, behavioral development, or language development in children exposed to TCAs in utero vs unexposed children (*NEJM.* 1997;336:258)

- **Other antidepressants**

  Limited data on mirtazapine, trazodone; larger data sets are required to determine risk of teratogenesis. MAOIs avoided in pregnancy; risk of hypertensive crisis with the use of obstetric interventions (ie, terbutaline)

Nonpharmacologic Treatment

- Psychotherapy: CBT, IPT, supportive psychotherapy. Consider for more mild cases of depression or in conjunction with medication for more severe cases
- ECT: Reserved for severe cases (ie, medication-resistant depression; psychotic features present). Considered safe in pregnancy with close collaboration with OB/GYN

ANXIETY DISORDERS IN PREGNANCY

Epidemiology (*J Affect Disord.* 2011;131:277; *Br J Psychiatry.* 2017;210:315)
- Up to 15% of pregnant women suffer from an anxiety d/o during pregnancy; 10% with GAD, ~4% with panic d/o
- Untreated maternal anxiety associated with poorer delivery outcomes, including ↑ rates of preterm birth and LBW infants

Clinical Presentation and Diagnosis
- No change in DSM-5 criteria when diagnosing GAD, OCD, panic d/o, social anxiety d/o in pregnancy
- Obsessional thinking more prevalent in anxiety d/o in pregnancy

Treatment
- Psychotherapy as 1st line for mild-to-moderate cases: CBT, supportive therapy
- Medication often required in more severe cases
- SSRIs considered 1st line medication; may also consider SNRIs or TCAs (see "Pharmacologic Treatment" under Unipolar Depression in Pregnancy for review of safety data for these medications)
- **Benzodiazepines** (*BMJ.* 1998;317:839)
  Studied as a class. Use of BZD can vary widely (ie, occasional PRN vs daily dosing). Aim for lowest effective dosing in pregnancy
  Risk for malformations: Some data suggest small (<1%) ↑ risk of oral cleft malformations in infants exposed to BZD in 1st tri vs risk in general population
  Neonatal outcomes: Infants exposed to high-dose BZD in 2nd/3rd tri may experience poor muscle tone, respiratory depression, BZD withdrawal sx at delivery. Infants are less likely to experience these outcomes at low doses
  Long-term outcomes: More data needed. Possible ↑ risk of internalizing behaviors (ie, emotional reactivity, anxiety) in young children exposed to benzodiazepines in utero, though unclear how maternal prenatal anxiety may confound this finding (*PLoS One.* 2017;12:e0181042)

BIPOLAR DISORDER IN PREGNANCY

Epidemiology (*Am J Psychiatry.* 2007;164:1817)
- Women with BPAD are at high-risk of recurrent mood episodes (depression > mania) during pregnancy
- Approx 2/3 of women who discontinue their mood stabilizer prior to conception will have recurrence of BPAD during pregnancy. Continuation of mood stabilizer in pregnancy ↓ rate of recurrence by 1/2
- Women with untreated BPAD in pregnancy are less likely to engage in prenatal care and are at ↑ risk for substance use

Clinical Presentation and Diagnosis
- Utilize same DSM-5 criteria as a major depressive episode or manic episode; can use qualifier "with peripartum onset" when episode occurs during pregnancy
- Be particularly mindful of any psychotic features present in episodes of BPAD in pregnancy

Treatment With Mood Stabilizers

Preferred Mood Stabilizers in Pregnancy

- **Lithium** (*NEJM. 2017;376:2245*)

  Carries some ↑ teratogenic risk, though the absolute risk remains low, and its teratogenic risk is much lower than some of the other mood stabilizing agents

  Risk of malformations: Sig ↑ risk of cardiovascular malformations (including Ebstein anomaly) with 1st tri exposure to lithium. Recent large retrospective study found ~2% of lithium-exposed infants with cardiac malformations vs ~1% of unexposed infants; 0.6% of lithium-exposed infants with right ventricular outflow tract defects (consistent with possible Ebstein anomaly) vs ~0.2% of unexposed infants. Risk of cardiac malformations likely dose-dependent. Recommend fetal echocardiography for screening

  Neonatal outcomes: Monitor for signs of toxicity

  Long-term effects: No established, overt consequences on child development, though data are limited

- **Lamotrigine** (*CNS Drugs. 2017;31:439*)

  Risk of malformations: Some past data suggest ↑ risk of cleft lip and palate malformations in infants exposed to lamotrigine in 1st tri vs unexposed infants, though more recent studies suggest no ↑ risk of malformations with 1st tri lamotrigine exposure. If ↑ risk is present, likely very low (<1%)

  Long-term effects: No established, overt consequences on child development, though more data are needed

Mood Stabilizers to Be Avoided in Pregnancy

- **Valproic acid** (*NEJM. 2009;360:1597; JAMA Neurology. 2018;75:663*)

  Avoided in pregnancy secondary to teratogenic risk and poor infant outcomes

  Risk of malformations: Infants exposed to valproic acid in pregnancy have ↑ risk of neural tube defects (up to 9% of exposed infants) vs unexposed population. ↑ risk of other congenital malformations (ie, cardiovascular, urogenital) found as well. Risk is likely dose-dependent

  Long-term effects: Children exposed to valproic acid in utero are at ↑ risk of poor neurocognitive outcomes (ie, lower IQ at 3 y/o, poorer school performance in early adolescence), ↑ ASD risk

- **Carbamazepine** (*NEJM. 1991;324:674*)

  Also avoided in pregnancy secondary to teratogenic risk

  Risk of malformations: Sig ↑ risk of neural tube defects (ie, spina bifida), also ↑ risk for other congenital malformations (ie, urogenital)

  Long-term effects: Some data to suggest poorer cognitive outcomes in exposed infants

- **Topiramate** (*Neurology. 2018;23:90*)

  Growing data suggest avoiding in pregnancy secondary to teratogenic risk

  Risk of malformations: Infants exposed to topiramate in the 1st tri more likely to have oral cleft malformations vs unexposed infants. Risk likely dose-dependent

Oxcarbazepine, gabapentin: limited safety data
- If a woman is taking an anticonvulsant, it is recommended she take 4 mg of folic acid daily while attempting conception and throughout the 1st tri of pregnancy. PNV typically only have max of 800 µg of folic acid

Treatment With Other Pharmacologic and Nonpharmacologic Treatments
- Antipsychotics: Atypical antipsychotics are often used in BPAD (see "Treatment" under Psychotic Disorders in Pregnancy for review of these agents)
- BZDs are often used in acute stabilization in mania (see "Treatment" under Anxiety Disorders in Pregnancy for review of these agents)
- Treatment of BPAD often requires multiple agents (ie, mood stabilizer and antipsychotic); there are minimal data on the effects of using multiple agents
- Consider ECT if the sx of mood episode are severe or unresponsive to medication tx

---

PSYCHOTIC DISORDERS IN PREGNANCY

Epidemiology (Psychiatr Serv. 1996;47:502)
- Women with chronic psychotic illness have more unwanted pregnancies, fewer planned pregnancies, and more often are victims of violence in pregnancy
- Women with psychosis at risk for numerous issues during pregnancy, including poor prenatal follow-up, poor delivery outcomes, substance use

Clinical Presentation and Diagnosis
- Important to identify if affective psychosis vs primary psychosis to target tx
- Screen for delusions around delivery and the baby
- Low threshold to consider hospitalization given potential for safety concerns

Treatment (JAMA Psychiatry. 2016;73:938; Am J Psychiatry. 2018;175:564; Psychosomatics. 2018;59:125)

Typical Antipsychotics
- Prefer high-potential typical agents (ie, haloperidol) over low-potency agents (ie, chlorpromazine)
  - *Risk for malformations:* No consistent, established ↑ risk of congenital malformations with use of high-potency typical agents, but some data to suggest ↑ incidence of malformations with low-potency agents
  - *Neonatal outcomes:* FDA warning in 2011 about potential risk of extrapyramidal sx and withdrawal sx in neonates exposed to antipsychotics in utero
  - *Long-term effects on children:* No established, overt consequences on child development, though more data needed

Atypical Antipsychotics
- *Maternal risk factors:* Growing concern over use of atypicals and weight gain/diabetes in pregnancy. Women on atypicals begin pregnancy with ↑ BMI

↑ risk of gestational diabetes with quetiapine or olanzapine

Risk for malformations: Limited, but growing data. Recent meta-analysis found no ↑ risk of congenital malformations with use of atypical antipsychotics as a class. When individual agents were evaluated, there was a small, but sig, ↑ risk of malformations with use of risperidone

Neonatal outcomes: FDA warning in 2011 about potential risk of extrapyramidal sx and withdrawal sx in neonates exposed to antipsychotics in utero

Long-term effects on children: Limited but growing data; requires more research

- Consider ECT if sx of psychosis severe and/or unresponsive to antipsychotic

PSYCHIATRIC ILLNESS IN THE POSTPARTUM PERIOD

General Considerations

- Women are at ↑ risk of psych illness in the postpartum, esp women with past psych hx
- Some mood changes are expected—a large majority of women (up to 85%) experience postpartum blues, or increased mood lability, tearfulness in the 2 wk following delivery. These symptoms self-resolve with no tx
- If the sx of postpartum blues worsen, persist beyond 2 wk, or interfere with a woman's functioning, she warrants full psych evaluation for PPD
- As in pregnancy, recs on tx of postpartum psych illness must be individualized and made on a case-by-case basis
- Treatment recs should weigh the risks of the proposed treatment vs the risks of untreated maternal postpartum psychiatric illness for mother and infant
- Women who choose pharmacologic tx for postpartum psych illness need to weigh the risks and benefits of breastfeeding as well (see "Breastfeeding and Psychotropic Medication" for more information)

UNIPOLAR DEPRESSION IN THE POSTPARTUM

Epidemiology (*Pediatrics.* 2006;118:659; *Am J Psychiatry.* 2007;164:1515)

- Approx. 10–15% of women are diagnosed with PPD
- Up to 1/2 of cases of PPD may start during pregnancy
- Risk factors: Hx of depression in pregnancy, hx of PDD, hx of MDD, hx of PMDD
- Untreated PPD is associated with poorer maternal bonding with infant, childhood emotional dysregulation, and changes in child brain development

Clinical Presentation and Diagnosis

- Same DSM-5 criteria as a major depressive episode, use "with peripartumonset" qualifier if onset of episode occurs within the 4 wk following delivery

- Most women experience onset of PPD within the first few months after delivery, but a smaller portion of women may experience later onset. Most clinicians will still consider depression to be PPD if the onset is within 12 mo of delivery
- PPD often presents with prominent anxiety sx
- Screen for any worries or intrusive thoughts around infant's safety, any thoughts of hurting the infant
- Assess suicide risk closely—suicide is a leading cause of death in perinatal women (Br J Psychiatry. 2003;279)

Treatment (J Clin Psychiatry. 2004;65:1236; Cochrane Database Syst Rev. 2014;11:CD002108; Lancet. 2017;390:480)
- Psychotherapy: CBT, IPT, supportive psychotherapy. Addition of couples therapy may be beneficial in some situations
- Pharmacologic Tx: SSRIs 1st line, SNRIs and bupropion also used (monitor for anyincreased anxiety on bupropion). Mirtazapine and TCAs beneficial to improve sleep when insomnia is prominent. MAOIs in refractory cases
- For most severe cases, consider ECT
- Recent focus on hormonal agents (allopregnanolone) for tx of severe PPD—while initial trials encouraging, still awaiting full FDA approval
- In women with severe hx of PPD, may consider prophylaxis with antidepressant near time of delivery in future pregnancies

ANXIETY DISORDERS IN THE POSTPARTUM

Epidemiology (J Clin Psychiatry. 2006;67:1285; Arch Gen Psychiatry. 2008;65:805)
- Up to 12% of women suffer from an anxiety d/o in the postpartum period
- Rates of GAD and OCD in postpartum women may be even higher than the rates in the general population

Clinical Presentation and Diagnosis
- Utilize usual DSM-5 criteria for these disorders, no peripartum specifier
- Screen for any obsessional thoughts around infant's safety and thoughts of harming infant. Obsessions will be intrusive, ego-dystonic, and distressing in postpartum OCD, with no true intent of harming the infant. Ego-syntonic thoughts or bizarre delusions should raise concern for postpartum psychosis
- Given high comorbidity with depression in the postpartum period, clinician should also screen for depression in women presenting with anxiety

Treatment (J Affect Disord. 2016;190:543)
- Psychotherapy: CBT as first-line, supportive psychotherapy
- Pharmacologic Tx: SSRIs considered 1st line; SNRIs also used; BZD may be introduced for short- or long-term course depending on severity of anxiety. TCAs may be particularly helpful in OCD (ie, clomipramine). Can consider atypical antipsychotics for refractory cases
- Combination pharmacologic and psychotherapy treatment in more severe cases

BIPOLAR AND PSYCHOTIC DISORDERS IN THE POSTPARTUM

Epidemiology (Am J Psychiatry. 2000;157:179; Am J Psychiatry. 2016;173(2):117)

- Women with BPAD are at high risk of recurrence in the postpartum period, with a recurrent mood episode occurring in a majority of women who have discontinued mood stabilizers
- Most concerning is the possible development of postpartum psychosis, which affects 1/1000 pregnancies
- In the majority of cases, postpartum psychosis arises in the setting of a manic episode, though psychosis can occur in the setting of a primary psychotic d/o or a major depressive episode as well
- Risk factors for postpartum psychosis: Hx of postpartum psychosis (up to 70% relapse), hx of BPAD, recent discontinuation of mood stabilizer
- Most feared consequence of untreated postpartum psychosis is infanticide—although infanticide is a rare event, the possibility of this consequence makes postpartum psychosis warrant immediate attention and treatment

Clinical Presentation and Diagnosis

- Postpartum psychosis is most likely to occur in the first 2 weeks following delivery, though can occur any time in postpartum, from immediately after delivery to several months postpartum
- Given the high prevalence of concurrent mania, important to screen for manic sx, like mood lability/irritability, ↓ sleep, ↑ activity
- Essential to ensure infant's safety: ask about delusional thinking regarding infant (ie, infant being evil) and any thoughts, plans, or command auditory hallucinations of harming the infant

Treatment (Am J Psychiatry. 1995;152:1641; NEJM. 2008;359:509; Am J Psychiatry. 2009;166:405)

- Postpartum psychosis is a psych emergency and requires immediate inpatient hospitalization for safety and stabilization
- Antipsychotics used 1st line for immediate tx of psychosis—usually prefer atypical antipsychotics over typical agents for additional mood stabilization
- For women with BPAD, initiate mood stabilizer—lithium often preferred as mood stabilizer, though need to consider pt's preference for breastfeeding (see "Breastfeeding and Psychotropic Medication")
- If unipolar depressive episode with psychosis, see "Treatment" under Unipolar Depression in the Postpartum for selecting antidepressant agent. However, given high incidence of BPAD in this population, will need to be mindful of possible activation on antidepressant
- BZDs often introduced for acute stabilization for agitation and restoration of sleep
- Consider ECT for most severe episodes unresponsive to medication
- In women who have a hx of postpartum psychosis in the setting of BPAD, strongly consider initiating prophylaxis with lithium near time of delivery in future pregnancies to reduce the risk of relapse

BREASTFEEDING AND PSYCHOTROPIC MEDICATION

General Considerations

- Recs on tx of postpartum psych illness must be individualized and made on a case-by-case basis. Recs will consider the pt's preferences regarding breastfeeding and weigh the benefits of breastfeeding vs the risks of medication exposure to the infant through breast milk
- The concentration of psych medication in mother's breast milk will depend on a number of factors: type of medication, dosing of medication, mother's drug metabolism
- The concentration of psych medication in the infant's system will depend on a number of factors: infant's drug metabolism, infant's own health, frequency of feedings. Breastfeeding while on psych medications is often avoided if infant was premature or has liver dysfunction. Close collaboration with the infant's pediatrician is recommended
- The decision to breastfeed should also consider how the maternal demands of breastfeeding will impact her own psych illness: breastfeeding may be discouraged in pts with BPAD as frequent disruptions in sleep may put them at ↑ risk of relapse

Antidepressants and Breastfeeding

- Although research studies have obtained infant serum levels of these drugs, there is no indication to do so clinically unless sig concern for toxicity. Mother and pediatrician should monitor infant for any signs of toxicity
- **SSRIs** (*Expert Opin Drug Saf.* 2015;14:413)
  As a class, infant exposure to SSRI from breast milk is considered low; rare cases of adverse events (ie, irritability, sleeping difficulties) in exposed breastfed infants. Sertraline and paroxetine most studied; considered 1st-line agents
- **Bupropion** (*J Clin Psychiatry.* 2002;63:910)
  Less data than those for the SSRIs. Minimal to nondetectable levels in infant serum. Mostly no sig events in exposed breastfed infants with exception of case report of seizure in infant exposed to bupropion from breast milk
- **SNRIs** (*Hum Psychopharmacol.* 2015;30:143)
  Venlafaxine (and metabolite, desvenlafaxine) present in higher levels in infant serum compared with other agents (ie, SSRIs), though no sig events noted in exposed breastfed infants. Much less data on duloxetine, although available data indicate low to undetectable drug levels in infants
- **TCAs**
  Nortriptyline preferred given low to undetectable levels in infant serum, reassuring safety data regarding infant tolerability. Other TCAs with reassuring data with exception of doxepin—long half-life, data suggest ↑ risk of sedation and adverse events in exposed breastfed infants

- **MAOIs**

  Minimal safety data, generally avoided in breastfeeding

Benzodiazepines and Breastfeeding (*J Pediatr.* 2012;161:448)

- Although research studies have obtained infant serum levels of these drugs, there is no indication to do so clinically unless sig concern for toxicity
- Infant exposure to BZD via breast milk appears to be relatively low
- One study found <2% of infants exposed to BZD via breast milk experienced oversedation; case reports of feeding difficulties, breathing difficulties
- To mitigate risk, typically rec using low doses of BZD and choosing short-acting agents over long-acting agents

Mood Stabilizers and Breastfeeding

- Choosing to breastfeed can be particularly difficult for women with BPAD. The frequent disruptions in sleep required for breastfeeding can put women at ↑ risk of relapse. Additionally, most mood stabilizers require infant serum level monitoring and infants may be at ↑ risk of toxicity
- Given the high relapse rate of BPAD in the postpartum period, it is critical for the mother to remain on a mood stabilizer during this period—benefits and risks of breastfeeding then need to be weighed accordingly
- **Lithium** (*J Clin Psychiatry.* 2000;61:79)

  Breastfeeding typically discouraged if mother is taking lithium as it is highly excreted in breast milk. Breastfed exposed infants often have ↑ serum levels of the drug and can be at risk of toxicity (ie, lethargy, dehydration)

  If mother does choose to breastfeed on lithium, close collaboration required with pediatrician—check infant CBC, BUN/Cr, TSH, lithium level at baseline and at least every 2 mo while breastfeeding
- **Lamotrigine** (*Pediatrics.* 2008;133:e223)

  Excreted in relatively high doses in breast milk; infant serum levels have been found to range widely. However, available safety data are reassuring with minimal adverse effects/toxicity for infant. One case report of apnea at very high maternal doses. Potential risk of Steven–Johnson syndrome, though no known cases
- **Valproic acid** (*Neurology.* 2010;30:1954)

  Relatively low excretion in breast milk; overall no consistent adverse effects in breastfed exposed infants, though at least one case of thrombocytopenia and anemia. No sig diff in childhood IQ in breastfed exposed infants. Given risk of potential hepatic dysfunction, thrombocytopenia, monitor breastfed infants closely with pediatrician; obtain infant CBC, LFTs, VPA level
- **Carbamazepine** (*J Clin Psychiatry.* 2000;61:79)

  Relatively high excretion in breast milk; some cases of hepatic dysfunction; sedation in exposed infants. Monitor breastfed infants closely with pediatrician; obtain infant CBC, LFTs, CBZ level
- **Topiramate, oxcarbazepine, gabapentin:** Limited information in breastfeeding

Antipsychotics and Breastfeeding

- Limited data in breastfeeding compared with other psychotropics
- **Typical antipsychotics**
  High-potency agents preferred over low-potency agents.
  Haloperidol excreted in low amounts; no adverse effects noted in
  case reports. Chlorpromazine exposure associated with oversedation in some cases
- **Atypical antipsychotics**
  Less data than for the typical antipsychotics. Olanzapine excreted in
  low levels; some cases of sedation in exposed infants. Quetiapine
  excreted in low levels as well. Caution with clozapine—high levels
  in breast milk, with a case of agranulocytosis in an exposed infant;
  monitor CBC closely

TREATING CHILDREN WITH PSYCHIATRIC ILLNESS

Epidemiology (Dialogues Clin Neurosci. 2009;11(1):7-20)

- Approximately 1/4 of youth have experienced a psychiatric disorder
  during the past year
- There is wide variation in prevalence estimates because of methodological differences, but median estimates of prevalence from
  meta-analyses are as follows:
  - Anxiety disorders 8% (range 2–24%)
  - MDD 4% (0.2–17%)
  - Bipolar disorder 0.5% (0–0.9%)
  - ADHD 3% (1.7–17.8%)
  - Disruptive behavior disorders (oppositional defiant or conduct
    disorder) 6% (5–14%)
  - Alcohol or substance use 5% (1–24%)
    - Dramatic variation by age—0.3% at age 13, 1.4% age 14, 5.3% age
      15, 7.6% age 16

General Principles for Clinical Practice

- **Children are not just small adults.** Although there is significant overlap in the psychiatric illnesses experiences by children
  with adults, children often display different symptoms for the
  same illness (eg, children with depression often display more
  irritability and/or somatic symptoms compared with adults with
  depression)
- **Safety comes first.** Whenever possible, interview the child both
  separately from and together with their parents/caregivers. Ensure that
  the child is in a safe environment. Health care workers are *mandated
  reporters* who need to report any concerns for child abuse or neglect
- **Involve and support families.** You are rarely treating a child in a
  vacuum. Maximize contact between child and family and consider all
  the dynamics at play in the family system
- **Broaden your differential** to child-focused diagnoses, such as
  learning disabilities, impulse control disorders, gender dysphoria.

However, you also need to screen for more conventionally adult diagnoses such as depression, trauma, and even substance abuse

- **Collateral** is essential: try to include not only parents and treaters but also teachers and guidance counselors whenever possible
- Double-check your medication doses (especially antipsychotics)! Children may have idiosyncratic reactions to medications that would be unexpected in adults. *Start low and go slow*
- Younger children tend to be more sensitive to adverse effects of medications

Adverse Childhood Experiences (ACEs) and Maltreatment
(Am J Prev Med. 1998;14:4)

- Includes physical abuse, psychological abuse, sexual abuse, as well as household dysfunction (eg, living with substance user, criminal, mentally ill)
- Linked to many adverse outcomes including poor academic performance, aggression, mental and physical health problems, as well as crime and violence
- There is a *dose–response* relationship; each exposure to abuse or household dysfunction increases risk of poor health outcomes, including heart disease and cancer
- Not all children who are maltreated experience negative consequences from early adversity—protective factors related to resilience have been identified

Protective Factors Related to Resilience	
Individual factors	Personality traits, intellect, self-efficacy, coping, appraisal of maltreatment, life satisfaction
Family factors	Family coherence, stable caregiving, parental relationships, spousal support
Community factors	Peer relationships, social supports, religion

Adapted from Can J Psychiatry. 2011;56:5.

Infant–Parent Attachment (Paediatr Child Health. 2004;9(8):551-555)

- Attachment is the way that we engage with others in times of stress. Infant–parent attachment explores the relationship between child and caregiver, wherein the child uses the caregiver as a secure base as they explore the world and encounter conflict
- Around 6 months of age is when infants begin to anticipate caregivers' response to their own distress and, accordingly, develop their own responses to distress

Attachment Styles	
Secure	Develops when an infant is confident that their caregiver will be available and responsive
Insecure— avoidant	Infants are uncertain whether caregiver will respond helpfully. Tend to avoid intimacy with the caregiver

Attachment Styles (continued)	
Insecure— resistant	Infants are uncertain whether the caregiver will be available in times of need. Theorized to develop because of inconsistently available parents
Insecure— disorganized	These infants display behavior that does not represent an organized strategy for maintaining closeness to their caregiver. They tend to demonstrate fear and confusion about the caregiver

Adapted from *Can J Couns Psychother*. 2012;45:2.

Developmental Milestones (Adapted from Centers for Disease Control and Prevention, *Milestone Moments Booklet*)

Key Developmental Milestones				
Age	Social/ Emotional	Language and Communication	Cognitive	Movement and Physical
6 mo	Knows familiar faces Responds to other's emotions Likes to look at self in mirror	Responds to sounds by making sounds Responds to name Vocalizations show joy and displeasure	Brings objects to mouth Begins to pass items from one hand to other Shows curiosity about things	Rocks back and forth Rolls over both front-to-back and vice versa
1 y	Nervous with strangers Cries when parent leaves Has favorite things/ people	Utilizes basic gestures (eg, waving bye) Says "mama" "dada"	Bangs two objects together Copies gestures Explores things in different ways	May take a few steps without holding on May stand alone Pulls to stand, cruises
2 y	Copies others Shows defiant behavior Starts to play with others, although mostly parallel play	Points to things or pictures when named Says sentence with 2–4 words Follows simple instructions	Builds tower of >4 blocks Names simple items in picture book Begins to sort shape/ color	Kicks a ball Begins to run Copies straight line

(continued)

Key Developmental Milestones (continued)				
Age	Social/ Emotional	Language and Communication	Cognitive	Movement and Physical
3 y	Dresses and undresses self Takes turn in games Shows range of emotions	Follows multistep instructions Can state first name, age, sex	Builds a tower of >6 blocks Can copy a circle Plays make-believe	Pedals tricycle Runs easily
4 y	Would rather play with other children than by self Can talk about likes/ dislikes	Can state first and last name Can sing and remember a short song or story	Can name some colors and numbers Uses scissors Starts to understand time	Catches a bounced ball most of time Hops and stands on one foot up to 2 s
5 y	Can differentiate real from make believe Awareness of gender Wants to be like friends	Can tell simple story with full sentences Can state name and address Uses future tense	Counts <10 things Draws person with >6 body parts	Hops Swings/ climbs Stands on one foot > 10 s

GENETIC DISORDERS

Psychiatric diagnoses overall do not have a single causative gene nor do they have a Mendelian inheritance pattern
- Many neurodevelopmental syndromes and one neurodegenerative syndrome are caused by particular genes with specific manifestations
- Other concepts
  - Anticipation: increasing number of triplet repeats with each successive generation, results in more severe disease (applies to Huntington disease)
  - Imprinting: methylation of the DNA causes selective silencing of either paternal or maternal homolog (ie, Prader–Willi, Angelman syndrome)

Disorder (Genetic Mutation)	Appearance	Incidence	Psychiatric manifestations	Treatment recommendations
Neurodevelopmental Disorders				
Angelman syndrome (15q11-q13 deletion due to loss of maternal gene (imprinting))	Microcephaly, can have hypopigmentation, strabismus, motor coordination issues	1 in 12,000 to 1 in 20,000	Social and happy, inappropriate laughter, fear of crowds and noise, disinhibition with strangers, hyperactivity, sleep disturbance	Melatonin (0.3–5 mg) before bed to improve sleep (J Child Neuro. 2008;23(6): 649) Minocycline 3 mg/kg daily improved communication (BMC Neurol. 2014;14(1): 1471)
DiGeorge syndrome or velocardiofacial syndrome (22q11.2 deletion)	Short stature, long, tapered fingers, hypotonia, long face, long nose, retrognathia, hooded eyes, palate malformed	1 in 3800 to 1 in 6000	Emotional dysregulation, anxiety, social withdrawal, autism, 30% with psychosis	Less responsive to antipsychotics than typical population
Down syndrome (trisomy chromosome 21)	Microcephaly, occipital flattening, midface hypoplasia, upslanting palpebral fissures, small nose and mouth, short neck, short height	~1 in 800 live births, more common with higher maternal age	Up to 1/3 with psychiatric disorder Hyperactivity, impulsive behavior, inattention, stubbornness, anxiety, depression 10% autism Increased rate and earlier onset Alzheimer disease	Risperidone 0.25–1.5 mg daily reduced aggression, self-injury, hyperactivity, and sleep quality (J Dev Behav Pediatr. 2008;29(2): 106)
Fragile X (CGG triplet repeat in the FMR1 gene, results in loss of FMR protein)	Macrocephaly, large and prominent ears, macroorchidism, long face	1 in 3000 births, carrier rate is 1% in females, 1 in 800 in males	ADHD, hyperarousal, social anxiety, 25–50% autism	Lithium titrated to 0.8–1.2 mEq/L resulted in global decrease in aberrant behavior (J Dev Behav Pediatr. 2008;29(4): 293)

(continued)

Common Genetic Disorders *(continued)*				
Lesch–Nyhan syndrome (hypoxanthine-guanine phosphoribo-syltransferase deficiency, X-linked, recessive)	Dystonia, dysarthria, choreo-athetosis Urate bulges in ears and joints	1 in 380,000 live births	Chronic compulsive self-injury, repeated ambivalent statements with anxiety and vulgarity, compulsive aggression toward others	Case report of bilateral globus pallidus deep brain stimulation stopping self-injury (*J Neurosurg.* 2003;98:414)
Prader–Willi (15q11-q13 deletion due to loss of paternal gene)	Central hypotonia, central obesity, short stature, small hands and feet, hypogonadism, fair pigmentation, almond-shaped eyes, bitemporal narrowing	1 in 10,000 to 1 in 15,000	Hyperphagia, self-injurious behavior, compulsive behavior, deficits in social cognition, cognitive inflexibility, poor affect regulation, depression, psychosis	Topiramate reduces self-injurious behavior (average 162 mg per day in adults) (*Am J Ment Retard.* 2004;109(4):301; *Int J Neuro-psycho-pharmacol.* 2002;5(2):141) Risperidone 1-3 mg/d reduces aggression, leads to weight loss, and improves global impression (*Acta Psychiatr Scand.* 2000;102(6):461)
Rett syndrome (MECP2 deletion)	No specific physical appearance, but characteristic loss of acquired developmental milestones, slowing of growth both linear and head circumference	1 in 10,000 females	Progressive disease, initially social withdrawal, autism-like, sleep distur-bance, eventually poor commu-nication and irritability	

Common Genetic Disorders (continued)				
Smith–Magenis syndrome (17p11.2 deletion)	Coarse features, prominent brow, deep set eyes, prominent mandible, hypotonia, diminished reflexes	1 in 25,000	Inverted circadian rhythm, self-injury, stereotypy, demanding of adults, delayed empathy	
Turner syndrome (loss of some or all of short arm of one X chromosome)	Lymphedema of hands and feet, short stature, delayed puberty, downslanting palpebral fissures, low-set ears, broad chest, wide neck	1 in 3000 infant girls	ADHD, social immaturity, hyperactivity, anxiety, depression	
Williams syndrome (7q11.23 deletion)	Short stature, bitemporal narrowing, long philtrum, wide mouth, stellate iris, full cheeks Hoarse voice, hypotonia, ligamentous laxity	1 in 10,000	Mild intellectual disability, superficially social, inattentive, impulsive, attention seeking, hyperactive, >50% ADHD, obsessions nonsocial fears, depression, sleep disturbance	
Neurodegenerative Disorders				
Huntington disease (CAG repeat in Huntingtin gene on chromosome 4q16) (Pringsheim et al., 2012)	Progressive neurodegenerative illness, no specific physical abnormalities until choreiform movements develop later in life (35–50)	2.71 per 100,000 worldwide, more common in Europe, US, Australia	Poor attention, cognitive impairment, dementia, rigidity	Case reports— fluoxetine 20 mg daily (Psychopharmacology. 2001;153(2): 264), aripiprazole 30 mg daily (J Neuropsychiatry Clin Neurosci. 2013;25(2): E3), quetiapine up to 600 mg daily (Psychosomatics. 2006;47(1): 70)

Common Genetic Testing			
Test	Method	Detects	Examples of Diseases Identified
Karyotype	Induce cells to replicate, halt in metaphase, stain chromosomes, compare banding patterns	Changes in chromosome number, chromosomal translocations	Trisomy 21, Turner syndrome
Fluorescence in situ hybridization (FISH)	DNA is denatured to single strand form, locus-specific DNA hybridizes to the patient's DNA If probe target is present, the probe binds and the binding is detected using florescent microscope	Gene deletions	22q11 deletion
Gene sequencing/ exon sequencing	Sequencing of particular regions known to cause a disorder	Gene deletions, single nucleotide polymorphisms	Fragile X

ELIMINATION DISORDERS

Overview (Pediatrics. 1999;103(3):e31)
- During toddlerhood (18 mo–3 y), a child usually becomes interested in mastering elimination
- Most children have achieved bowel and bladder continence by age 4
- Acquiring continence usually proceeds in the following order:
  Nighttime bowel → Daytime bowel → Daytime bladder
    → Nighttime bladder
- 1/3 of children in the US are completely toilet trained by age 24 mo
- Females achieve continence earlier than males

ENURESIS

Definition
When a child fails to successfully achieve toilet training by the age of 5 and has repeated voiding of urine into the bed or clothes at least twice per week for at least 3 consecutive months

Classification of Enuresis Adapted from J Clin Child Adolesc Psych. 2017;46(6):767-797		
Time of day	Nocturnal	Voiding while asleep; most common type
	Diurnal	Voiding while awake
	*Some children have both nocturnal and diurnal enuresis	

Classification of Enuresis (continued)		
Timing with regard to development	**Primary**	Primary enuresis indicates that a child has never accomplished continence through the night. This type is usually due to maturational and/or physiological delays
	Secondary	A child who has achieved continence for at least 6 consecutive months but began wetting again. This type may be caused by psychological factors or an underlying medical condition

Prevalence (Urology. 2010;76(2):265-270)
- Between 5 and 10% of 5-year-olds meet criteria for enuresis, but up to 20% of 5-year-olds have bedwetting problems
- 5–7 million US children have primary nocturnal enuresis
- Enuresis is more common in African-Americans and Asian immigrants in the US
- There appears to be genetic influence:
  - 77% incidence of enuresis in offspring of parents who have had enuresis, 44% incidence in children who have one parent who had enuresis, and 15% incidence in children without an enuretic parent
  - Twin studies have shown 68% concordance with monozygotes and 36% with dizygotes
- Notably, only 5–10% of all cases have an underlying medical cause

Differential Diagnosis Adapted from Curr Opin Pediatr. 1998;10(2):167-173	
Anatomical abnormalities	Weak bladder, detrusor overreactivity, detrusor areflexia, stress incontinence, giggle incontinence
Endocrine	Diabetes mellitus, diabetes insipidus, hyperthyroidism, abnormal release of nighttime vasopressin
Neurologic	Loss of consciousness, seizure disorder, spinal cord disease, cerebral palsy, sleepwalking
Medications	Lithium, diuretics, valproic acid, clozapine, antipsychotics, SSRIs, theophylline, caffeine, alcohol
Psychological	Stress, divorce, death, new sibling, hospitalization, abuse, school stress; more commonly seen in children with ADHD and selective mutism
Other	Malnutrition, urinary tract disease

Diagnostic Workup
- History (onset of sx, timing, frequency, family hx, developmental hx)
- Physical exam (neuro exam, skin exam, abdominal exam, routine blood draw, UA)
- Consultation—particularly if repeated UTIs or diurnal enuresis

Treatment (*J Urol.* 2010;183(2):441-447)
- Education for families and normalization of behaviors if developmentally appropriate
- Watchful waiting (15% annual spontaneous remission rate)
- Nonpharmacologic management ("bell and pad" is most successful)
- Medication management: desmopressin and imipramine are FDA-approved for nocturnal enuresis
  - Desmopressin is an ADH analog that decreases nocturnal urine output
  - Imipramine is a tricyclic with anticholinergic and antidiuretic actions
- Therapeutic interventions (CBT, biofeedback, psychodynamic psychotherapy)

ENCOPRESIS
Definition
Repeated passage of feces in inappropriate places (usually undergarments); can be voluntary or involuntary
- Unlike enuresis, encopresis rarely occurs during sleep. When it does, it is a poor prognostic indicator

Classification of Encopresis *Adapted from DSM-V*	
Primary	• Soiling in a child >4 y who has never gained bowel continence for 6 mo or more
Secondary	• Encopresis in a child who had previously acquired bowel control • When due to psychological stress (birth of sibling, parent divorce, abuse), referred to as regressive enuresis
Retentive	• Encopresis with constipation and overflow incontinence
Nonretentive	• Encopresis without constipation and overflow incontinence • More common in children with oppositional defiant disorder or conduct disorder

Prevalence (*Arch Dis Child.* 2007;92(6):472-474; *Gastroenterology.* 2003;125(2):421-428)
- Secondary encopresis more common than primary
- Between ages 7 and 8 y, prevalence is 1.5%
- 3:1 male to female ratio
- Retentive type in 80–95% of cases

Etiology
- Delay in maturation
- Underlying medical condition (anismus, IBS, rectal hypersensitivity, spinal cord injury, Hirschsprung disease, lead poisoning, hypothyroidism, hypokalemia, hypercalcemia)
- Psychological/behavioral
- Constipation

Diagnosis (Curr Opin Pediatr. 2002;14(5):570-575)
- History (onset, timing, frequency, location of soiling, melena/hematochezia, pain, dietary habits, mental health, stressors)
- Physical exam (abdominal exam, neuro exam, skin exam, rectal exam, XR abdomen, stool studies, rectal biopsy/barium enema in some cases)

Treatment (Pediatr Clin North Am. 1992;39(3):413-432)
- Unlike enuresis, watchful waiting is not an option
- Education (dietary change, fluid intake, toilet training)
- Nonpharmacologic (CBT, biofeedback, psychodynamic psychotherapy)
- Pharmacologic (laxatives, suppositories, enemas, mineral oil, fecal disimpaction)

PLAY THERAPY

Background and Philosophy
- The importance of play has been recognized since time of Plato, but was more formally developed in the mid-20th century, with Anna Freud and Melanie Klein implementing play in psychoanalysis
  - Melanie Klein saw play as the child's equivalent to the adult's free association in psychoanalysis, with interpretations based strongly on S. Freud's ego theory (J Infant Child Adolesc Psychother. 2006;5(3):259-267)
  - Anna Freud believed that analyst observation of the child over multiple sessions was necessary to make sense of the child's play in the context of their development and that play can sometimes be an imitation of things witnessed rather than always based on underlying desires/urges (Freud A. The Ego and the Mechanisms of Defense. London: Hogarth Press; 1954; J Infant Child Adolesc Psychother. 2006;(3):259-267)
- Play can be incorporated into a variety of treatment modalities, building on the natural way that children learn about themselves, others, and the world around them
- Play therapy is a developmentally/age appropriate application of other treatment modalities so as to become accessible to the child patient

Principles and Techniques (Encyclopedia of Children's Health, www.healthofchildren.com; Lilly J, et al. Play Therapy Makes a Difference, www.a4pt.org)
- Play is activity free from the constraints of reality
- Play is often thought of as self-amusement, as it is enjoyable to the child, but it is also a crucial factor for normal development
- Play is "the work of children," and a space in which the child develops physically, emotionally, cognitively, socially, and morally
- Jean Piaget: "play provides the child with the live, dynamic, individual language indispensable for the expression of [the child's] subjective feelings for which collective language alone is inadequate" (Piaget J. Play, Dreams, and Imitation in Childhood. New York: W.W. Norton & Company, Inc.; 1962:166)
- Imagination and fantasy are child's natural medium of self expression, provides clues about child's conscious and unconscious states
- Through play, child creates a safe psychological distance from what is distressing them and is able to express their thoughts and feelings in a developmentally appropriate way

- Play therapy is not exclusively self-directed, as the therapist may use the play the child engages in to develop an understanding of the child and modify the play in order to bring about healing and to work through the child's problems
- Play is a metaphoric or symbolic expression of the child's core issues; the role of the therapist is to help the child understand what they are trying to communicate
- Understanding and symptom improvement may happen whether the play is interpreted or left in displacement

Techniques
- Provide developmentally/age appropriate toys for child (typically age 3–12)
- Use psychodynamic psychotherapy theories to make sense of the child's play
- Includes elaboration (± interpretation) from the therapist to guide play in order to allow the child to express their thoughts/feelings regarding their current difficulties
- May work through the expression in displacement or provide interpretations to the child

Evidence-Based Applications
- Frequency and duration of child's pretend play with an adult correlates to greater emotion regulation ability, adaptive affect displays, empathy, and emotional self-awareness (*Early Child Dev Care.* 2001;166:93-108)
- Play has been shown to decrease anxiety (self-report and biometrics) following a stressor (*Leis Sci.* 1981;4(2):161-175)
- Play provides children with opportunities for emotional expression, cognitive understanding, and behavioral or fantasized change following a traumatic experience and allows for organization of memories, integration of fragmented sensory experiences, and creation of coherent and meaningful narrative. Play can become maladaptive posttrauma, and several trauma-specific play-based interventions have been developed and demonstrated efficacy (*Child Adolesc Psychiatr Clin North Am.* 2013;22:51-66; *Curr Psychiatry Rep.* 2018;20(5):31)

FAMILY THERAPY

Background and Philosophy (*J Child Psychol Psychiat.* 2002;43:573-586)
- Many types of family therapy, ranging from psychoanalytic to systemic
- Psychoanalytic family therapy can be based on attachment (focuses on the degree of security of attachments between individuals, problems arise because attachment needs are not met) or object relations (adult relationships are the product of prior infant–parent relationships, difficulties arise from differences between "reality" of a person and assumptions about how that person should be in a relationship)
- Other types: systemic therapy (family is a group of living organisms that forms a stable system that maintains homeostasis), structural (family problems result from issues in family relationship structure and boundaries), brief solution-focused (problems are maintained by beliefs surrounding problems and from repetitive behavioral sequences surrounding problems)

Principles and Techniques (J Child Psychol Psychiat. 2002;43(5):573-586)

- Families are their own ecosystem with individual members having patterns of dependency and relationships with each other
- Patterns of communication and family structure maintain problems within the family
- Family therapy is often centered upon a child, but the child's problems are assumed to be related to the family system as a whole, rather than due to an individual family member
- Focused on changing the interactions between family members as a means to improve function of the family as a whole and/or the functioning of individual family members
- Differs from psychoeducation or behavioral parent training in the focus on interactions, rather than on educating/training the family
- Therapist is present to point out patterns of interaction between family members and to provide interventions

How to Start? (J Child Psychol Psychiat. 2002;43:573-586; J Child Psychol Psychiat. 1978;19:57-62; Fam Proc. 1969;8:280-318)	
Ideal therapeutic candidate	Family with systemic issues resulting in a behavioral problem, capacity for reflection on communication and actions in family, less helpful with young children compared with teenagers
Relative contraindications	Domestic violence, abuse, safety issues If individuals in therapy do not feel safe, may not be able to bring up issues in therapy, could result in abuse or retaliation outside of therapy
Frequency, number of sessions	q1w, can be indefinite versus time-limited based on type of problem
Therapeutic stance	Therapist typically fairly active, depending on the type of therapy, may do more interventions versus just drawing attention to a problem

Evidence for Effectiveness (J Marital Fam Ther. 1995;21(4):585-613; J Marital Fam Ther. 2003;29(4):547-570)

- Based on meta-analysis, clinically significant effect in 40–50% of those treated
- In most studies, at least as good as individual psychotherapy, problem-solving training, or group therapy
- No significant differences in efficacy by type of family therapy
- For children: more helpful for conduct disorder, behavioral issues, communication problems, and global family issues; less helpful for substance use or academic underachievement
- For adults: more helpful for substance use, schizophrenia, dementia
- Evidence within major psychiatric disorders:
  - Schizophrenia: psychoeducational family therapy—more effective than medication alone, reduces relapse rate, reduces blame, provides problem-solving strategies

- Mood disorders: inpatient family therapy improves global functioning upon discharge
- Autism: family therapy highly effective, also more cost-effective than other interventions such as institutionalization

GERIATRIC PSYCHIATRY

Background (Census 2000 Summary File 1 and Vintage 2016 Population Estimates; Am J Geriatr Psychiatry. 2009;17(9):769-781)
- Number > 65 y old ↑ rapidly (35 million in 2000; 49.2 million in 2016); predominantly Caucasian and ♀ but becoming more diverse
- **Prevalence of psychiatric disorders:** Most common symptoms include sleep issues, anxiety, depressive symptoms; most common disorders: dementia, anxiety disorders
- Expected cognitive changes w/ aging: slower processing speed, ↓ recall of names/faces, ↑ trials needed for learning, ↓ in divided attention, ↓ abstract thought
- When medically ill, elderly can quickly lose ability to remain independent (↓ functional reserve)

Evaluation (Budson. Memory Loss. 2nd ed.; 2016:47-50; J Am Geriatr Soc. 2015;63(6):1214-1238)
- See "Major Neurocognitive Disorders" section for memory loss evaluation
- Use standard diagnostic interview (HPI, PMH, FH, medication trials, etc) **with focus on context of symptoms, medical comorbidities, MSE, functional status (eg, ADLs, iADLs);** capacity/decision-making ability
- Collateral from family/caregiver is often key (esp. if concern for cognitive impairment)—focus on history, services provided, how available they are to aid patient, tolerance of psychiatric symptoms, etc
- Consider rating scale(s) for cognitive functioning, depression, general assessment: useful to have caregivers fill out as well
- Monitor for elder abuse (physical, sexual, psychological, financial, neglect, etc): prevalence range: 10–47%, dementia and > 80 = highest risk (↑ risk w/ cognitive and physical impairment, psychosocial distress, social isolation); abuser is usually a family member; **requires mandatory reporting to Adult Protective Services**

Psychopharmacology (JAMA Intern Med. 2016;176(4):473-482; J Am Geriatr Soc. 2018;66(5):916; Br J Clin Pharmacol. 2004;57(1):6-14)
- Aging causes ↓ renal + hepatic clearance w/ effect on volume of distribution (eg, ↓ lean body mass and ↓ total body water → in ↓ volume for hydrophilic drugs; ↑ body fat → in ↑ volume for lipophilic drugs)
  - Many medications have ↑ elimination half-life/↑ plasma drug concentrations → ↑ medication sensitivity (mantra "Start low and go slow") (Curr Drug Metab. 2011;12(7):601-610)
- Side effects of medications commonly used in the elderly:

Antipsychotics + anticoagulants most cited medications in preventable adverse drug reactions (*Am J Med.* 2005;118(3):251); TD risk ↑ w/ age; dosages of risperidone > 2 mg have similar EPS side effects as typical antipsychotics, **FDA Black Box warning**: ↑ risk of death with antipsychotics for treatment of behavioral disorders in the elderly (still often used with caution)

Sedation: BZDs (can also cause paradoxical agitation), TCAs, anticholinergics

Orthostasis: quetiapine, trazodone, clozapine, chlorpromazine, TCAs

- **Risks of polypharmacy** (various definitions; commonly 5+ prescribed medications)
  - Common > 1/3 adults 65+ prescribed 5+ medications; highest risk in nursing homes
  - ↑ use of herbal/dietary supplements
  - Consequences: ↑ adverse effects, drug–drug interactions, medication nonadherence, falls, urinary incontinence, cognitive impairment, delirium, hospital admissions
  - Avoid unnecessary medications, use nonpharmacologic treatment (eg, behavioral interventions, therapy); use ↑ dosages of an already prescribed medication 1st for PRNs

Delirium (*Lancet.* 2014;383(9920):911-922)
- In those >65 **most frequent complication of hospitalization**; risk ⇑ with existing cognitive impairment; sensory impairment; post-cardiac surgery; burn victims; substance use; autoimmune diseases
- Associated with ↑ morbidity and mortality; loss of ADLs and iADLs; ↑ nursing facility placement
  See Delirium chapter for additional treatment

Example Acute Agitation Meds for Delirious Elderly Patients		
Trazodone	12.5–25 mg PO	
Olanzapine	2.5–5 mg PO, IM or SL	If IM, avoid concurrent BZDs
Quetiapine	12.5–25 mg PO	Preferred if parkinsonism
Risperidone	0.25–0.5 mg PO, SL, liquid	
Haloperidol	0.5–1 mg PO, IM	
Lorazepam	0.25–0.5 mg PO, IM	Increases risk of falls
Note: No difference in efficacy between haloperidol and atypical antipsychotics olanzapine and risperidone; no official guidelines for dosing exist; antipsychotics in elderly should be used with caution		
Cochrane Database Syst Rev. 2007;(2):CD005594.		

GERIATRIC 9-25

Anxiety (*J Affect Disord.* 2015;172:24-29)
- **Prevalence:** GAD is common, 25% of cases have late-life onset; other anxiety disorders also common (eg, simple phobias, panic disorder, OCD, anxiety associated w/ chronic illness, disability, bereavement)
- **Comorbid anxiety common with depression:** worse prognosis
- **Treatment:** similar as adults, use caution when prescribing BZDs

Bipolar Disorder (*Bipolar Disord.* 2004;6(5):343; *J Affect Disord.* August 1, 2017;217:266-280; *Am J Psychiatry.* 2017;174(11):1086-1093)

- **Prevalence:** <0.5% in community; ↑ in clinical settings (~10% elderly inpatient psych admissions); less likely to have comorbid SUD (~30%); ↑ risk of suicide ~12× (*J Affect Disord.* 2002;68(2-3):167)
- **Secondary mania:** ↑ probability of medical condition (eg, multiple sclerosis, stroke, HIV, hyperthyroidism, neurosyphilis, neurodegenerative disorders) or medication side effects (eg, steroids) causing manic symptoms (*Am J Psychiatry.* 2005;162(11):2033)
- **Treatment:** Guidelines based on adults; *lithium* first-line; some suggest targeting lower plasma levels (<0.6 mmol/L); caution in renal or thyroid disorders; ↑ concentrations w/ thiazide diuretics, NSAIDs, ACEi, physiologically ↓ renal clearance

  Also commonly used: valproate, carbamazepine, lamotrigine (may have fewer cognitive symptoms); limited data on antipsychotics

Depression (*N Engl J Med.* 2014;371(13):1228-1236; *Am Fam Physician.* 2004;69(10):2375)

- Depression not considered a normal part of aging; often underdiagnosed/not treated
- **Prevalence:** Rates vary based on criteria used; depressive episodes ↓ frequency compared to other life stages; ↑ in hospitalized patients and those w/ medical comorbidities
- **Risk factors:** ♀; social isolation, ↓ SES, widowed/divorced/separated, pain, insomnia, functional/cognitive impairment (*Am J Psychiatry.* 2003;160(6):1147); **late-life depression may be a prodrome of dementia**
- **Evaluation:** more somatic complaints (GI—nausea + constipation; chest pain, headaches, arthritic pain, dizziness, fatigue, weight loss); may have anhedonia or apathy > dysphoric mood; may ruminate on subjective cognitive impairment; elderly men have highest rate of suicide in the US; **attempt suicide less often but are more successful at completion**
- **Treatment:** therapy effective; all FDA-indicated antidepressants effective; consider ECT/other neurotherapies

Possible Side Effects of Medication Options for Depression in the Elderly	
SSRIs (1st line)	Sedation, weight gain, GI sx, risk for bruising/GI bleed, hyponatremia
TCAs	Anticholinergic side effects, orthostatic hypotension, cardiac side effects
SNRIs	Hypertension, anxiety, insomnia, cardiac issues
Mirtazapine	Weight gain and sedation; small risk for neutropenia
Bupropion	Insomnia
Stimulants	Possible exacerbation of anxiety, psychosis, anorexia, hypertension
Note: Patients will often end up needing similar dosages of medication as younger patients	
Drugs Aging. 2001;18(5):355; *Prim Care Companion J Clin Psychiatry.* 2001;3(1):22-27.	

Psychosis (*J Cell Mol Med.* 2012;16(5):995; *Psychosomatics.* 2000;41(6):519; *Int J Endocrinol.* 2015;2015:615356)

- **Prevalence:** Psychosis most commonly caused by **dementia or delirium** (may be related to sensory impairments) > mood disorders > primary psychotic disorders
- *Late-onset schizophrenia:* onset after 40 y; ~1/5th of pts; predominantly ♀ (hypothesis: estrogen may act like an endogenous antipsychotic, estrogen replacement not effective tx); higher functioning w/ better cognition
- *Very late onset schizophrenia:* onset after 60 y; rare; may be caused by neurodegenerative process
- **Treatment:** Atypical antipsychotics; recommend starting dosages 50%/maintenance dosages 25–30% lower than for adults, typical antipsychotics less used 2/2 ↑ risk of EPS
- Adjuvant psychosocial treatments are important

Substance Use (*Clin Geriatr Med.* 2014;30(3):629-654)

- **Prevalence:** Often unreported/overlooked; alcohol misuse most common, ↑ risk of suicide, malnourishment, dementia; medication misuse (prescribed + OTC) ↑ w/ age; illicit substance use less common but ↑
- **Recommendation:** ≤7 standard drinks/wk (↑ blood alcohol concentration relative to amount ingested compared to younger adults)
- Intensive treatment options geared toward general population have been shown to be effective for elderly

GENDER AND SEXUAL MINORITY POPULATIONS

GENDER MINORITY PATIENTS

Terminology (*Am J Public Health.* 2013;103:5)

Gender minority: those w/ gender identity/expression that differs from sex assigned at birth; include, but NOT limited to, *transgender woman, transgender man, transfemale, transmale, genderqueer, nonbinary gender, gender fluid,* **does not imply medical/psychiatric pathology**

Gender dysphoria: clinical diagnosis describing significant distress; ↓ functioning due to discordance between current gender identity/expression and assigned sex

- NOT present w/ gender minority identities
- Often resolved through gender affirmation (eg, changing name/physical appearance), social transition (eg, using bathroom congruent w/ gender identity), and individual +/− family psychotherapy

Caring for Gender Minority People

- Gender identity and expression may change over time, critical to do regular check-ins about identity/names/pronouns. Intake forms and electronic records can be standardized to be inclusive and can prompt staff to check in about changes

- Several steps can be taken to ensure clinical spaces are safe and welcoming for gender minority people
  1. Training providers/staff in inclusive care (eg, calling pts by last name, avoiding Mr/Ms)
  2. Inclusive clinical forms (eg, ?s of natal sex and current gender identity)
  3. Pamphlets/pt material depicting gender diverse pts
  4. Creating clinic spaces that welcome all genders (eg, designating all gender restrooms)

DSM History and Gender (Int Rev Psych. 2016;28:1)
- **DSM-I and II (1952, 1968):** No gender-related dx
- **DSM-III (1980):** Transexualism, Gender Identity Disorder of Childhood (GIDC), and Atypical GID listed under Psychosexual d/o
- **DSM-IIIR (1987):** Transexualism and GIDC moved under Disorders Usually First Evidence in Infancy, Childhood, or Adolescence; Gender Identity Disorder of Adolescence and Adulthood (GIDAA) + Nontranssexual Type (GIDAANT) and Gender Identity Disorder Not Otherwise Specified (GIDNOS) added under the same category
- **DSM-IV (1994):** Transexualism and GIDAANT removed; GIDC and GIDAA retained, under Sexual and Gender Identity Disorders, Gender Identity Disorder NOS added
- **DSM-5 (2013):** Dx roots changed from "disorder" to "dysphoria," w/ "Gender Dysphoria in Adolescents or Adults," "Gender Dysphoria in children," "Other Specified Gender Dysphoria," and "Unspecified Gender Dysphoria"

Mental Health in Gender Minority People (Prof Psychol Res Pr. 2012;43:5; Am J Public Health. 2013;103:5; J Sex Res. 2015;52:3; J Adolesc Health. 2015;56:3; Providing Care for Addictions in the LGBT Community, Fenway Health. 2016; The Report of the 2015 U.S. Transgender Survey. 2016)
- > prevalence of mental illness related to ↑ discrimination, violence, and rejection associated w/ gender identity/expression
- **Affective and anxiety disorders:** Transgender women: ~49% w/ depression, 33% w/ anxiety, 23% w/f somatization (via Brief Symptom Inventory); transgender men: ~37% w/ depression, 33% w/ anxiety, 34% w/ somatization; **youth:** ~1/10 identify as gender minority; age 13–18, ↑ odds of past 1 y EtOH use, MJ use, illicit use; if experienced bullying/harassment, age 12–29, 2-3× ↑ risk of depression, anxiety disorder, SIB, SI, suicide attempt
- Transgender people ↑ AUD/SUD
- **Suicide:** 40% have attempted, rate ~9x > US population (4.6%)

SEXUAL MINORITY PATIENTS

Terminology (LGBTQ and Allies at Harvard Medical School/Harvard School of Dental Medicine, Terminology Related to Sexual Orientation, Gender Identity, and More 2017)

Sexual minority: people who have a sexual orientation other than heterosexual/straight; include, but NOT limited to, asexual, bisexual, gay, lesbian, pansexual, and queer
- Knowing a pt's sexual orientation or attractions does not provide detailed information about sexual practices or partners

DSM History and Sexual Orientation (Behav Sci. 2015;5)
- **DSM-I (1952):** Homosexuality listed as a disorder, under sociopathic personality disturbance
- **DSM-II (1968):** Homosexuality reclassified under sexual deviation
- **1973 APA Decision:** In response to published reports noting homosexuality to be common in general pop + gay and lesbian activists disrupting 1970/1971 APA mtgs, APA voted to remove Homosexuality and was replaced w/ Sexual Orientation Disturbance (SOD), sparked ongoing debate regarding impact of the DSM in pathologizing experience
- **DSM-III (1980):** SOD was replaced w/ Ego Dystonic Homosexuality (EDH)
- **DSM-IIIR (1987):** EDH was removed

Mental Health in Sexual Minority People (Psychol Bull. 2003;129:5; JAMA. 2016;176:9; Providing Care for Addictions in the LGBT Community, Fenway Health. 2016; Crisis. 2018;15:1-6)
- Complicated by the classification of homosexuality as a mental disorder until 1973 confounding reasons for ↑ prevalence of mental illness in sexual minority people
- ↑ experiences of stigma, prejudice, and discrimination
- **Affective and anxiety disorders:** Report of moderate psychological distress > in lesbian women than straight women (OR, 1.34; 95% CI, 1.02–1.76); report of severe psychological distress > in gay men (OR, 2.82; 95% CI, 1.55–5.14) and bisexual men (OR, 4.70; 95% CI, 1.77–12.52) than straight men
- **SUD:** universally at > risk for AUD + SUD than heterosexual counterpart
- **Suicide:** 14% of sexual minority individuals have attempted suicide, 45% of sexual minority individuals report SI in past 1 y

HOMELESS PATIENTS

Background (Am J Public Health. 2004;94:103; Curr Psychiatry Rep. 2012;14:259)
- ↓ in psychiatric funding + bed availability ongoing since the mid-1950s 2/2 multifactorial process of deinstitutionalization
- Intent of deinstitutionalization was transition from long-term psychiatric hospitals to enhanced community care, which was never fully realized
- Evidence suggests corresponding ↑ in the number of homeless w/ mental illness
- **Transinstitutionalization:** ↑ number of people w/ mental illness now in jail/prisons or nursing homes
- Community + public psychiatry = subspecialty most directly associated w/ population care

Epidemiology (US Dept. of HUD 2017 Annual Report to Congress)
- Diverse, significant differences between those who live on the street (~1/3) and those who stay in shelters (~2/3); majority = single adult men (families/children/women between 1/4 and 1/3 of population)

- Systemic racism (housing segregation, War on Drugs) plays a major role in the disproportionate number of homeless AA (40.6 vs ~13% in the general population)
- More likely to have SUDs, trauma exposure, SMI, and poor physical health
  - SUD most common disorder (*Lancet.* 2014;384:1529)
  - A survey of 966 homeless patients found ~20% past-year physical or sexual assault (*Am J Public Health.* 2010;100:1326).
  - A review of 10,340 patients w/ SMI in San Diego County found 15% were homeless (*Am J Psychiatry.* 2005;162:370)
  - Mortality up to 9× > age 25–44 + 4.5× > age 45–64 than general population; drug overdose, cancers, + heart disease were leading causes of death (*JAMA Intern Med.* 2013;173:189)

Wrap-Around Service Models
- **Intensive Case Management (ICM):** Emphasizes small caseloads + time-unlimited services, 2014 Cochrane review found ↓ hospitalizations, ↑ cate retention, globally ↑ social functioning for those w/ SMI (*Cochrane Database Syst Rev.* 2010;10:CD007906)
- **Assertive Community Treatment Teams (ACT or PACT):** Multidisciplinary team w/ shared caseloads, 2007 meta-analysis demonstrated 37% ↓ + 26% ↓ in symptom severity (*Am J Psychiatry.* 2007;164:393). Also known as PACT teams
- **Health Care for the Homeless Programs:** Integrated system providing primary, specialty, + mental health care in the community w/ "street teams" and embedded shelter clinics

Housing First
- Provides housing without requiring sobriety/employment/treatment adherence
- **The At Home/Chez Soi Trials:** Two large RCTs across 5 Canadian cities comparing housing first (with ICM/ACT services) against usual care. ICM trial: 5% never housed in intervention group vs 31.5% in control. ACT trial: 73% stably housed at 1 y vs 31% in control (*JAMA.* 2015;313:905; *Psychiatr Serv.* 2015;66:463)
- **The Pathways to Housing Trial:** RCT in NYC comparing sobriety first against housing first. 80% stably housed at 2 y vs 30% in sobriety group (*Am J Public Health.* 2004;94:651)

TRANSPLANT PATIENTS

Overview of Transplantation (*Am Fam Physician.* 2016;93:203-210)
- Longitudinal, multidisciplinary endeavor including highly invasive surgical tx of end-stage dz
- **Team** includes transplant recipient *plus* (potentially) surgery, anesthesia, medical subspecialties, psychiatry, psychology, palliative care, social work, chaplain, pharmacy, PT, OT, nursing, financial advisor, nutritionist, aides, donor, family, supports/community
- USA allocations managed by a division of the United Network for Organ Sharing, called the Organ Procurement and Transplant

Network. Allocation influenced variably (for different organs) by location, length of time on waitlist, acuity of condition, clinical progression, age, and HLA compatibility
- Demand (US waitlist >100 k pts) **>>>** Supply (~40 k solid organ transplants/y in the US)
- **Ethics**
  Duties to: Patient (beneficence, respect autonomy) and public (graft protection/stewardship)
  Allocation: Egalitarian (=) **vs** Utilitarian (most social value) **vs** Maximizing (best prognosis)?
  Challenge: Holding one's own morals + affects amid hard cases and varied medical cultures

Psychiatric Evaluation (*Indian J Med Res.* 2015;141:408-416; *Transplantation.* 2017;101:S8)
- **Overall goals** include (1) develop rapport and longitudinal relationship; (2) education and expectation clarification; (3) identify and treat any psychiatric illness, which may interfere with transplant success; (4) graft protection; and (5) capacity assessment
- **Exclusion criteria:** *disabling* psychiatric sx (no national consensus on precise criteria; may include acute psychosis, active SI, active HI, active substance use, dementia, h/o multiple suicide attempts). Many centers strict on SUDs (eg, require 6 mo of sobriety) but this is increasingly controversial (*J Hepatol.* 2014;60:866-871)
- **Recipient**
  PM hxH: End-stage dz hx, comorbidities, tx/meds (eg, O$_2$, dialysis, warfarin), tx adherent?
  Psych hx: Diagnoses, severity (SI/SA? violence? hospitalizations?), active sx screens, tx (meds? therapy? ECT? adherent? no shows?), *substance use* (esp. tobacco, EtOH, IV)
  Social Hx: Housing, finances, *relationships* (characterize closeness, supportiveness, alliance/tension), transportation, medical literacy, spirituality/faith, cultural background(s)
  Collateral: Regarding as much of the above as able, from family/friends/treaters/records
  Physical: Stigmata of substance use, SIB, debility, expected stigmata of end-stage dz
  Data: UTox, EtOH metabolites, nicotine metablt (cotinine), extended tox (r/o false +/−ives)
  Mental status: Hygiene/self-care, reliability, cooperation/guardedness, capacity to consent, active s/sx (eg, depressed affect, response to internal stimuli, speech latency/pressure/slurring, agitation, disorganization, SI), coping/personality style
  Cognitive: Level of alertness, orientation, intoxication, intelligence, general+med fluency
  (*+ive Prognostic Factors:* h/o perseverance over adversity, strong social support, solid connection to care system, motivation to improve health)
- **Living donors (15% of transplants)**
  Evaluation *must* be performed by separate team other than the recipient to avoid conflict of interest. Similar evaluation, plus:
  - *Motivation:* exclude coercion (eg, if family/friend is recipient)

- *Capacity:* include discussion of potential lifelong consequences of donating given organ
- **Pediatrics**
  Similar eval; plus additional ethical/legal issues (eg, assent, substituted judgment)
  (See also dedicated chapter on "Children")

Useful Scales *(Glob Cardiol Sci Pract. 2016;2016:e201626)*

- **Psychiatric assessment:** PHQ-9, BDI, GAD-7, AUDIT, MOCA/ MMSE, etc (see also chapters on "Neuropsychiatric Assessment" and "Commonly Used Rating Scales")
- **Psychological assessment:** Variety of neuropsychological and personality assessments have been used to predict outcomes; non-standardized currently
- **Psychosocial screening/risk stratification:** No consensus regarding acceptable level of psychosocial risk in transplant candidates; varies per transplant center discretion. Several validated scales help assess and communicate psychosocial risk for poor outcome
  - Transplant Evaluation Rating Scale (TERS)
  - Psychosocial Assessment of Candidates for Transplantation (PACT)
  - Stanford Integrated Psychosocial Assessment for Transplantation (SIPAT)

Psychopathological Considerations *(Crit Care Clin. 2008;24:949; Indian J Med Res. 2015;141:408-416)*

- Psychological concerns
  Waiting and uncertainty
  - Indeterminate waitlist and dz course: may wait yrs, get a call today, or die tmrw waiting
  Anxiety, depressed mood
  - Reactive (ie, normal) or pathological? +if abnl: 1° or 2°? Eg, endocrinopathy, anemia
  - Neuroveg sx and depression may affect >50% of end-stage pts (varies per organ). Fx may already be very limited. Assessing Δ in psych sx and fx status can be challenging
    (1 strategy: "If it weren't for your [end-stage dz], would you [insert PsychROS]?" Depressed pt may, for example, report hypothetical anhedonia indep of disability)
  Facing mortality
  - Existential +/− spiritual distress; +logistical complexities of ?death (eg, will, funeral)
  - Provider/pt avoidance/denial of advance care planning *(Mayo Clin Proc. 2017;92:940-946)*
  - Was end-stage dz status sudden/unexpected?
  - Note: many pts w/ SUDs or other stigmatized dz may not be told that they are progressing to a transplant requirement. Trajectory may seem obvious, but be a shock to the pt. If such pts aren't warned, they *will not* be transplant candidates; if they *are* warned, they *may* have that chance, even if odds seem against it
  - Demoralization due to graft failure—in the setting of nonadherence or despite adherence
  Maladaptive coping (Transplant Proc. 2010;42:3149-3152)

- Eg, **denial**, regression, displacement, projection, intellectualization
- Utilizing destructive, addictive, or alienating behaviors to manage distress/distract

Damaged self-image
- Potential changes in hair, skin, weight/habitus; disfigurement; progressing disability

Trauma
- Posttransplant, 10–17% incidence of clinician-ascertained transplant-specific PTSD (*Gen Hosp Psychiatry*. 2015;35:387-398) Can be d/t ICU stays, delirium memories, surgeries, pain, SOB

Striving for normalcy
- Denial/guilt/disappointment about (in)ability to return to work/ school/parenting/sex, etc
- "Feeling fine again" and ↑ risk of noncompliance w/ meds or monitoring
- Feeling tethered to meds/tx (pre- and/or posttransplant)

- **Biological concerns**
  Delirium and cognitive dysfunction
    Common (1) in end-stage dz (eg, uremic/hepatic encephalopathy, drugs/withdrawal); (2) perioperatively (eg, pain, nausea, withdrawal, anesthetic, infection); and (3) posttransplant period (eg, medications, infections, malignancies, graft failure, PRES, dysfunction of oxygenation/ventilation/perfusion) (see dedicated "Delirium" chapter.)
  Pain, nausea, disability, etc
    Very common pre- and posttransplant; can cycle w/ anx and depression
  Antirejection medication effects
    Eg: corticosteroids and calcineurin inhibitors (tacrolimus, cyclosporine)
    - *Tacrolimus* can cause delirium, depression, anorexia, insomnia, vivid dreams/nightmares, vision changes, PRES, neuropathy, tremor, seizures and catatonia
    - *Cyclosporine* can cause delirium, neuropathy
    - See discussion of *corticosteroids* in chapter on "Autoimmune Psychiatry"

Treatment Considerations (*Crit Care Clin*. 2008;24:949; *Indian J Med Res*. 2015;141:408-416)
- **Take uniqueness of psychosocial stressors into account**
  As noted, existential and spiritual issues may feature uniquely in transplant pt's suffering, which overall may differ significantly from problems seen more commonly in psychiatry
  - Explore meaning and don't rush to pathologize pt's process. Normalize, validate, support
  - Acknowledge unknowns and personal limitations
  - Enlist multidisciplinary team support and pt's support system as allowed
  - Find pt support for practical/logistical issues attendant to transplant and possible death
  - Employ supportive, cognitive, and behavioral psychotherapeutic approaches

- Consider narrative, dignity, person-centered and other psychotherapy modalities that may offer less-utilized tools to cope with existential uncertainty and distress
- **Dosing modifications**
  - Impairments in renal/hepatic/GI function affecting clearance/metabolism/kinetics?
  - Cardiac/neuro vulnerabilities? (eg, QTc prolongation; BZD/anticholinergic deliriogenicity)
  - Interactions w/ antirejection meds? (SSRIs and mood stabilizers often affect/are affected)
  - Under/overweight? Cachectic? Cushingoid? Δs in tissues affecting bioavailability?
- **Rational pharmacology** (*J Am Acad Dermatol.* 2017;77:1068-1073.e7)
  When indicated, choose psychopharm w/ side effects that treat comorbid problems
  Pain: SNRIs, TCAs, gabapentin, carbamazepine, oxcarbazepine
  Nausea: Antipsychotics, BZDs, cannabinoids
  Anorexia: Antipsychotics, mirtazapine, cannabinoids
  Pruritus: Hydroxyzine, doxepin (and other TCAs), SSRIs, mirtazapine
  Fatigue: Bupropion, psychostimulants, fluoxetine, aripiprazole
- **If available, involve palliative care as needed**

ONCOLOGY PATIENTS

Background
- **History:** Stigma was a significant barrier to discussions of psychological distress and mental illness in cancer pts until the 1970s; "psycho-oncology" has since emerged as a distinct and growing subspecialty of oncology and consultation-liaison psychiatry (*Psychosomatic Med.* 2002;64:206)
- **Distress:** Common as pts cope with questions about illness tx/sx, mortality, meaning/purpose, spirituality. Most cancer centers now required to screen for distress (using scales) at initial and/or critical appts as per ASCO guidelines (*J Clin Oncol.* 2014;32:1605)
- **Coping and denial:** Cancer often tests and amplifies pts coping skills/defenses (eg, denial, avoidance, rumination, taking control). Degree of denial often fluctuates throughout the illness; can aid pts in maintaining hope and relationships, but can also be detrimental
- **What's normal?:** Psychiatrists can play key role in helping to distinguish normal range of emotional reactivity from psychopathology, the latter of which can lead to: ↓ QOL, poor access/adherence to tx, ↑ physical sx, ↑ hospital LOS, and ↓ survival rates

General Tips
- **Allow adequate space for pts to process negative or "shameful" emotions**
- **Try not to make assumptions** about how pts feel in and about their cancer experience; avoid such statements as "I can imagine" or "I totally understand"

- **Be judicious about reassurance;** when used globally ("You're going to be fine") rather than specific to a certain issue/problem ("You'll be out of the MRI machine soon"), it can be received as invalidating and counterproductive
- **Don't entirely gloss over terminality and mortality;** try to balance awareness and preparation for death with a maintenance of hope
- **Distress doesn't necessarily end when the cancer is "cured."** Survivors of cancer face unique challenges (physical/cognitive/emotional sequelae, reentry into life)

Psychosocial Interventions

Adaptations of Existing Therapeutic Approaches	Novel Therapeutic Approaches	Complementary and Alternative Medicine
Support groups, CBT, mind-body, stress-reduction, problem-solving, supportive-expressive (psychodynamic)	Dignity-based, meaning-centered	Acupuncture, massage, pet therapy, expressive writing

Depression (J Oncol Pract. 2016;12:747)
- **Epidemiology:** Cancer ↑ risk of minor and major depressive disorders (adjustment d/o, MDD). Prev varies depending on multiple factors (cancer type, psych hx, type of tx, stage of tx), but overall estimates approx. 10–20%. Male = female
- **Risk factors:** Certain cancers, degree of physical debilitation/disability, prior psych and SUD hx, family hx, chronic med illness, psychosocial vulnerabilities (limited supports/isolation, financial/housing stress, unstable relationships, maladaptive defenses)
- **Evaluation:** Many sx overlap between cancer and MDD; look for nonsomatic sx (hopelessness, anhedonia, tearfulness, isolation, self-pity) in addition to less specific somatic sx (fatigue, anorexia, insomnia) (Cancer. 1984;53:2243). Rule out other medical contributors to sx (pain, low B_{12}/folate/D, anemia, thyroid dz, CNS dz) and consider impact of various cancer treatments
- **Treatment approach** (J Clin Oncol. 2014;32:1605):
  - *All pts* → Screen using scale (PHQ-2, if + → PHQ-9; ASCO recommends cutoff score 8), normalize distress/nonpathologic sadness, provide psycho-ed/support, optimize somatic sx control, collaborate with medical teams, monitor for worsening sx
  - *For mild to mod depression (including adjustment d/o)* → Equivocal evidence for psychosocial vs pharm interventions, usually try psychosocial first and meds if refractory sx
  - *For MDD* → combined psychosocial + pharm; if severe +/− safety concerns (eg, suicidality, psychosis, self-neglect) should consider inpatient psych, ECT

Medications for Depression in Oncology Patients (*J Clin Oncol.* 2012;30:1187)

Choice of med(s) guided by combination of sx, tx side effects, and possible drug–drug interactions. Limited availability of placebo-controlled studies in onc pts

SSRIs: First-line, as w/ typical MDD. Sertraline, citalopram, escitalopram common first choices given tolerability and low likelihood for drug–drug interaction. Paroxetine also useful, but w/ risk of discontinuation syndrome. Avoid paroxetine, fluoxetine, sertraline in pts on tamoxifen (CYP2D6 inhibition can ↓ tamoxifen levels)

SNRIs: Venlafaxine first-line for pts on tamoxifen because no CYP2D6 inhibition; may also help w/ hot flashes/menopause sx; avoid in cardiac dz. Duloxetine useful if comorbid neuropathic pain; avoid in hepatic dz

TCAs: May confer additional benefit in pts with pain, but anticholinergic toxicity, drug–drug interactions, and risk for lethality in OD limit utility

Bupropion: Avoid bupropion in pts on tamoxifen (CYP2D6 inhibition can ↓ tamoxifen levels) and pts with seizure risk (CNS involvement, electrolyte derangements, EDs)

Mirtazapine: Useful for pts with insomnia, anorexia/weight loss. Paradoxically more sedating at lower doses. Generally safe in geri pts and few drug–drug interactions

Stimulants: Useful for sx palliation in severe neurovegetative MDD; quick onset of action. Modafinil confers less side effects. Caution in pts with anorexia/weight loss. Avoid in pts with cardiac dz, seizure risk

ECT: Consider for severe, refractory depression. Requires medical clearance; contraindicated with CNS lesions

Anxiety (*J Clin Oncol.* 2012;30:1197)

- **Types:** Situational (eg, "scan-xiety"), psychiatric, organic, existential
- **Epidemiology:** Heterogenous (adjustment d/o, phobias, GAD, acute stress d/o, PTSD, panic, SAD, OCD); in a large-scale study, 34% of oncology outpts reported clinically sig levels of anxiety. Meta-analysis rates of adjustment d/o in cancer settings = 20%; other anxiety disorders = 10%. M = F, no age diff
- **Risk factors:** Premorbid anxiety, temperament/coping style(s), psych hx, trauma hx, illness severity, dependent children
- **Evaluation:** As w/ depression, many sx overlap between cancer and anxiety. Look for pt w/ specific anxiety d/o sx (panic, phobias) and worries disproportionate to cancer-related risk. Rule out medical contributors, incl common and serious complications of cancer: pulmonary embolism/hypoxia, cardiac dz/toxicity, complex partial seizure, withdrawal (opioids, benzos). Consider impact of various cancer treatments
- **Treatment approach** (*J Clin Oncol.* 2014;32:1605):
  - *As w/ depression, all pts* → Screen using scale (GAD-7; ASCO recommends cutoff score 10), normalize distress/nonpathologic nervousness, provide psycho-ed/support, optimize somatic sx control, collaborate with medical teams, monitor for worsening sx

- For mild to mod anxiety → psychosocial interventions +/− medications
- For severe anxiety → combined psychosocial interventions + medications

---

Medications for Anxiety in Oncology Patients (*J Clin Oncol.* 2012;30:1197)

Choice of med(s) guided by combination of sx, tx side effects, and possible drug–drug interactions. Limited availability of placebo-controlled studies in onc pts

SSRIs: First-line for longer treatment of anxiety (PTSD, GAD, SAD), as w/ general popul. Same considerations as in table above

SNRIs, TCAs, mirtazapine: Same considerations as in table above

Buspirone: Safe option for a nonhabit-forming medication for longer treatment of anxiety; can be used on its own or as augmentation

Benzodiazepines: Commonly used; lorazepam PRN for panic, anticipatory anxiety (eg, chemo, scans) and/or nausea; clonazepam for longer treatment of anxiety. Habit-forming, serious withdrawal and OD risk. Caution in pts: >65, fall risk, delirium risk, compromised respiratory status. Advise pts to arrange transportation to/from the clinic or hosp if using preprocedure/tx

Atypical antipsychotics: Evidence primarily from general popul, but increasingly used for sx palliation: insomnia, anxiety, anorexia/nausea. Monitor metabolic profile. Olanzapine for anxiety/nausea frequently given in high antimanic or antipsychotic doses when unnecessary; watch for this and provide feedback to tx teams accordingly

Gabapentin: Useful in pts with anxiety, neuropathic pain, alcohol use (can reduce cravings), menopausal sx. Caution in pts w/ renal dz or getting nephrotoxic chemo

---

Cognitive/Neuropsych Complications

- Many cancer-related syndromes can impact cognitive fx and cause neuropsych sx: hypoNa, hyperCa, CNS involvement (tumors/LMD), chemo, hormone therapy, RT
- Can be permanent or may resolve w/ correction of abnormality and/or completion of tx

Neuropsychiatric Effects of Common Cancer Treatments			
Medication(s)	Side Effects	Risk Factors	Tx Considerations
Note that this table reviews more common sx/agents and is not exhaustive.			
Antiandrogens	Hot flashes, fatigue, mood sx		
Antiestrogens	Menopausal sx, cognitive sx	↑ confusion w/ higher doses	SSRI/SNRI can be useful for menopausal sx

(continued)

Neuropsychiatric Effects of Common Cancer Treatments *(continued)*			
Medication(s)	**Side Effects**	**Risk Factors**	**Tx Considerations**
Asparaginase	Depression, fatigue, delirium		
Bevacizumab	Fatigue, rare PRES		
Carboplatin	Neurotoxicity	High doses	
Cisplatin	Peripheral neuropathy, sensorineural hearing loss, rare PRES, cortical blindness	High doses, duration of exposure	
Cytarabine	Cognitive sx, sz, cerebellar dxfx, leukoenceph	Renal dxfx, ↑ age	
Fludarabine	Somnolence, delirium, rare progressive leukoenceph		
5-Fluorouracil	Fatigue, cerebellar dxfx, parkinsonism, enceph	Deficiency of DPD (inhibits 5FU metabolism)	
Glucocorticoids	Insomnia, ↑ appetite/energy, mood sx (mania, depression), psychosis	Neuropsych sx usually assoc. w/ pred. >60 mg, dex. >9 mg	Mood/psychotic sx responsive to antipsychotics and mood stabilizers
Ifosfamide	Delirium, fatigue, cerebellar dxfx, parkinsonism	Renal/liver dxfx	Can make pts look "drunk"
Imatinib	Fatigue, confusion		
IL-2	Fatigue, "flu"-like, delirium, neurotoxicity	Neurotox = dose dependent	Monitor thyroid fx
Methotrexate	Neurotoxicity (common and can be severe, usually reversible)	IV and intrathecal admin, LMD, ↑ peak level, ↑ exposure time	Monitor MTX levels, folinic acid (leucovorin) = "rescue"

Neuropsychiatric Effects of Common Cancer Treatments *(continued)*			
Medication(s)	**Side Effects**	**Risk Factors**	**Tx Considerations**
Procarbazine	Delirium, disulfiram-like effect w/ ETOH		Weak MAOI (wash out other serotonergic meds before use!)
Paclitaxel	Fatigue, depression, peripheral neuropathy, encephalopathy, rare sz		Usually given w/ steroids
Rituximab	Insomnia, headache, dizziness		
Trastuzumab	Insomnia, asthenia, rare PRES		

Adapted from *MGH Handbook of General Hospital Psychiatry*. 2018:351.

Delirium *(J Clin Oncol.* 2012;30:1206)
- **Epidemiology:** Most common neuropsych complication in onc pts (particularly HSCT). Prevalence 10–30% in hospitalized and up to 85% in terminally ill pts w/ cancer (*JAMA.* 2008;300:2898)
- **Etiology:** Usually multifactorial in onc pts (eg, direct CNS effects of cancer, infections, organ failure, chemo, opioids)
- **Risk factors:** Dementia/cog impairment, old age/frailty, renal or liver dxfx, opioids/benzos, visual/hearing impairment, polypharmacy, dehydration/malnutrition
- **Evaluation:** Clinical sx same as general popul. Look for reversible causes, taking into account vulnerabilities in onc pts (hyperCa, hypoNa, DIC, infection, brain mets)
- **Treatment:** Limited data on onc pts, though generally support short-term use of low-dose haloperidol (IV>PO) and atypical antipsychotics (quetiapine, olanzapine, risperidone)

Drug–Drug Interactions/Special Pharmacologic Considerations		
Note that this table reviews more common sx/agents and is not exhaustive.		
Cancer Medication(s)	**Psychiatric Medication**	**Interaction/Risks**
Tamoxifen	Paroxetine, fluoxetine, bupropion	CYP2D6 inhibition from these meds can ↓ tamoxifen levels
Cisplatin	Lithium	Nephrotoxicity

(continued)

Drug–Drug Interactions/Special Pharmacologic Considerations *(continued)*		
Note that this table reviews more common sx/agents and is not exhaustive.		
Cancer Medication(s)	**Psychiatric Medication**	**Interaction/Risks**
	Carbamazepine	Bone marrow suppression
Methadone (for pain), ondansetron (for nausea)	Citalopram/ escitalopram, antipsychotics	Risk for QTc prolongation, monitor EKG regularly
Procarbazine	Serotonergic medications	Serotonin syndrome (procarbazine = weak MAOI)

Survivorship *(NCCN Guidelines. 2014;v2)*
- Cancer survivors often face late effects and long-term psychosocial problems
- Close monitoring for anxiety, depression, sleep, substance use disorders is recommended, particularly at transition points, surveillance visits and with major life events, losses, isolation

HIV PSYCHIATRY

Diagnosis and treatment of psychiatric symptomatology in the patient with HIV/AIDS requires careful consideration of unique risk factors and disease processes. The most important categories on differential diagnosis are *comorbid primary psychiatric illnesses*, *adverse effects of antiretroviral medication*, and *discrete psychiatric syndromes associated with HIV*

Comorbid Psychiatric Illness and HIV
- **Major depressive disorder** appears to be about twice as common in HIV patients compared with at-risk HIV-negative controls, and risk increases further with disease progression (eg, at onset of an AIDS-defining illness)
  - Suicide is twice as likely to because of death in HIV patients compared with general population. 19% of HIV patients report suicidal ideation in the past week *(AIDS. 2007;21:1199-1203)*
  - MDD is associated with increased risk of HIV progression and mortality *(JAMA. 2001;285:1466)*
  - Treatment of depression in HIV patients improves both adherence to ART and clinical outcomes of HIV disease *(JAIDS. 2008;47:384)*
  - Depressive symptoms in HIV patients also often occur in the setting of demoralization, bereavement, and/or survivor guilt
  - No antidepressant has shown particular efficacy or inefficacy in HIV patients; even more than in general population, agent selection should be based on adverse effect profile and interactions with other drugs. Sertraline and escitalopram are commonly used because they have fewer drug–drug interactions

- Avoid bupropion at high doses (>300 mg), as HIV/AIDS may lower the seizure threshold
- Melatonin interacts with many substrates of the immune system and may alter the effectiveness of other immunomodulating drugs
- **Chronic mental illness (schizophrenia and bipolar disorder, type I)**
  - No evidence suggests that HIV has a causal relationship with schizophrenia or bipolar disorder, but severe mental illness may contribute to risk factors for HIV transmission
  - HIV patients are highly sensitive to extrapyramidal adverse effects of neuroleptic drugs 2/2 early damage to subcortical dopaminergic neurons; low-potency atypicals may be better-tolerated because of weaker D2 binding
  - HIV is not a contraindication for clozapine use, and standard monitoring protocols for agranulocytosis may be used
  - Be aware that some antiretrovirals cause metabolic adverse effects similar to atypical antipsychotics, and patients using both classes of drugs should be carefully monitored for insulin resistance, hypercholesterolemia and weight gain
  - Carbamazepine should be avoided because of interactions with many antiretrovirals
  - Lithium can be challenging to manage in HIV patients because of the narrow therapeutic window, increased sensitivity to adverse effects, and potential to precipitate delirium
- **Substance use disorders** are strikingly common in HIV patients: 48% of a large multisite cohort met criteria for 1+ SUD and 20% showed polysubstance use (AIDS Behav. 2017;21:1138). These disorders are also an important vector for HIV transmission (eg, unclean needles, disinhibited sexual behavior, prostitution)
  - The most commonly implicated drugs are marijuana, alcohol, methamphetamine, cocaine, and opiates
  - Methamphetamine, in particular, is highly associated with HIV transmission in the MSM population
  - After acute detoxification, treatment in the willing patient can include psychotherapeutic, pharmacotherapeutic, and social interventions for maintenance and relapse prevention, similar to the general population
  - In patients not ready for sobriety but at risk of HIV transmission, consider harm reduction with pre-exposure prophylaxis for HIV (emtricitabine/tenofovir)
- **Personality disorders** are also highly prevalent in HIV patients, and key elements of personality pathology (affective instability, impulsivity, volatile relationships) likely account for risk-taking behavior that may lead to HIV transmission
  - Early ART-era data suggest that over a third of HIV patients meet criteria for a personality disorder (Am J Psych. 1995;152:1222), most commonly antisocial PD and/or borderline PD
  - Substance users with ASPD have riskier behavior than substance users without ASPD and may show an attenuated response to counseling on HIV risk reduction (Drug Alcohol Depend. 2000;58:247)

Psychiatric Adverse Effects of Antiretrovirals

- **Efavirenz**, an NNRTI, causes mood changes, insomnia, and vivid dreams in about half of patients started on the drug and may be associated with increased suicidality (*AIDS.* 2011;15:1803; *Ann Int Med.* 2014;161:1). In smaller reports, efavirenz has been reported to provoke psychosis and mania
- As a general rule, **efavirenz should be avoided in patients with comorbid severe psychiatric illness or those at risk**, and treaters should strongly consider discontinuing the drug in patients who develop significant psychiatric complaints. Note that efavirenz is present in a commonly used one-pill combination of ART drugs
- **Zidovudine** (AZT), an NRTI, can cause mania at high doses
- **Corticosteroids** are commonly used for secondary infections, putting patients at risk for their characteristic psychiatric side effects
- **Ritonavir and cobicistat**, used to increase bioactivity of ART drugs, can also increase the availability of the psychiatric drugs metabolized through CYP3A4, including aripiprazole and other antipsychotics, most TCAs, pimozide, and importantly the BZDs alprazolam, triazolam and midazolam, which are contraindicated for concomitant use

Discrete Neuropsychiatric Syndromes Associated With HIV

- **HIV infects the nervous system early in infection** and can contribute directly to the experience of psychiatric symptoms
- Most of these syndromes manifest when the CD4 count is low (eg, below 200). However, antiretrovirals variably penetrate the CNS and it is possible for viral replication to proceed in the CNS while suppressed in the bloodstream, a rare phenomenon called **"CNS escape."** Preferentially selecting antiretrovirals that penetrate the CNS may be useful in the right clinical situation (*Arch Neurol.* 2008;65:65)
- **AIDS mania** is rare in the ART era but presents as a manic syndrome (usually irritable more than euphoric) in a patient with advanced HIV. Treatment involves symptom control with mood stabilizers and/or antipsychotics, as well as ART
- Neurocognitive disturbances are grouped as **HAND (HIV-associated neurocognitive disorder)**, which is a diagnosis of exclusion after rule-out of reversible causes of delirium or dementia in the HIV patient. Clinically, HAND is characterized by psychomotor slowing, anhedonia, dysphoria, diffuse impairments in multiple domains of cognition, and impaired coordination and gait. Notably, a large proportion of HIV patients without cognitive complaints show abnormalities on formal neuropsychological testing. HAND is classified using the **Frascati Criteria** based on severity of symptoms and functional impairment:

Stage	Functional Impairment	Neuropsychological Testing	Estimated Prevalence (Among all HIV Patients)
Asymptomatic neurocognitive impairment (ANI)	None	>1 SD below mean in at least 2 cognitive domains	33%
Mild neurocognitive disorder (MND)	Impairment in ADLs	>1 SD below mean in at least 2 cognitive domains	12%
HIV-associated dementia (HAD)	Marked impairment in ADLs	>2 SD below mean in at least 2 cognitive domains	2%

Neurol. 2010;75:2087.

- The differential diagnosis for any psychiatric or mental status change in a person with advanced HIV should include the **AIDS-defining illnesses** toxoplasmosis, cryptococcal meningitis, CMV encephalitis, CNS lymphoma, and progressive multifocal leukoencephalopathy

Comprehensive Care of Patients at Risk for HIV
- Psychiatrists can reduce the public health burden of HIV by **testing at-risk patients for the virus** and referring seropositive patients for primary HIV care. Be aware that current guidelines are to initiate ART as soon as the diagnosis is made, a departure from previous practice of waiting until the CD4 count dropped
- In patients receiving psychiatric but not general medical care, psychiatric providers may wish to consider counseling and prescribing **pre-exposure prophylaxis (emtricitabine/tenofovir)** in at-risk and interested patients

(dys)fx	(dys)Function
+ive	Positive
1°	Primary
2/2	Due to
2/t	Due to
2°	Secondary
5-HT	5-Hydroxytryptamine (serotonin)
a/w	Associated with
A1c	Hemoglobin A1c
AA	African Americans
AA	Alcoholics Anonymous
Ab	Antibody
ABC	Airway, breathing, circulation
ABG	Arterial blood gas
abnl	Abnormal
ABX	Antibiotics
ACE	Angiotensin converting enzyme
ACEis	ACE inhibitors
ACT	Acceptance and commitment therapy
ACT	Assertive community treatment
AD	Alzheimer's dementia
ADH	Antidiuretic hormone
ADHD	Attention deficit hyperactivity disorder
adj	Adjunct
ADLs	Activities of daily living
AE	Autoimmune encephalitis
AED	Antiepileptic drug
aff	Affinity
a. fib	Atrial fibrillation
AH	Auditory hallucinations
ALS	Amyotrophic lateral sclerosis
AML	Acute myeloid leukemia
AMP	Amphetamine
AMS	Altered mental status
AN	Anorexia nervosa
ANA	Antinuclear antibody
ANCA	Antineutrophil cytoplasmic antibody
angio	Angiography
anx	Anxiety
APOE	Apolipoprotein E
ARB	Angiotensin receptor blocker
ARDS	Acute respiratory distress syndrome
ASD	Autism spectrum disorder
ASPD	Antisocial personality disorder
AUD	Alcohol use disorder
AUDIT	Alcohol Use Disorders Identification Test
B/c	Because
B12	Vitamin B12
BA	Bioavailability
BBB	Blood–brain barrier
B-blocker	Beta blocker
BDD	Body dysmorphic disorder
BDI	Beck Depression Inventory
BED	Binge eating disorder
BETA	Best practices in Evaluation and Treatment of Agitation
BF	Bifrontal
BID	Twice daily (dosing)
BMI	Body mass index
BMP	Basic metabolic panel
BN	Bulimia nervosa
BP	Blood pressure
BPAD	Bipolar affective disorder
BPD	Borderline personality disorder
BT	Bitemporal
BUN	Blood urea nitrogen
bvFTD	Behavioral variant frontotemporal dementia
bx	Biopsy
BZDs	Benzodiazepines
C3	Complement 3
C4	Complement 4
Ca	Calcium
CA	Cancer
CADASIL	Cerebral autosomal dominant arteriopathy with subcortical infarcts and leukoencephalopathy
CAM	Complementary and alternative medicine
CART	Chimeric antigen receptor T-cells
CATIE	Clinical Antipsychotic Trials of Intervention Effectiveness
CBC	Complete blood count
CBT	Cognitive behavioral therapy
CBZ	Carbamazepine
CD	Conduct disorder
CFS	Chronic fatigue syndrome
CKD	Chronic kidney disease
clin	Clinical
CMP	Complete metabolic panel
CNS	Central nervous system
CO	Carbon monoxide
cog	Cognitive
COMT	Catechol-O-methyltransferase

COPD	Chronic obstructive pulmonary disease	**EPS**	Extrapyramidal side effects/extrapyramidal symptoms
CPAP	Continuous positive airway pressure	**ER**	Extended release
CPT	Cognitive processing therapy	**ERP**	Exposure response prevention therapy
Cr/CR	Creatinine	**esp**	Especially
CRP	C-reactive protein	**ESR**	Erythrocyte sedimentation rate
CS	Corticosteroids		
CSF	Cerebrospinal fluid	**EtOH**	Ethyl alcohol/ethanol
CT	Computed tomography	**eval**	Evaluate/evaluation
		ex	Example
CV	Cardiovascular	**excr**	Excretion
CVA	Cerebrovascular accident (stroke)	**F/M**	Female/male
		F	Female
CVD	Cardiovascular disease	**FDA**	United States Food and Drug Administration
CYP(###)	Cytochrome p450 (isoenzyme #)		
d/o	Disorder	**FGA**	First-generation antipsychotic
d/t	Due to		
d	Day(s)	**FH(x)**	Family history
D	Dopamine receptor	**FLAIR**	Fluid-attenuated inversion recovery
D2	Dopamine receptor subtype 2		
		FLE	Frontal lobe epilepsy
D3	Vitamin D3	**FLP**	Fasting lipid panel
DA	Dopamine	**FM**	Fibromyalgia
d-AMP	Dextroamphetamine	**FND**	Focal neurologic disorder
DAT	Dopamine transporter		
DBS	Deep brain stimulation	**Freq**	Frequency
DBSA	Depression and Bipolar Support Alliance	**FTA-ABS**	Fluorescent treponemal antibody absorption
DBT	Dialectical behavioral therapy		
		fx	Function
DC	District of Columbia	**GABA**	Gamma-aminobutyric acid
DDx	Differential diagnosis		
depr	Depression/depressed mood	**GAD**	Generalized anxiety disorder
		GAD-7	Generalized Anxiety Disorder 7-Item Scale
DKA	Diabetic ketoacidosis		
DLB	Dementia with Lewy bodies		
		GAF	Global Assessment of Functioning
DLPFC	Dorsolateral prefrontal cortex		
		GBS	Guillain–Barré syndrome
DM	Diabetes mellitus		
d-MPH	Dexmethylphenidate	**GCS**	Glasgow Coma Scale
DNA	Deoxyribonucleic acid		
DSM	Diagnostic and Statistical Manual of Mental Disorders	**GDD**	Global developmental delay
		GED	General Education Diploma
dx	Diagnosis		
dz	Disease	**Gen**	Generation
Δ	Change	**GERD**	Gastroesaphogeal reflux disease
eg	Exempli gratia		
ECG (or EKG)	Electrocardiogram	**geri**	Geriatric
ECT	Electroconvulsive therapy	**GHB**	Gamma-hydroxybutyrate
		GI	Gastrointestinal
ED	Emergency department	**GPM**	Good Psychiatric Management
EEG	Electroencephalogram/electroencephalography		
		GPS	Global positioning system
		GU	Genitourinary
EMDR	Eye-movement desensitization and reprocessing	**H&P**	History and physical
		h/o	History of
EMR	Electronic medical record	**HA**	Headache
Epi	Epinephrine		

hCG	Human chorionic gonadotropin
HCR-20	Historical Clinical Risk Management-20
HD	Hemodialysis
HDRS	Hamilton Depression Rating Scale
HEENT	Head/eyes/ears/nose/throat
HI	Homicidal ideation
HIV	Human immunodeficiency virus
HLA	Human leukocyte antigen
HLD	Hyperlipidemia
HPA	Hypothalamic pituitary adrenal axis
HPI	History of present illness
HR	Heart rate
HSV	Herpes simplex virus
HTN	Hypertension
hx	History
iADLs	Instrumental activities of daily living
IBD	Inflammatory bowel disease
IBS	Irritable bowel syndrome
ICD	Impulse control disorder
ICD-10	International Classification of Diseases, tenth edition
ICI	Immune checkpoint inhibitor
ICM	Intensive Case Management
ICU	Intensive care unit
ID	Intellectual disability
IED	Intermittent explosive disorder
IL(-##)	Interleukin(-number)
IM	Intramuscular
IN	Intranasal
Inc/incl	Including
infxn	Infection
inpt	Inpatient
INR	International normalized ratio
IPT	Interpersonal psychotherapy
IQ	Intelligence quotient
IR	Immediate release
IRIS	Immune reconstitution inflammatory syndrome
IV	Intravenous
IVDU	Intravenous drug use
-ive	Negative
IVIG	Intravenous immunoglobulin
KUB	Kidney/ureter/bladder X-ray
LA	Long acting
l-AMP	Levoamphetamine
LBW	Low birth weight
LFTs	Liver function tests
LGBTQ	Lesbian/gay/bisexual/transgender/queer
Li	Lithium
LLD	Late life depression
LOC	Level of consciousness
LP	Lumbar puncture
M	Male
maint	Maintenance
MAO	Monoamine oxidase
MAOI	MAO inhibitor/monoamine oxidase inhibitor
MAS	Mixed amphetamine salts
MAT	Medication-Assisted Treatment (for substance use)
MBCT	Mindfulness-based cognitive therapy
MBRP	Mindfulness-based relapse prevention
MBSR	Mindfulness-based stress reduction
MBT	Metallization-based therapy
Mcg	Microgram
MDD	Major depressive disorder
ME	Myalgic encephalomyelitis
Meds	Medications
MELAS	Mitochondrial encephalopathy, lactic acidosis, and stroke-like episodes
met	Metabolic
Mg	Magnesium
mg	Milligrams
mgmt	Management
MI	Motivational interviewing
MI	Myocardial infarction
MIBG	Metaiodobenzylguanidine
MJ	Marijuana
mL	Mililiter
MMSE	Mini-Mental State Examination
MND	Major neurocognitive disorder
mo	Month(s)
MoCA	Montreal Cognitive Assessment
MPH	Methylphenidate
MRI	Magnetic resonance imaging
MS	Multiple sclerosis
MSE	Mental status exam
MSK	Musculoskeletal
MTX	Methotrexate

MVA	Motor vehicle accident
MVI	Multivitamin
N/V/D	Nausea/vomiting/diarrhea
N/V	Nausea/vomiting
NDRI	Norepinephrine and dopamine reuptake inhibitor
NE	Norepinephrine
NET	Norepinephrine transporter
NICU	Neonatal intensive care unit
NIMH	National Institute of Mental Health
NINDS-CSR	National Institute of Neurological Disorders and Stroke Center for Scientific Review
NK	Natural killer
nl	Normal
NMDA	N-Methyl-D-aspartate
NMS	Neuroleptic malignant syndrome
NNH	Number needed to harm
NNRTI	Non–nucleoside reverse transcriptase inhibitor
NNS	Number needed to screen
NNT	Number needed to treat
NP	Neuropsychiatric
NPD	Narcissistic personality disorder
NSAIDs	Nonsteroidal anti-inflammatory drugs
NT	Neurotransmitter
OB/GYN	Obstetrician/gynecologist
OCD	Obsessive-compulsive disorder
OCP	Oral contraceptive pill
OCPD	Obsessive-compulsive personality disorder
OD	Overdose
ODD	Oppositional defiant disorder
OFC	Olanzapine Fluoxetine Combination therapy (Symbyax® brand name)
OR	Odds ratio
OROS	Osmotic-controlled release oral delivery system
OSA	Obstructive sleep apnea
Osm	Osmolality
OT	Occupational therapy
OTC	Over-the-counter (medications)

PACT	Program for Assertive Community Treatment
Palp	Palpitations
PANDAS	Pediatric autoimmune neuropsychiatric disorders associated with Streptococcal infections
Path	Pathology
PCP	Phencyclidine
PCP	Primary care physician
PD	Panic disorder
PD	Parkinson disease
PD	Personality disorder
PDD	Pervasive developmental disorder
PDP	Psychodynamic psychotherapy
PE	Physical examination
ped	Pediatric
PET	Positron emission tomography
Phos	Phosphorous
PHQ	Patient Health Questionnaire
PHQ-9	Patient Health Questionnaire, 9 question depression screen
plt	Platelets
PM	Poor metabolizer
PMDD	Premenstrual dysphoric disorder
PMH(x)	Past medical history
PML	Progressive multifocal leukoencephalopathy
PMT	Parent management training
PNV	Prenatal vitamin
PO	By mouth/orally/per oral/per os (oral)
pop	Population
PPA	Primary progressive aphasia
PPD	Postpartum depression
PPHN	Persistent pulmonary hypertension of the newborn
ppx	Prophylaxis/prevention
Pref	Perference
PRES	Posterior reversible encephalopathy syndrome
PRN	pro re nata (as needed)
PRNs	As-needed medications
PSG	Polysomnography
pt(s)	Patient(s)
PT	Physical therapy
PT	Prothrombin time
PTs	Patients
PTSD	Posttraumatic stress disorder
QD	Daily (dosing)

QIDS	Quick Inventory of Depressive Symptomatology	SS	Serotonin syndrome
		SSRIs	Selective serotonin reuptake inhibitors
QOL	Quality of life	STAR*D	Sequenced Treatment Alternatives to Relieve Depression
RA	Rheumatoid arthritis		
Rad	Radiology		
RBD	REM behavior disorder	SUD	Substance use disorder
RCT	Randomized controlled trial	sx(x)	Symptom(s)
		sz	Seizure
Ref	Reference	T	Temperature
REM	Rapid eye movement	$t_{1/2}$	Half-life
RF	Rheumatoid factor	TBI	Traumatic brain injury
RF	Risk factor	TCAs	Tricyclic antidepressants
RLS	Restless legs syndrome		
ROS	Review of systems	TD	Tardive dyskinesia
RPR	Rapid plasma reagin	TdP	Torsades de Pointes
RR	Respiratory rate	TDS	Transdermal delivery system
RUL	Right unilateral		
Rx	Medication	TF-CBT	Trauma-focused cognitive behavioral therapy
rxn	Reaction		
s/sx	Signs/symptoms		
SA	Suicide attempt	TFP	Transference-focused psychotherapy
SAD	Seasonal affective disorder		
		TID	Three times daily (dosing)
SAD	Social anxiety disorder		
SAM	Sympathetic adrenal medullary system	TLE	Temporal lobe epilepsy
		tmrw	Tomorrow
		TNF	Tumor necrosis factor
SAPROF	Structured Assessment of Protective Factors for Violence Risk	Tox	Toxicity
		tox	Toxicology (screen)
		TRD	Treatment-resistant depression
SCAD	Schizoaffective disorder		
SCD	Sudden cardiac death	TSH	Thyroid stimulating hormone
SCM	Structural clinical management		
		TTE	Trans thoracic echocardiogram
SCZ	Schizophrenia		
SE	Side effects	tx	Treatment/therapy
SEID	Systemic exertion intolerance disease	Tyr	Tyramine
		UA	Urinalysis
SERT	Serotonin transporter	UC	Ulcerative collitis
SES	Socioeconomic status	UD	Use disorder
SFT	Schema-focused therapy	URI	Upper respiratory infection
SGA	Second-generation antipsychotic	US	United States
		USPSTF	US Preventive Services Task Force
SI	Suicidal ideation		
SIADH	Syndrome of inappropriate antidiuretic hormone	Utox	Urine toxicology screen
		VaD	Vascular dementia
SIB	Self-injurious behavior	VBG	Venous blood gas
SIBO	Small intestinal bacterial overgrowth	VH	Visual hallucinations
		VPA	Valproic acid
SJS	Stevens–Johnson syndrome	VRAG	Violence Risk Appraisal Guide
SL	Sublingual	VS	Vital signs
SLE	Systemic lupus erythematosus	VSD	Ventricular septal defect
		w/	With
SMD	Standardized mean difference	w/i	Within
		w/o	Without
SMI	Severe mental illness	Wk/wk	Week(s)
SNRIs	Serotonin and norepinephrine reuptake inhibitors	WNL	Within normal limits
		wt	Weight
SOB	Shortness of breath	XR	X-ray
SPECT	Single-photon emission computed tomography	Y-BOCS	Yale-Brown Obsessive Compulsive Scale
		YR/yr	Year(s)